Restorative Neurology of Spinal Cord Injury

Restorative Neurology of Spinal Cord Injury

EDITED BY ■

MILAN R. DIMITRIJEVIC, MD, PhD
PRINCIPAL INVESTIGATOR OF
THE FOUNDATION FOR MOVEMENT RECOVERY
OSLO, NORWAY
EMERITUS PROFESSOR
BAYLOR COLLEGE OF MEDICINE
HOUSTON, TEXAS

BYRON A. KAKULAS, MD, FRACP, FRCPA, FRCPath
MEDICAL DIRECTOR
AUSTRALIAN NEUROMUSCULAR RESEARCH INSTITUTE
CENTRE FOR NEUROMUSCULAR AND NEUROLOGICAL DISEASES
UNIVERSITY OF WESTERN AUSTRALIA
AUSTRALIA

W. BARRY MCKAY, BS
RESEARCH SCIENTIST
NORTON NEUROSCIENCE INSTITUTE
LOUISVILLE, KENTUCKY

GERTA VRBOVÁ, MD, PhD, DSc
EMERITUS PROFESSOR
DIVISION OF DEVELOPMENTAL NEUROSCIENCE
UNIVERSITY COLLEGE LONDON
VISITING PROFESSOR
ROYAL VETERINARY COLLEGE
LONDON, UNITED KINGDOM

OXFORD
UNIVERSITY PRESS

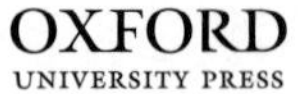

Oxford University Press, Inc., publishes works that further Oxford University's objective of excellence in research, scholarship, and education.

Oxford New York
Auckland Cape Town Dar es Salaam Hong Kong Karachi
Kuala Lumpur Madrid Melbourne Mexico City Nairobi
New Delhi Shanghai Taipei Toronto

With offices in
Argentina Austria Brazil Chile Czech Republic France Greece
Guatemala Hungary Italy Japan Poland Portugal Singapore
South Korea Switzerland Thailand Turkey Ukraine Vietnam

Published by Oxford University Press, Inc.
198 Madison Avenue, New York, New York 10016
www.oup.com

Library of Congress Cataloging-in-Publication Data

Restorative neurology of spinal cord injury / [edited by] Milan R. Dimitrijevic ... [et al.].
p. ; cm.
Includes bibliographical references and index.
ISBN 978-0-19-974650-7 (hardcover : alk. paper)
1. Spinal cord—Wounds and injuries. 2. Spinal cord—Wounds and injuries—Diagnosis.
I. Dimitrijevic, Milan R.
[DNLM: 1. Spinal Cord Injuries—physiopathology. 2. Movement—physiology.
3. Spinal Cord Injuries—therapy. WL 403]
RD594.3.R47 2012
617.4'82044—dc23 2011019144

9 8 7 6 5 4 3 2 1
Printed in the United States of America
on acid-free paper

This book is dedicated to Vivian L. Smith (1908-1989), founder of the Vivian L. Smith Foundation for Restorative Neurology, Houston, Texas, USA. Thanks to her continuous support and the understanding of William Butler, MD, then President of Baylor College of Medicine, the Division of Restorative Neurology and Human Neurobiology was created within the college (1987-1996). The Division housed clinical and research programs from which many new assessment and restorative treatment strategies emerged to help people suffering from weakness, paralysis, spasticity, or pain. This Division also trained many clinicians from around the world who have gone on to install the principles of Restorative Neurology into their own clinical and research environments to improve the quality of life for people who have suffered the effects of neurological injury or disease.

FOREWORD

This is a textbook that has opinions, so be prepared to be pleased or irritated depending on your prior views. Hopefully, it will change at least some of these. The authors are pragmatic from the start. Despite the huge surge of interest in high technology solutions to SCI, such as spinal repair or brain machine interfaces, they recognize that these will take several more years to develop and may fail to yield as high an expectation as is sometimes portrayed. They concentrate squarely on current problems of individual patient management, always stressing the need to assess patients' remaining functional capacities with the greatest care possible. In particular they emphasize the so-called "discomplete" lesion, in which there may be no clinical sign of volitional control of muscles caudal to the lesion yet in which careful EMG monitoring may reveal activation of small numbers of individual motor units, or where volitional input can change spinal reflexes below the lesion. Both are signs of remaining connectivity and the authors highlight how these can be harnessed with appropriate techniques.

The approach is always to base treatments on remaining functional capacity in order to exploit the remarkable capabilities of the existing spinal circuitry to control function. The intrinsic circuitry of the spinal cord together with its sensory inputs and motor outputs is a remarkable machine that can produce fully functional patterns of motor output. The authors view this machinery as a "spinal brain" that can operate in a variety of different modes depending on the patterns of input that it receives. In this view, which reflects that of the neuroscience community at large, descending commands from the brain do not consist of patterned sets of instructions for individual movements and muscles, but are "biases" or "presets" that tune spinal circuits to operate in different modes and produce required patterns of output. The most remarkable demonstration of this is the spinal stimulation method pioneered by Dimitrijevic in which stimulation of the lumbar dorsal root inputs at different frequencies can result in different patterns of output to leg muscles varying from cocontraction to alternating "gait-like" patterns at other frequencies. Thus, just by changing the frequency of an input, we can change the pattern of motor output that is obtained.

The recognition of the intrinsic abilities of the cord below a lesion leads to the conclusion that more invasive interventions such as baclofen pumps or botulinum toxin, or even surgical intervention, must be used in a way that opens possibilities for control rather than simply for treating symptoms.

The chapters cover material from both the basic science perspective as well as the practical approach to treatment. The former contain sections on spinal locomotor generators in different species and discussions on possibilities of new treatments involving techniques from spinal regeneration with stem cells to nerve grafting. The latter cover the examination of remaining function as detailed in the Brain Motor Control Assessment (BMCA) Protocol and the individual approach to patient care. In addition there are sections on surgical monitoring of spinal function, on surgical prevention of early complications of injury and on functional electrical stimulation from neuromuscular stimulation to spinal cord stimulation.

Throughout, the emphasis is on remaining capabilities of the damaged system and developing methods to maximise its potential for restoration of function. The spinal cord itself contains the best circuitry for control of our muscles, and only by harnessing that in the most effective way will we be able to optimize individual patient function.

John Rothwell, MA, PhD
Professor of Human Neurophysiology
Institute of Neurology
Sobell Department of Motor Neuroscience
and Movement Disorders
University College London
Queen Square, London, UK

PREFACE

Today, between 721 and 1,009 people per million in the United States are estimated to be living with a spinal cord injury (SCI), and each year, 20 to 50 per million more are newly injured.[1] Significant progress has been made in the development of treatments for spinal cord injuries, prevention of medical complications, and improvement of mobility and independence. Today, patients with SCI have a similar life expectancy to that of non-injured people. Rehabilitation engineering and robotics continue to develop devices that enhance the ability of people with SCI to perform activities of daily living, participate in community activities, and achieve a better quality of life than was possible even 10 years ago. However, these methods and devices have been designed to replace lost movement rather than to take advantage of and strengthen surviving, residual neural control of movement that often exists caudal to the injury.

Parallel studies of motor control in animals and humans have contributed to our knowledge of how the central nervous system generates and controls movement. In animal models of SCI, studies examining neurons and the circuits they form, the loss of connections between nerve cells, and the processes by which anatomical and neurochemical reorganization occurs after injury have told us that recovery is a complex and dynamic process that begins in the acute phase and continues throughout the patient's life. Furthermore, findings from these animal models have begun to suggest and test potential interventions to protect and restore neural circuitry affected by SCI. Thus the stage has been set for treatment of SCI in humans to transition from replacing mechanical function to restoring neural control of movement. However, in order to accomplish this paradigm shift successfully, it is essential that we recognize and respect the neural circuitry that survives after SCI.

The development and application of neurophysiological assessment methods in humans with intact and damaged central nervous systems have made it possible to advance our understanding of the nature of neural circuits that produce reflexes and perform automatic and volitional movement. Thus, in human SCI, it has become possible to assess the features of altered motor control below the level of the lesion. This approach, the testing of neural circuits, has contributed to the translation of clinical neurological findings from the large variety of neurological motor deficits

1. Cripps, R. A., Lee, B. B., Wing, P., Weerts E., Mackay, J., Brown, D. A. "GA global map for traumatic spinal cord injury epidemiology: Towards a living data repository for injury prevention." *Spinal Cord*. Published ahead of print. DOI: 10.1038/sc.2010.14949(2011):493–501.

found in people with SCI into information about their motor control and the underlying mechanisms of its disruption.

The assessment of motor control below the spinal cord injury allows us to monitor the modified functional relationships within the hierarchical network of motor control in such a way that absent or partially preserved brain control over the lumbar locomotor network can be substituted for or improved by artificial external electrical control. This is only one of numerous examples where the newly established functional relationship between the brain and the lumbar cord can be modified by additional external control. Therefore, it was important to assess SCI-altered neurocontrol to determine the underlying mechanisms responsible for the changed performance and clinically unrecognized residual function in order to design appropriately tailored intervention strategies.

This approach to the treatment of spinal cord injury through the assessment and modification of surviving motor control has led to the establishment of a *restorative neurology* program for spinal cord injury that is described and discussed in this book. Emerging over the past 50 years, this program recruited established multidisciplinary teams to demonstrate the efficacy of such a clinical practice.

This book is written for health care professionals to provide them with theoretical and practical information about restorative neurology in spinal cord injury. Here, for the first time, we describe the underlying principles of restorative neurology in one comprehensive text. These principles are supported by a wide variety of clinical applications. For this purpose we invited active health care professionals and scientists to contribute their knowledge of and experience with the application of these principles in their specific fields.

This volume is structured into four parts. Part I is dedicated to the clinical practice of restorative neurology (Chapters 1–3). Part II deals with the experimental animal work that has been done on the neurocontrol of locomotion and repair of the injured spinal cord (Chapters 4–5). Part III focuses on practical aspects of reconstructive neurosurgery (Chapters 6–7). Part IV is devoted to the assessment of motor control in chronic and acute spinal cord injury and includes restorative methods that focus on the lumbar spinal cord network such as posterior root stimulation (Chapters 8–10).

In Chapter 1, Dimitrijevic introduces the concept that, following traumatic injury, spinal cord neural circuitry and its connections to and from supralesional centers are altered and highly individualized. He draws from his experience with a large number of patients who were neurophysiologically examined during decades of work on identifying and characterizing subclinical aspects of neural function while developing restorative neurology in Houston, Texas. In this chapter, he makes the point that, once physiologically characterized, this new anatomical organization created by the injury and biological recovery becomes available for selective, targeted intervention. He also stresses the clinical and subclinical criteria that need to be applied when examining the resulting "residual motor control" and the role of each in the selection and adjustment of restorative procedures applied to upgrade function in the chronic phase of recovery.

In Chapter 2, Kakulas, Tansey, and Dimitrijevic describe and discuss the specific clinical and neurophysiological principles that underlie the assessment of residual motor control caudal to a spinal cord injury in humans. They extensively describe clinical, laboratory, and neurophysiological criteria for recognizing subclinical neurocontrol of movement in chronic spinal cord injury. This chapter also reviews published work that describes and supports the neurophysiologically differentiated "discomplete syndrome" that exists within the paralyzed, clinically motor-complete patient population. Finally, they cover the examination of motor control in gait and introduce the lumbosacral locomotor central pattern generator circuitry, its behavior and modification after SCI.

The third chapter in this section, by Tansey, Dimitrijevic, Mayr, Bijak, and Dimitrijevic, describes the clinical practice of restorative neurology using neurophysiologically based interventions to improve motor function in chronic SCI. They cover the specific treatment modalities used to adjust residual motor control and produce improved function, including: physiotherapeutic techniques; neuromuscular, functional, and spinal cord electrical stimulation methods; intrathecal and peripheral nerve pharmacological interventions.

In the second part of this book, Vrbová, Sławińska, and Majczyński (Chapter 4) present animal models of SCI and discuss how an understanding of the mechanisms responsible for producing the locomotor pattern, rhythmic limb movements associated with locomotion, is useful for the development of interventions to repair the damaged spinal cord. They provide an extensive review of the work performed in cat and rat models of SCI describing the contributions of supraspinal, spinal, and peripheral neural circuitry to the generation of spinal motor output, organized to perform functional standing and stepping movements. Their review includes models of complete transection, selective focal lesions, and generalized diffuse injury and covers the effects of a wide array of ablative and pharmacological manipulations. Finally, they review what is known about the different neurotransmitter systems at work in the spinal neural circuitry and how they are impacted by SCI.

In Chapter 5, Vrbová and Sławińska explore recent intervention approaches being tested on patients in relation to the experimental work performed to encourage regeneration within the central nervous system. They review studies that have elucidated the neurobiological basis for the difficulties faced by neurons attempting to survive, grow, and interconnect within the damaged spinal cord. Their comprehensive review includes results from studies that examined the success of neural grafts made from a wide variety of cell types and sources that have been implanted in attempts to replace lost cells and bridge lesions within an array of support strategies.

The next part of this book focuses on the surgical treatment of chronic SCI in humans. In Chapter 6, Brown describes "reconstructive" neurosurgery as the functional neurosurgical counterpart to restorative neurology and reviews its use in SCI. He presents a conceptual framework for understanding the "new anatomy" caused by trauma to the spinal cord and how interventions must capitalize upon its unique features. This chapter covers neurosurgical methods to reduce spasticity and augment function in upper and lower limbs by decreasing pathological input to spinal motor structures. It also covers peripheral nerve and tendon transfer techniques and treatment to improve control.

Tansey and Kakulas review, in Chapter 7, the pathophysiological status of the spinal cord after injury and establish criteria for biological intervention. They detail the pathological cascade that occurs during the acute phase of the injury in which damaged axons swell, excitatory neurotransmitters trigger excitotoxic injury, reactive oxygen species are generated, and inflammation develops, leading to further loss of neurons and glia. They describe the application of agents to impede this cascade and reduce the damage expressed in the finally established lesion. This chapter also reviews the effectiveness of pharmacological agents and neuronal grafts and provides guidelines for what should be done for a patient with chronic post-traumatic spinal cord injury if neurobiological interventions are available.

The fourth part of this book begins with Chapter 8: by McKay, Sherwood, and Tang, in which they present the practical aspects of assessing human motor control and describe changes caused by spinal cord injury. It focuses on the use of spinal motor output, recorded as surface electromyographic activity from multiple muscles during specifically selected reflex and volitional motor tasks to develop a profile of surviving motor control. This chapter is supplemented by Appendix I, a manual for conducting the brain motor control assessment (BMCA) protocol. Expected multi-muscle patterns from non-injured people and disrupted patterns typical of those with SCI are described and quantification methods presented that offer a sensitive, validity-tested method that generates a reproducible profile of motor control. The profile produced is then available for use in clinical research, and evaluation of changes in motor control induced by treatment.

In Chapter 9, Deletis, Sala, and Costa provide detailed descriptions of methods used for the intraoperative neurophysiological assessment of spinal cord function, including the epidural, scalp, and electromyographic recording methods, to evaluate ascending and descending long-tract conduction. They review the neurophysiological, killed-end potential that indicates the site of traumatic injury and markers that have been established as indicators of transient and permanent surgically induced loss of function.

Chapter 10, by Minassian, Hofstoetter, and Rattay, describes the selective stimulation of posterior root fibers through surface electrodes to produce reflex responses recorded from multiple muscles. They discuss the use of these responses that, like H-reflexes, are used to monitor changes in spinal motor excitability resulting from conditioning stimuli or motor task attempts, in the assessment of post-SCI function. Finally, they describe the use of this noninvasive transcutaneous approach to modify spinal motor control that is being expressed as spasticity and thus, to improve function.

Much of the work presented in this volume and the concepts that underlie the definitions and principles of restorative neurology are the result of contributions made by many individuals working in many laboratories around the world. It relies heavily on the development of tools that measure electrical activity and neurophysiological methods for examining the neural circuits in humans that has occurred over nearly a century. Appendix II by Zupanič Slavec provides the historical context in which the perspective presented in this book was developed.

The book concludes with an epilogue, prepared by Andresen, Kakulas, Vrbova, and Dimitrijevic, which critically evaluates the significance of considering residual neural function at the subclinical level in clinical practice to enhance the control of movement after spinal cord injury.

The development of this neuroscientific approach to human motor control after spinal cord injury was made possible by the continuous support of foundations for research and science in Slovenia, United States, Austria, and Norway. We would like to thank Craig Panner and Kathryn Winder from Oxford University Press for their continuous support while working on this book. We would like to express our appreciation to Dr. Meta M. Dimitrijevic for her development and successful application of the clinical practice of restorative neurology. We would also like to thank Dr. Martin Grabois for maintaining a place for restorative neurology within Baylor College of Medicine in Houston, Texas, USA. A special expression of gratitude is owed to Dr. Heinrich Binder for many fruitful discussions. Also, we appreciate deeply Kent Waldrep and his National Paralysis Foundation for always being around to provide creative, intellectual, and financial support to sustain the development of Restorative Neurology for spinal cord injury. The editors are also grateful for the efforts of assistant editor Simon M. Danner, who made this otherwise complex endeavor fluid and coherent. Finally the contents of this book are a result of contributions made by many professionals from many disciplines, but most importantly, from the people with injured spinal cords who so willingly supported and joined us in our process of learning about the motor control that survived their injuries.

CONTENTS

Contributors xvii

PART I The Clinical Practice of Restorative Neurology

1. Residual Motor Function after Spinal Cord Injury 1
   Milan R. Dimitrijevic

2. Neurophysiological Principles for the Assessment of Residual Motor Control Below the Spinal Cord Injury in Humans 10
   Byron A. Kakulas, Keith Tansey, and Milan R. Dimitrijevic

3. Restorative Neurology of Motor Control after Spinal Cord Injury: Clinical Practice 43
   Keith Tansey, Meta M. Dimitrijevic, Winfried Mayr, Manfred Bijak, and Milan R. Dimitrijevic

PART II Neurocontrol of Locomotion and Repair of the Injured Spinal Cord

4. Neural Control of Locomotion 65
   Gerta Vrbová, Urszula Sławińska, and Henryk Majczyński

5. Summary of Strategies Used to Repair the Injured Spinal Cord 93
   Gerta Vrbová and Urszula Sławińska

PART III Practical Aspects of Reconstructive Neurosurgery

6. The Reconstructive Neurosurgery of Spinal Cord Injury 134
   Justin M. Brown

7. Criteria for Biological Interventions for Spinal Cord Injury Repair 169
   Keith Tansey and Byron A. Kakulas

PART IV Assessment of Motor Control in Chronic and Acute Spinal Cord Injury

8. Neurophysiological Assessment of Human Motor Control and Changes Caused by Spinal Cord Injury 181
   W. Barry McKay, Arthur M. Sherwood, and Simon F. T. Tang

9. Neurophysiological Monitoring of the Human Spinal Cord Functional Integrity during Surgical Interventions 200
Vedran Deletis, Francesco Sala, and Paolo Costa

10. Transcutaneous Lumbar Posterior Root Stimulation for Motor Control Studies and Modification of Motor Activity after Spinal Cord Injury 226
Karen Minassian, Ursula Hofstoetter, and Frank Rattay

Epilogue 256
Nils G. Andresen, Byron A. Kakulas, Gerta Vrbová, and Milan R. Dimitrijevic

Appendix I: A Manual for the Neurophysiological Assessment of Motor Control: The Brain Motor Control Assessment (BMCA) Protocol 261
W. Barry McKay, Arthur M. Sherwood, and Simon F. T. Tang

Appendix II: Academic Environment for the Development of Human Motor Control in Ljubljana 285
Zvonka Zupanič Slavec

Index 301

CONTRIBUTORS

Nils G. Andresen, MS
Foundation for Movement Recovery
Oslo, Norway

Manfred Bijak, PhD
Center for Medical Physics and Biomedical Engineering
Medical University Vienna
Vienna, Austria

Justin M. Brown, MD
Division of Neurosurgery
Center for Neurophysiology and Restorative Neurology
University of California at San Diego School of Medicine
San Diego, California

Paolo Costa, MD
Section of Clinical Neurophysiology
Department of Neurosurgery
CTO Hospital
Torino, Italy

Simon M. Danner, MSc
Institute for Analysis and Scientific Computing
Vienna University of Technology
Vienna, Austria

Vedran Deletis, MD, PhD
Albert Einstein Colleague of Medicine
Institute for Neurology and Neurosurgery
St. Luke's–Roosevelt Hospital
New York, New York

Meta M. Dimitrijevic, MD
Foundation for Movement Recovery
Oslo, Norway

Milan R. Dimitrijevic, MD, PhD
Foundation for Movement Recovery
Oslo, Norway
Department of Physical Medicine and Rehabilitation
Baylor College of Medicine
Houston, Texas

Ursula Hofstoetter, PhD
Institute for Analysis and Scientific Computing
Vienna University of Technology
Center for Medical Physics and Biomedical Engineering
Medical University Vienna
Vienna, Austria

Byron A. Kakulas, MD, FRACP, FRCPA, FRCPath
Australian Neuromuscular Research Institute
Centre for Neuromuscular and Neurological Diseases
University of Western Australia
Perth, Australia

Henryk Majczyński, PhD, DSc
Nencki Institute of Experimental Biology PAS
Department of Neurophysiology
Laboratory of Neuromuscular Plasticity
Warsaw, Poland

Winfried Mayr, PhD
Center for Medical Physics and Biomedical Engineering
Medical University of Vienna
Vienna, Austria

W. Barry McKay, BS
Norton Neuroscience Institute
Louisville, Kentucky

Karen Minassian, PhD
Institute for Analysis and Scientific Computing
Vienna University of Technology
Center for Medical Physics and Biomedical Engineering
Medical University Vienna
Vienna, Austria

Frank Rattay, PhD
Institute for Analysis and Scientific Computing
Vienna University of Technology
Vienna, Austria

Francesco Sala, MD
Institute of Neurosurgery
University Hospital
Verona, Italy

Arthur M. Sherwood, PhD
Department of Physical Medicine and Rehabilitation
Baylor College of Medicine
Houston, Texas

Urszula Sławińska, PhD, DSc
Nencki Institute of Experimental Biology PAS
Department of Neurophysiology
Laboratory of Neuromuscular Plasticity
Warsaw, Poland

Simon F. T. Tang, MD
Department of Physical Medicine and Rehabilitation
Chang Gung Memorial Hospital
Chang Gung University
Taipei, Taiwan

Keith Tansey, MD, PhD
Director, Spinal Cord Injury Research and Restorative Neurology Programs
Crawford Research Institute, Shepherd Center
Departments of Neurology and Physiology
Emory University School of Medicine
Spinal Cord Injury Clinic
Atlanta Veterans Administration Medical Center
Atlanta, Georgia

Gerta Vrbová, MD, PhD, DSc
Division of Developmental Neuroscience
University College London
Royal Veterinary College
London, United Kingdom

Zvonka Zupanic Slavec, MD, MA, PhD
Institute for the History of Medicine
Medical Faculty, University of Ljubljana
Ljubljana, Slovenia

1

Residual Motor Function after Spinal Cord Injury

MILAN R. DIMITRIJEVIC

CONTENTS

1. Clinical and Subclinical Function
2. Neurophysiological Assessment—Restoration of Function
3. Subclinical Motor Control
4. Extent of Motor Control Recovery
5. Conclusion
References

1. CLINICAL AND SUBCLINICAL FUNCTION

Spinal cord injury (SCI) divides the spinal cord, disconnecting, to varying degrees, the caudal portion from supraspinal structures that include the brain, brain stem, and cerebellum. When neural circuitry belonging to the motor system is involved, then we must focus our interest on residual motor functions, the abilities that survive, and how motor control has been altered. Residual motor control may produce clinically obvious movement or be subclinical, able to modify motor excitability in ways that are only recognizable through neurophysiological recording. Persons with SCI whose residual motor function can produce clinically obvious movements also experience subclinical alterations in control that are relevant to treatment planning and can only be identified through neurophysiological means. The existence of clinical and subclinical residual descending input to spinal motor processing centers also provides some of the biological resources needed for repair of the injured spinal cord and restoration of its function. Thus, neurophysiological assessment to illuminate the subclinical aspects of residual neural function and neurophysiological intervention targeting this surviving motor control are the essential components of "restorative neurology."

The ability to perform a desired movement depends on the residual motor control that is present after SCI. Figure 1–1 illustrates this relationship by showing the dependence between movement capabilities and the degree of residual brain motor control.

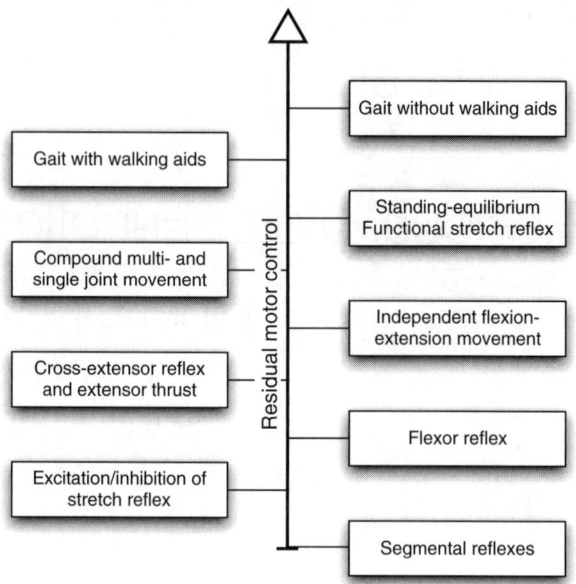

Figure 1–1 Motor capability depends on the degree of residual motor control.

Spinal reflex responses can be modified by residual brain influence: with an increase in brain motor control, more components of movement become available. For example, while weak residual control may provide only for whole-limb flexion-extension movement, greater residual control would support standing and walking.

Restorative neurological intervention would seek to augment residual motor control through external methods that increase the central state of excitability within the cord to enhance weakened brain motor control to improve function. This can be accomplished, for instance, by utilizing neuromuscular stimulation, functional electrical stimulation, and spinal cord stimulation.

2. NEUROPHYSIOLOGICAL ASSESSMENT—RESTORATION OF FUNCTION

Neurophysiology of human neurocontrol for volitional, automatic, and reflex movement and alteration of motor control after traumatic spinal cord injury has made significant progress in the past 20 years. Not long ago, manual muscle testing was the only method for assessing the severity of an incomplete spinal cord lesion (Little et al., 1990). Thanks to developments in human neurophysiological assessment of motor activity below the spinal cord injury, it has become possible, not only to assess clinical motor activity of incomplete SCI, but also to identify and record subclinical motor function (Eccles & Dimitrijevic, 1985). The possibility of adding subclinical, neurophysiogically recorded motor activity to the assessment of the spinal cord injured patient opened a new approach in the clinical practice of restorative neurology. Laboratory studies confirmed that subclinical residual motor activity can be used to augment basic excitatory and inhibitory CNS functions below the level of the injury, thus enhancing motor control. The clinical practice of restorative neurology is built upon the subclinical discovery and measurement of residual function and the application of interventions that neurophysiologically enhance this residual motor control.

Injury of the multi-parallel system—the descending motor, ascending sensory spinal cord tracts, and spinal gray matter networks—results in altered or lost motor and sensory spinal cord functions. Months after the injury, between 10% and 20% of spinal cord injury subjects recover the ability to stand and walk (Ducker et al., 1983; Young, 1989). However, the rest may be wheelchair-bound, depending on their SCI and the degree of residual motor function present below the spinal cord lesion. The fact that residual motor functions are present in practically all chronic spinal cord injured people prompts the questions: how do we identify and characterize motor control; and then, how can this surviving control be externally modified?

3. SUBCLINICAL MOTOR CONTROL

An example, shown in Figure 1–2, illustrates how a patient recovered well-organized volitional activity for ankle movement five months after injury, and slightly improved motor control over the following years, even in the presence of paralysis in all other parts of his body. In the polyelectromyographic recording performed two and a half months after injury, there was no volitional activity, even at the level of motor units. Five months after injury, the beginnings of well-organized dorsal plantar flexion of the right ankle showed the return of volitional activity, and there were simultaneous clinical findings for traces of dorsal foot movement. During the next four months, the activity became organized, with increased amplitude, better reciprocity, and a

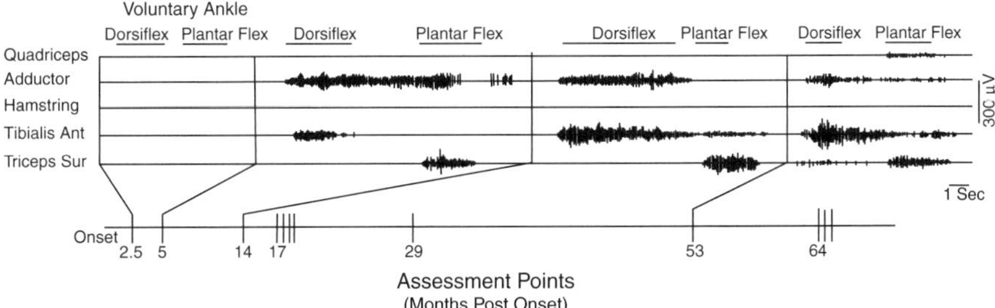

Figure 1–2 Recovery and improvement of volitional motor function in a quadriplegic patient. Four polyelectromyographic recordings of EMG activity recorded by surface electrodes from the right quadriceps, adductors, hamstrings, tibial anterior, and triceps surae muscle groups during the patient's attempt to perform ankle dorsal and plantar flexion (first recording 2.5 months after injury). Ankle movement task cuing is marked above the EMG traces. Calibration signal for EMG amplification of 0.3 mV is shown to the right of the figure. This figure summarizes the findings of 12 subsequent polyelectromyographic recordings acquired during 64 months, emphasizing that once volitional activity was recovered at five months after injury, it was maintained throughout the observation period (from Dimitrijevic, 1988).

more rapid onset and cessation of electromyographic (EMG) activity. These findings remained unchanged even after 14, 17, 29, 53, and 64 months, clearly illustrating that the right ankle had maintained the same degree of function throughout the observation period of five years.

In the clinically paralyzed leg, polyelectromyography can sometimes record volitional activation of motor units as illustrated in Figure 1–3, which shows the recording of attempted volitional activity in the same patient as was shown in Figure 1–2. Both lower limbs at that time were completely paralyzed. Two and a half months after onset, in contrast with the volitional clinical and neurophysiological activity present in the right ankle (Figure 1–2), the left leg recovered activity in isolated motor units in the adductor muscle groups, minute activity in the tibialis anterior and triceps surae, and the co-activation of the contralateral quadriceps, hamstrings, and triceps surae. The activation of motor units was subclinical, and there was no movement during this maneuver, but the patient described a feeling of stiffness.

When the patient performed preserved volitional activity of the right ankle (Figure 1–2), induced motor unit activity was present only in the right leg. However, when he attempted to move the left (Figure 1–3), minimal, subclinical EMG activity was present ipsi- and contralaterally, but there was no activation of muscles with residual volitional control. Therefore, the patient was able to generate motor unit activity in the absence of actual clinical movement and to maintain this ability for years. The patient in Figure 1–2 and Figure 1–3 also had incomplete impairment of sensory function immediately after injury. Three months later, a degree of recovery was documented, together with the presence of altered cortical somatosensory evoked

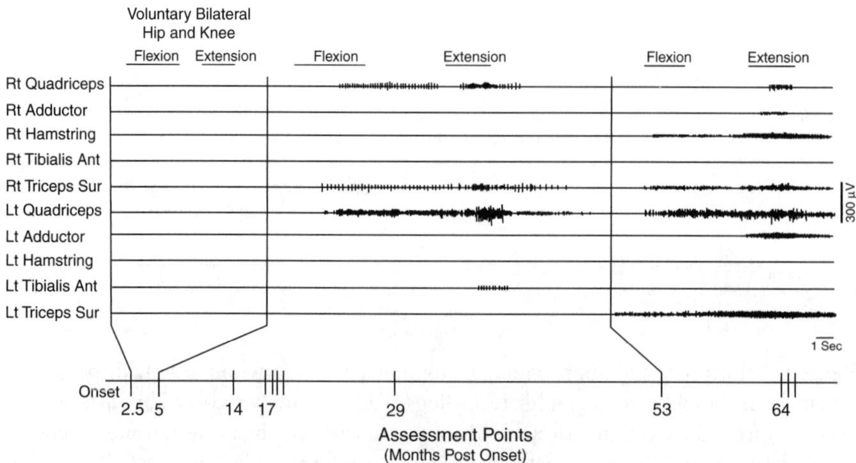

Figure 1–3 Subclinical improvement of residual motor function after SCI. Polyelectromyographic recording of motor unit activity during attempts to perform bilateral hip and knee flexion and extension. The patient was unable to produce any visible movement during the attempts. However, five months after injury, the patient activated the motor unit potential of 100 µV–150 µV, which was maintained four and five years following the onset of injury (from Dimitrijevic, 1988).

potentials from tibial nerve stimulation. Twenty-eight months after injury, sensory functions were nearly normal and were maintained throughout an observation period of seven years. Therefore, in this patient, the degree of injury to the sensory structures was less marked than that to the motor circuitry.

Analysis of this data showing the recovery of isolated and well-organized volitional activity for right ankle movement and the poorly organized motor-unit activation of the left leg, along with the nearly full recovery of sensory function, indicated that the ascending and descending functions of the central nervous system, which had been integrated before the onset of injury, were differentiated by the severity of the lesion, which resulted in different degrees and rates of recovery. These findings further illustrate that recovery of well-organized motor functions can begin even four months after injury. Therefore, nonfunctional recovery of suprasegmental control is also possible, and such residual influence can be present even in the absence of clinical activity.

Another example, which we studied at the end of the first week after onset of injury and repeated assessments throughout a year at regular monthly intervals, is the case of a gunshot lesion, which resulted in an immediate clinical neurological finding of a complete motor and sensory lesion of the spinal cord. Within the first week, the patient developed diffuse and severe muscle hypertonia, which persisted throughout the observation period. Within two months, the patient began to show signs of recovering sensory functions, but no clinically obvious evidence of motor recovery. However, the patient had preserved suprasegmental influence over segmental reflex excitability, and showed well-developed vibratory tonic reflexes and responses to reinforcement maneuvers in the paralyzed muscles of the lower limbs. Spasticity, in this case, developed within the first week after injury, so it could not be attributed to sprouting, synaptogenesis, or any other mechanism below the level of the lesion. It was probably caused by partial preservation of the descending facilitory and suppressive influence on lumbar spinal cord networks.

Residual central nervous system (CNS) axonal activity can help explain the clinical neurophysiological findings for subclinical evidence of brain influence in patients with clinically complete spinal cord injury. Therefore, by examining a large population of complete spinal cord injured patients, it might be possible to record the activity of single motor units in the corresponding, otherwise clinically paralyzed muscle groups that would be contracted during a specific motor task in subjects with intact CNS motor function. Actually, after examining 211 clinically completely paralyzed patients, this was found to be the case in six individuals, showing that volitional activation of only single motor units in paralyzed spinal cord injured subjects is rare, but possible. One of these six patients was able to activate very few motor units of the tibialis anterior when attempting ankle dorsal flexion, but a much larger number of motor units were activated when attempting a multi-joint flexion movement (Figure 1–4). The other five subjects showed a similar phenomenon of activation of single motor units during attempted dorsal or plantar ankle flexion, but only two of them had the ability to respond to multi- and single-joint volitional command with differentiated motor unit activity.

It was possible to repeat the above-described finding after several months and without training the subject to generate such motor unit activity through biofeedback or any other procedures. This suggests that, occasionally, in the fully paralyzed spinal cord injured patient, it is possible to document the function of the long

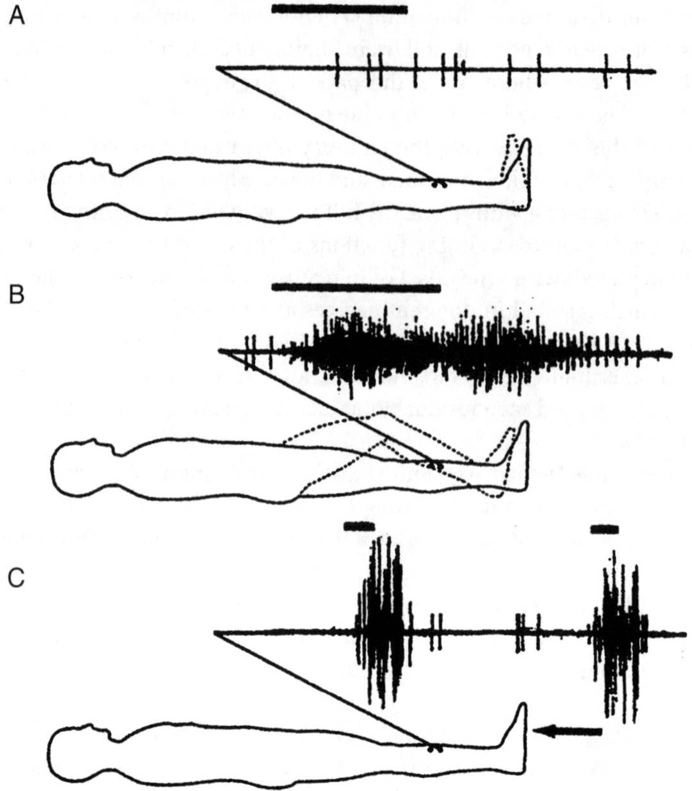

Figure 1–4 Rare finding of volitional motor control of single motor units in a clinically motor and sensory complete SCI subject. Summary of a recording with surface EMG electrodes from the right tibialis anterior muscle in a 19 year-old male, 42 months after onset of a C-5 spinal cord injury. Neurophysiological evaluation showed the presence of vibratory tonic reflexes and suprasegmental activation of motor units by reinforcement maneuvers. This particular patient was able to activate single motor units in the paralyzed tibialis anterior muscle when attempting dorsiflexion of the ankle (A). When he attempted to elicit multi-joint movement of the whole right limb (flexion of the hip, knee, and ankle), he was able to generate a much larger motor unit output (B). Plantar stimulation also activated the same tibial anterior muscle during a withdrawal flexion reflex (C) (from Dimitrijevic, 1995).

descending tract involved in the volitional control of isolated motor activity (Dimitrijevic, 1995).

Thus, if 10% to 20% of patients with traumatic spinal cord injury can expect a significant functional recovery, the remaining 80% to 90% will manifest numerous spinal cord dysfunctions with varying degrees of incomplete recovery.

4. EXTENT OF MOTOR CONTROL RECOVERY

In order to expand our knowledge of extended recovery after traumatic spinal cord injury, we examined 581 SCI subjects, both clinically and neurophysiologically

(Dimitrijevic et al., 1990). They were 116 women and 465 men whose time since injury ranged from two to 64 years. One hundred and eighteen of them were seen within the first six months after injury. Seventy were assessed between seven and 12 months, 111 between one and two years, 63 from two to three years, and 219 were assessed three or more years after onset. We were able to build three different illustrative groups. The first group consisted of 58 SCI subjects, whom we used for our clinical observation of their recovery. From those, 55 subjects showed evidence of motor complete spinal cord injury, and 13 of those 55 partially recovered and became motor incomplete after one or more years from initial injury.

The second group was composed on the basis of subclinical observations and consisted of 20 subjects who were initially motor complete, 12 of whom showed evidences for subclinical motor incompleteness by being able to activate motor units caudal to the lesion through reinforcement tasks or sustained response to vibration, or volitional suppression of withdrawal from plantar surface stimulation, five to seven years after injury. Thus, in this group, there was a large proportion of discomplete (see Chapters 2 and 8 and Appendix I) and incomplete subjects.

The third group is illustrated in Figure 1–5, which summarizes results of volitional multi-joint flexion and extension of lower limbs in six incomplete spinal cord injury subjects. We can see in this illustration that the strategy for performing this multi-joint task was different when compared to subjects with intact nervous systems and across those with altered function due to the spinal cord injury.

Another group of 18 subjects was selected from the original 581 subjects because they suffered complete lesions and were studied two to three years after injury. Their neurological deficit had not changed, but they developed spasticity between one and 17 months after injury. Thus, there is no specific time window within which spasticity can appear in an initially clinically complete injury.

5. CONCLUSION

According to the observations described in this chapter, it is obvious that SCI produces a diverse population with a wide range of recovery that can occur years after injury. The majority of individuals with clinically complete lesions will, in time, regain at least some of their nervous system functions, even in the absence of clinical evidence of such. Others will reveal clinical signs of trace or gross but not functionally useful movement, while there are also some who can even recover the ability to stand and walk. Thus, in the majority of initially clinically complete SCI subjects, recovery of impaired functions can occur spontaneously, but the extent of this recovery varies. Therefore, surviving or residual motor control and that recovered after clinically complete SCI should be regarded as an available neurobiological resource for use in the restoration of spinal cord function and the upgrading of nonfunctional translesional interaction to a modest degree of functional motor control.

In summary, after SCI, residual brain motor function can develop with neurocontrol features that are quite different across individuals, and those features suggest the presence of conducting translesional axons and the locations of their endings within the spinal gray matter.

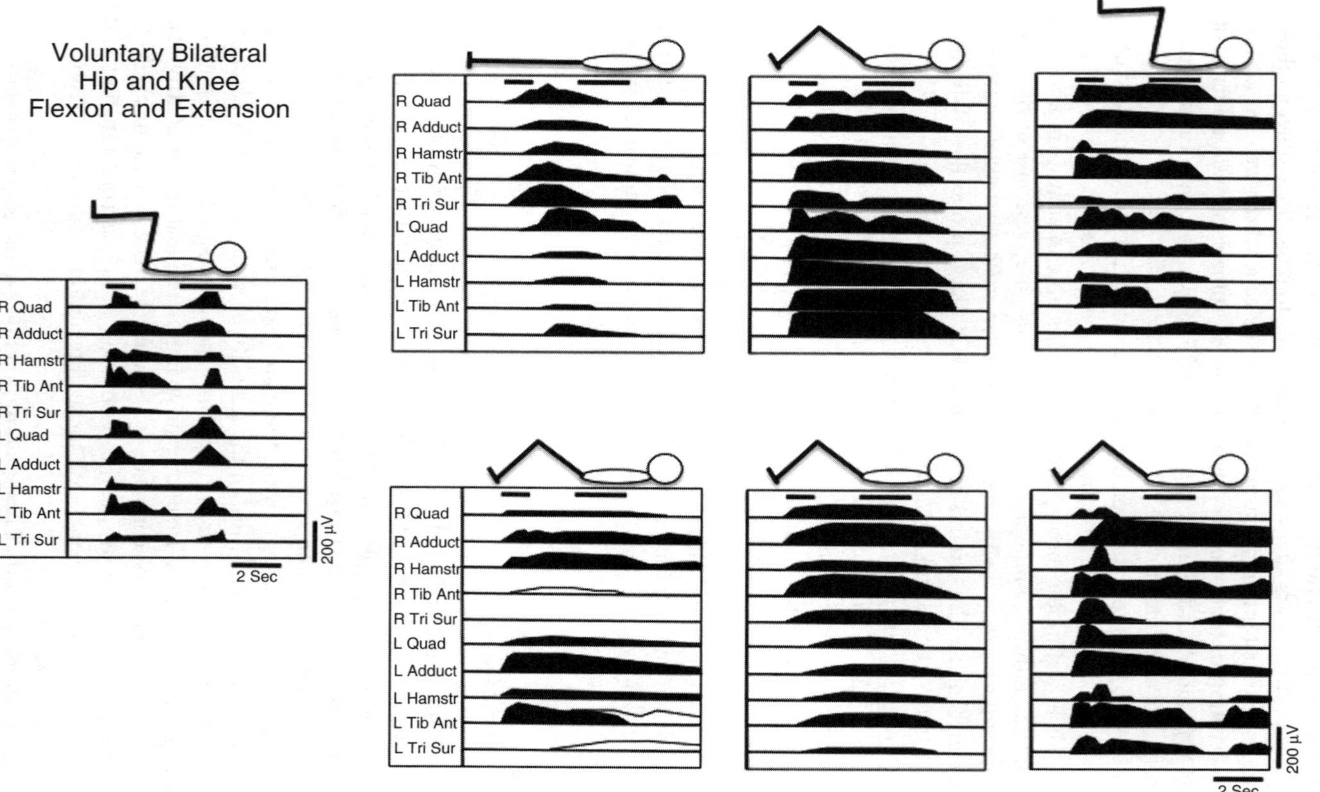

Figure 1–5 Schematic of EMG pattern recorded during the performance of a voluntary multi-joint motor task by a healthy subject (*left*). Three different SCI subjects (T8, C3, T7) attempt to perform the same task with different degrees of clinical movement (*top right*). Three other SCI subjects (T5, C6, C4) accomplish the same clinical movement with very different neurocontrol strategies (*bottom right*) (from Dimitrijevic, Lissens & McKay, 1990).

References

Dimitrijevic, M. R. "Clinical aspects of traumatic injury to central nervous system." In *The Axon: Structure, Function and Pathophysiology*, edited by S. G. Waxman, J. D. Kocsis, P. K. Stys, 669–679. New York: Oxford University Press, 1995.

Dimitrijevic, M. R., Lissens, M. A., McKay, W. B. "Characteristics and extent of motor activity recovery after spinal cord injury." In *Advances in Neural Regeneration Research*, edited by F. J. Seil, 391–406. New York: Wiley-Liss, 1990.

Ducker, T. B., Lucas, J. T., Wallace, C. A. "Recovery from spinal cord injury." *Clinical Neurosurgery* 30 (1983): 495–513.

Eccles, J., Dimitrijevic, M. R., eds. *Recent Achievements in Restorative Neurology: 1 Upper Motor Neuron Functions and Dysfunctions*. Basel, Switzerland: Karger, 1985.

Little, J. W., Ditunno, J. F., Stiens, S. A., Harris, R. M. "Incomplete spinal cord injury: Neuronal mechanisms of motor recovery and hyperreflexia." *Archives of Physical Medicine and Rehabilitation* 80 (1990): 587–599.

Young, W. "Recovery mechanisms in spinal cord injury: Implications for regenerative therapy." In *Neural Regeneration and Transplantation*, edited by F. J. Seil, 157–169. New York: Raven Press, 1989.

2

Neurophysiological Principles for the Assessment of Residual Motor Control Below the Spinal Cord Injury in Humans

BYRON A. KAKULAS, KEITH TANSEY, AND MILAN R. DIMITRIJEVIC

CONTENTS

1. Introduction
2. Principles of Neurological Evaluation
    2.1. Phasic Stretch Reflex
    2.2. Tonic Stretch Reflex
    2.3. Withdrawal Reflex
    2.4. Volitional Motor Activity
    2.5. Summary and Recommendation
3. Principles of Neurophysiological Evaluation
    3.1. Spasticity and Spasms
    3.2. Individual Stereotype Responses
    3.3. Central State of the Spinal Cord
    3.4. Tendon Jerk after Discharge
    3.5. Cutaneo-Muscular Reflex Organization
    3.6. Repetitive Tendon Jerks
4. Residual Brain Influence and Motor Control Below the Injury
    4.1. Presence of Exaggerated Tendon Jerks in Spastic SCI
    4.2. The Characteristics of the Vibratory Tonic Reflex in the Clinically Complete SCI Syndrome
    4.3. Volitional Suppression of Withdrawal Flexor Plantar Reflex
    4.4. Suprasegmentally Induced Motor Unit Activity in Paralyzed Muscles of Patients with Established Spinal Cord Injury
5. Modification of Volitional Motor Task Output Below Level of Incomplete SCI

6. Neurocontrol of Human Locomotion
6.1. Gait after Spinal Cord Injury
6.2. Spinal Cord CPG; Spinal Cord Stimulation
References

1. INTRODUCTION

The behavior patterns of spinal motor activity above and below a spinal cord lesion are diverse. The muscles below the level of the lesion, lacking varying degrees of volitional control, may show altered reflex, automatic, postural, and positioning regulation of the body and limbs. This altered spinal motor activity results in both loss of power, coordination, dexterity, and endurance (the so-called negative phenomena of paresis), and the emergence of uncontrolled and non-coordinated movements and/or muscular contractions (the so-called positive phenomena of spasticity). More often than not in spinal cord injury, it is not the presence or absence of movement that is the issue, but rather the quality and control of that movement. Fundamentally, the movements of normal stepping are similar to the movements in extensor or flexor spasms, but they differ in their magnitude, duration, rhythmicity, and modifiability.

Increased excitability of motor unit activity, exaggerated stretch reflexes, increased muscle tone, loss of cutaneo-muscular local responses. and impairment of volitional control are the sequelae of disordered or impaired supraspinal control and are collectively often referred to as the "upper motoneuron syndrome," or in clinical use, the "gestalt of 'spasticity.'" These effects are the more significant components of our noninvasive neurophysiological studies, which we have applied to patients with spinal cord injury (SCI) who show the clinical features of spasticity. The study of each of these phenomena contributes to our understanding of the neurophysiology of SCI. Our deeper, scientific understanding of these neurological abnormalities has been derived originally from animal experiments used to investigate the afferent and central mechanisms involved in mono- and polysynaptic segmental reflex activity. Lundberg (1967) described the contribution of different primary afferents and central inputs derived from the descending tracts, which converge on the spinal interneurons of the premotor network of the spinal cord (Dimitrijevic & Faganel, 1985; Dimitrijevic, 1987; Dimitrijevic, 1992).

Advances in animal neurophysiology, in parallel with the development of spinal cord neurology and human neurophysiology, have made it possible to introduce the assessment of motor control of the spinal cord below the level of lesion into the clinical practice of restorative neurology. Figure 2–1 illustrates the neurophysiological approach used for the assessment of spinal cord motor control in the human (Figure 2–1A).

Three major motor clinical syndromes are recognized in the human with SCI:

- Firstly, there is *incomplete SCI* with clinical evidence of altered but to some extent retained motor functions below the level of injury;
- Secondly, there is the clinical syndrome of *discomplete SCI* with absence of all voluntary motor function below the level of the lesion but with demonstrable neurophysiological evidence of residual conscious—i.e.,

volitional—influence upon spinal reflex activity below the level of injury;

- Thirdly, and the least common outcome of SCI, is the "absolute" *complete SCI syndrome* recognized as meeting all clinical and neurophysiological criteria for total absence of voluntary movement or sensation below the lesion and complete absence of any neurophysiological evidence of supraspinal influence or consciously directed influences on the spinal reflexes below the level of the lesion.

Figure 2–1 illustrates these three syndromes diagrammatically. *A* shows the impairment of transmission in the three syndromes. *B* shows the tests for stretch and cutaneo-muscular reflexes below the level of the lesion under specific paradigms with and without effort to elicit residual brain influence and volitional motor control. Depending on the severity of the lesion, additional assessment of volitionally controlled motor unit activity is reordered during the performance of motor tasks involving discrete and diffuse movements in order to delineate the features of altered motor unit activity resulting from the SCI.

In this chapter we describe the neurological and neurophysiological protocols for the assessment of motor control in the human spinal cord after injury and the basic principles applied when measuring an individual's spatiotemporal coordination of the activity of the motor neuron pools during reflex activity and volitional motor tasks.

2. PRINCIPLES OF NEUROLOGICAL EVALUATION

In the clinic it is common practice to carry out clinical assessment and classification of SCI according to the American Spinal Injury Association (ASIA)/International Spinal Cord Society (ISCoS) neurological standard scale (American Spinal Injury Association, 2002; Steeves et al., 2007). The ASIA classification is composed of the following:

1. The neurological level of the lesion based on volitional motor and conscious somatosensory (light touch and pain) testing
2. Whether it is clinically *complete* or *incomplete* SCI (loss or sparing of the lowest sacral levels' sensorimotor function)
3. ASIA impairment scale (AIS) Grade A, B, C, D, or E
4. Zone of partial preservation (ZPP) in complete SCI

Protocols for ASIA assessment are widely accepted and are the present tools used to describe the functional and clinical characteristics of post-traumatic SCI syndromes (American Spinal Injury Association, 2002).

Clinical neurological examination of motor function includes testing the maximal strength of volitional contractions, signs of neurological deficits in upper and lower motor neuron function, and corresponding clinical changes such as altered muscle tone resulting in spasticity and reflex changes secondary to the affected motor pathways.

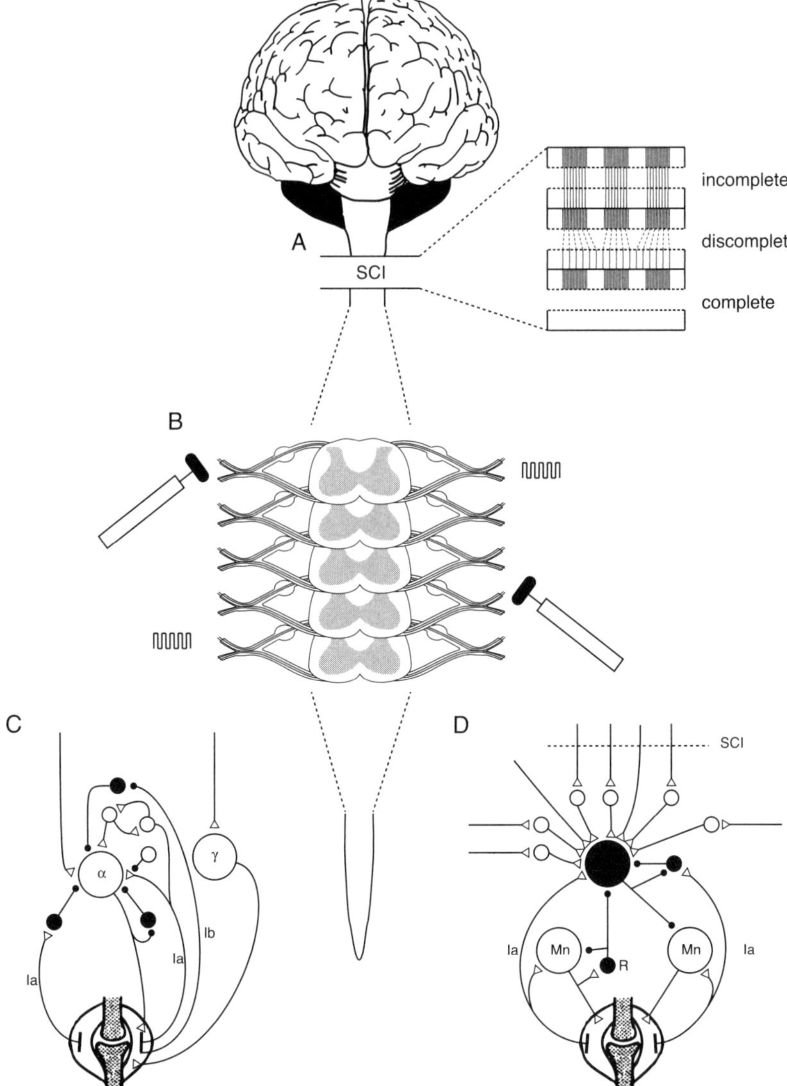

Figure 2–1 Sketch of (*A*) spinal cord injury, dividing rostral from caudal portions of spinal cord. (*B*) Sketch of plurisegmental networks illustrates simultaneous surface poly-EMG recordings of motor outputs during stretch, cutaneous-muscular reflexes, and brain-controlled motor task. (*C*) Sketch of circuits for stretch and cutaneo-muscular reflex. (*D*) Sketch of circuitry for premotor spinal cord center (adapted from Dimitrijevic, 1992).

Neurological definitions of *complete* and *incomplete* spinal cord injury syndromes were provided by Guttmann in 1976. The *complete* clinical syndrome included what was believed to be a clear-cut transverse spinal injury causing the complete loss of all voluntary and sensory functions caudal to the lesion. The *incomplete* clinical syndrome resulted when there was partial sparing of the spinal cord so that some functions were retained below the level of injury. The incomplete designation was subdivided into two main subgroups: (1) a diffuse injury affecting more or less all of the central gray matter as well as the sensory and motor tracts again at any level but not resulting in complete loss of neurological functions below; (2) anatomically circumscribed lesions affecting distinct parts of the spinal cord resulting in incomplete deficits of dissociated type with the clinical picture being determined by which part of the spinal cord is involved as viewed in cross section. These incomplete syndromes are subclassified as being lateral, anterior, posterior, central, or mixed; or as pure motor, sensory, and cauda equina syndromes (Eidelberg, 1987).

However, our intention here is to draw the attention of the reader to several new clinical spinal cord injury syndromes that are based on neurophysiological criteria. First, in neurologically complete patients who supposedly have a transverse lesion of the spinal cord lacking all voluntary movement and conscious sensation below the level of the injury, we have identified individuals in whom neurophysiological evidence can be found of the transmission of signals passing though the injury zone. The resulting supraspinal influence on spinal motor function can be detected as changes in recorded patterns below the level of injury. These signals can only come from above, being induced either by conscious effort by the patient or by reflex-enhancing maneuvers such as neck flexion. This newly identified SCI syndrome may be considered to be subclinically incomplete. That is to say, there exists a spinal cord syndrome characterized by the retention of non-volitional residual brain excitatory and inhibitory activity with impulses traversing the lesion and thereby influencing reflex activity of the spinal cord below the level of injury.

We have coined the term *discomplete* to describe this new spinal cord injury syndrome, which can only be identified by neurophysiological assessments. Thus we point out that there are some patients who are thought to be clinically "complete" but who in reality are subclinically incomplete. This finding implies the theoretical supposition that there is a small population of axons that have survived the injury and are able to conduct signals through the injury zone. In this way properties of spinal reflex activities are modified by brain influence arising from supraspinal inputs (Sherwood et al., 1992). Neither the ASIA exam nor our neurophysiological assessments described above necessarily capture all supraspinal influences on infra-injury neural circuitry. For instance, it takes rather "complete" cervical lesions to release the phenomenon of autonomic dysreflexia, which probably reflects the loss of hypothalamic influence on preganglionic sympathetic neurons of the intermedial lateral cell column of the thoracic cord.

Considerable anatomical postmortem evidence exists in support of the concept of a clinically *discomplete* SCI syndrome as the phenomenon of the continuity of a small number of axons surviving the injury and passing through the lesion in an uninterrupted fashion is now well known (Kakulas, 1999).

The second, less-known, spinal cord syndrome is an *incomplete lesion with distinct biomechanical characteristics* resulting from diffusely distributed or patchy surviving and conducting axons of sufficient number to elicit similar alterations in reflex motor performance implemented through different motor tasks below the level of the lesion and showing neurocontrol features of functional muscle synergies (Dimitrijevic et al., 1990). Figure 2–2 is a sketch of these two new spinal cord injury syndromes: *A* showing a population of surviving, conducting axons which, during brain-controlled volitional effort, can modify the central state of spinal cord excitability expressed as increased tone or as long-delayed involuntary movement and/or spasms below the level of the lesion; and *B* showing brain-induced volitional movement or the performance of a specific motor task eliciting a discrete or diffuse movement through activation of motor units—this being a feature of neurocontrol of so-called residual brain control in clinically incomplete spinal cord injury syndromes mentioned above and in Figure 2–2B.

Thus there are two situations wherein suprasegmental influences may be detected in otherwise neurologically complete SCI. The first is detected by surface polyelectromyography (sPMG) in the lower limbs when the SCI patient performs the Jendrassik reinforcement maneuver or makes some postural change; for example, neck flexion. The second is a change in tone and postural reflexes resulting from the same inputs and referred to as *biomechanical effects*. Both are due to a small number of descending axons traversing the injury site having survived the injury. The clinical and neurophysiological parameters of these discomplete syndromes correlate exactly with postmortem reports of humans wherein about a third of clinically complete patients were shown to have a small number of surviving axons in continuity from above to below the injury site.

These cases have been referred to as being *anatomically discomplete* (Kakulas, 1999). In these individuals, the number of preserved axons is insufficient for volitional movements or to conduct conscious sensation; that is, they are clinically complete, but nevertheless, residual axons are able to carry signals and influence the spinal cord below the level of the lesion, which manifest either as surface polyelectromyographic (sPEMG) changes or as biomechanical effects as described above.

In the clinical practice of restorative neurology, we have learned that it is essential to extend the neurological evaluation of upper motor neuron activity in SCI to include the following paradigms: (1) the stimulus-response paradigm to determine if the response to a test stimulus input is *present, altered, or absent;* (2) the conditioning paradigm in which peripheral or central input is added to determine if a response to a test stimulus can be modified and if so, by how much and in what ways and can the change be clinically observed; (3) repetitive task performance in which motor response behavior to stimuli delivered to the same site at a constant repetition rate, and strength of stimulation produce consistent responses, or do attempts to perform repeated volitional motor tasks produce identical movements or is there a the developing trend of increase, decrease, or disruption over time (Figure 2–3).

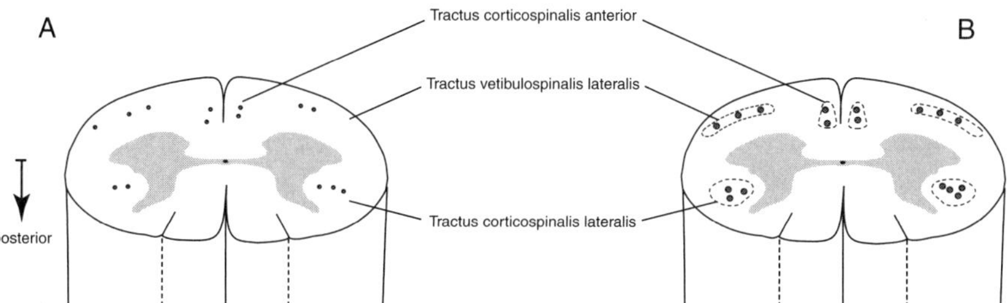

Figure 2–2 Schematic drawings of (*A*) spinal cord with surviving axons within descending long tracts, (*B*) spinal cord with reduced population of functional axons still present in the long, descending tracts.

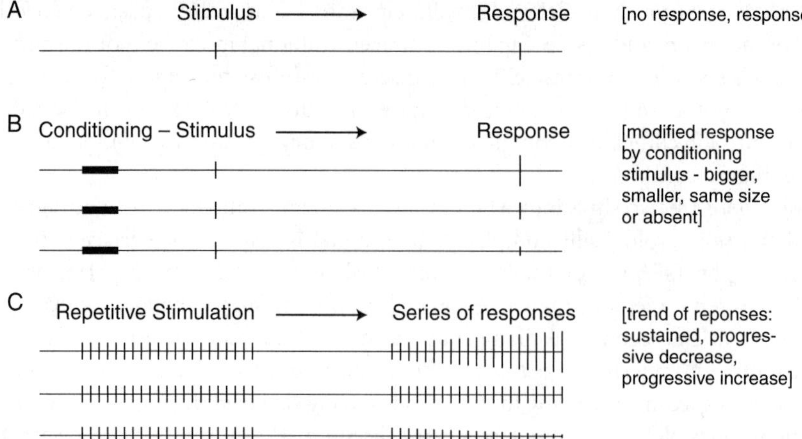

Figure 2–3 Sketch for three testing paradigms to be used in clinical testing of neurological signs for spinal cord motor function impairments. (*A*) Test stimulus and response. (*B*) Condition to test stimulus and response. (*C*) Series of repetitive stimulation and monitoring behavior of motor responses.

When the researcher is neurologically evaluating motor function in clinically complete and incomplete syndromes in post-traumatic SCI, the above parameters may disclose additional evidence of clinically non-obvious brain influence and residual motor control below the injury zone. This extra information contributes to the appreciation of spinal cord motor control below the level of the SCI and is pertinent to restorative neurological interventions designed to augment functional performance of residual motor control. As shown in Figure 2–4, it is useful to use the *stimulus-response paradigm*, with tendon taps to elicit phasic stretch reflex responses (*A*); to perform passive movement, shortening or lengthening of the whole limb to elicit tonic stretch reflexes (*B*); to request that the subject under examination perform selected volitional movements, shortening and lengthening of the limb as much as possible (*C*). Also, asking the subject to perform the task repetitively, for at least five times, depending on the person's capabilities shows the consistency of their ability to perform and control movement. All of these parameters should be systematically tested and recorded.

2.1. Phasic Stretch Reflex

In post-traumatic chronic SCI, whether clinically complete or incomplete, the response to phasic stretch is expected to be exaggerated or greater than in non-injured people. The phasic stretch reflex can be easily elicited by percussion of the tendon with a reflex hammer, especially so for the Achilles, patellar, triceps, biceps, and triceps tendons. When muscle hypertonia is present, percussion with the reflex hammer on various muscles below the spinal cord lesion can be effective. One should add the short flexors of the toes, the abductors, the adductor of the thigh, and abdominal, paraspinal, styloradial, deltoid, pectoralis, rhomboid, and trapezius muscles to those most often tested.

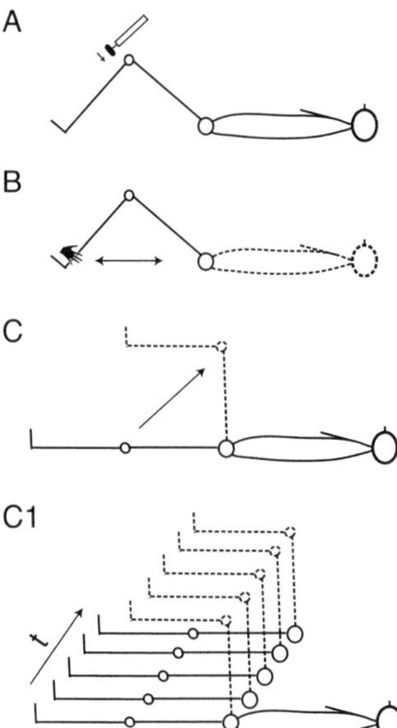

Figure 2–4 Sketch illustrating clinical maneuvers for testing (*A*) phasic stretch by tendon tap, (*B*) manual passive flexion/extension movement of the whole limb for eliciting tonic stretch reflex, (*C*) single volitional multi-joint limb flexion and extension, and (*C1*) repeated volitional flexion and extension movements at regular intervals while monitoring the behavior of motor control.

It is essential to describe the *threshold of the phasic stretch reflex* and the definitive threshold level for brisk reflex contraction induced by repetitive percussion to the tendon (or muscle belly, for muscles without a tendon). While performing repetitive taps, it is possible to have reflex responses in non-tapped muscles in addition to reflex responses restricted to the tapped muscle, a "radiation" or "spread" of stretch reflex responses. A proposed mechanism, which may be responsible for radiation, is muscle spindle hypersensitivity to mechanical wave resonance secondary to bone conduction of the tap (Lance & De Gail, 1965). There is also the possibility for radiation arising from spinal cord central mechanisms as suggested by the recording of a silent period, which may occur without preceding synchronized motor unit activity and/or brisk muscle contraction. This phenomenon is illustrated in Figure 2–5.

Finally, there also exists the possibility that, with the loss of descending modulation of dorsal horn inputs, sensory input can activate synergist motoneuron pools. It is known in the cat that individual Ia afferents project to a majority of homonymous motoneurons and many heteronymous motoneuron pools. This could explain why, in the spastic condition, stretch of a thigh adductor can activate the contralateral adductor, and why biceps tendon percussion can elicit finger flexion.

2.2. Tonic Stretch Reflex

Sustained passive movement of the whole upper or lower limbs or of one joint is part of the clinical evaluation of stretch reflex responses to differing but constant rates of

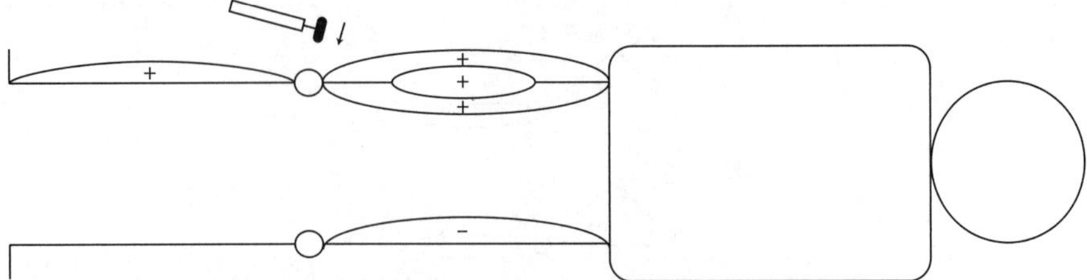

Figure 2–5 Surface electromyographic (sEMG) recording from thigh and leg muscle groups in a spastic SCI subject. Tapping of right quadriceps can elicit simultaneous phasic stretch reflexes in thigh and right tibialis anterior muscle due to peripheral mechanisms. The appearance of an inhibitory effect on the contralateral hamstring is the result of a central mechanism, through mediation of inhibition via the lumbar cord network (adapted from Dimitrijevic & Nathan, 1967b).

movement. The test goal is to find out if and how much resistance is present, starting from the slowest rate and proceeding without any gap to the fastest. The strongest resistance to passive stretch is encountered at the fastest rate. This technique tests the threshold for rate-dependent muscle hypertonia. During the same maneuver, we should record how much the unstretched, ipsi- and contralateral muscles respond, with visible contractions observed. Naturally, again we should at least repeat the manual muscle tonic movement test five times, observing whether the stretch reflex response causes decreased, normal, or increased muscle tone, as well as paying attention to the effects of repetition on the features of persistent, declining, or increasing muscle tone.

An essential prerequisite for the examination of muscle tone is for the patient to be placed in a *comfortable supine* position in a quiet environment (Figure 2–6). The examination of muscle tone and its possible modification through changes of the body posture, from supine to sitting, standing, stepping, and even, when possible, walking on the floor or treadmill with weight support, should be part of protocol for assessment of the effects of posture on phasic, tonic stretch reflexes and volitional

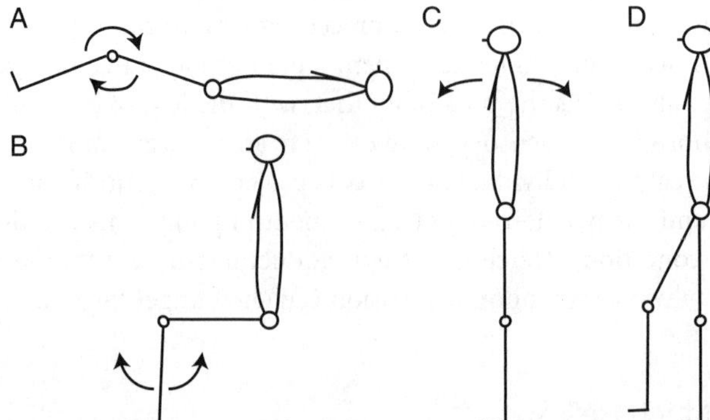

Figure 2–6 Sketch of body position testing of the influence to tendon jerk response. (*A*) testing in supine position, (*B*) testing in sitting position, (*C*) testing in standing position and leaning forward and backwards, and (*D*) testing during stepping in place.

activity. Also, the examiner should systematically evaluate how the subject's position and posture may modify muscle tone, looking for postural deformities and/or volitional, automatic, or involuntary movements in the form of so-called spasms.

2.3. Withdrawal Reflex

The *withdrawal reflex* is an avoidance movement induced by cutaneous stimulation. Withdrawal from plantar stimulation may be brisk or long-lasting, consisting of as little as flexed or extended toes, or larger with toe and ankle movements, or larger yet including movement of the ankle, knee, and hip, or largest involving both legs. These degrees of plantar reflex intensity and whether it declines in amplitude, remains constant, or even progressively increases with repeated stimulation characterize the response (see Figure 2–3; Dimitrijevic, 1973). It is also possible to show "spread" of this response to cutaneous/noxious inputs. Toe-pinching, for instance, can trigger dorsiflexion of just the ankle, or it can trigger a triple flexion response with ankle, knee, and hip flexion movements.

2.4. Volitional Motor Activity

The presence of intact, altered, or absent volitional motor activation; the performance of a variety of motor tasks, discrete, rhythmic, combined, skillful, or postural; and their control of accuracy, force, and endurance are other factors that describe motor control in SCI syndromes. There can be paralysis and/or paresis with different degrees of severity of muscle hypertonia and frequency of spasms (i.e., powerful involuntary movements) (Dimitrijevic et al., 1989). Therefore, the description of the degree of volitional activity during single and multi-joint movements and their scoring is recommended as a standard for widespread clinical application. The paradigms of stimulus-response, conditioning-testing, and repetitive stimulation, as well as the examination of repeated volitional motor acts as described above, provide the additional information needed for restorative neurological assessment.

2.5. Summary and Recommendation

Extending the usual detailed, clinical neurological evaluation of upper motor neuron function to include the additional paradigms of stimulus-response, conditioning-test stimulus-response, repetitive stimulation, and observing behavior of sequential responses should be part of clinical testing of motor control in a program for the restorative neurology of chronic SCI. Sustained and not-sustained features of elicited spinal cord reflexes, and their modification by conditioning of peripherally controlled sensory or residual supraspinal inputs, should be part of the protocol for evaluation of motor control of the injured spinal cord. Simple and logical descriptions of the findings for all three of these paradigms should be part of the medical record. There is also the potential to develop a scoring system in order to improve communication between different spinal cord injury centers (Dimitrijevic, 1991). While examining the residual volitional control of movement, we should evaluate volitional movement on command, even when such performance is impaired and incomplete. This approach uses the application of reinforcing supraspinal maneuvers in the assessment of clinically complete spinal cord syndromes as well as to a variety of incomplete syndromes in order to elicit "involuntary" movements; that is, spasms.

A summary of the neurological principles for the assessment of motor control is shown in Figure 2–7. This is a sketch of the approach we use in seeking information, not only about the strength at the threshold of response, but also about the immediate and late effects according to the kind of afferent input applied. These late effects may be in the form of afterdischarges or certain behaviors in evoked motor responses modified by progressive habituation or dishabituation.

3. PRINCIPLES OF NEUROPHYSIOLOGICAL EVALUATION

Following the acute period of suppressed spinal reflexes, the injured spinal cord recovers with progressively increased spinal reflex responses, with or without partial

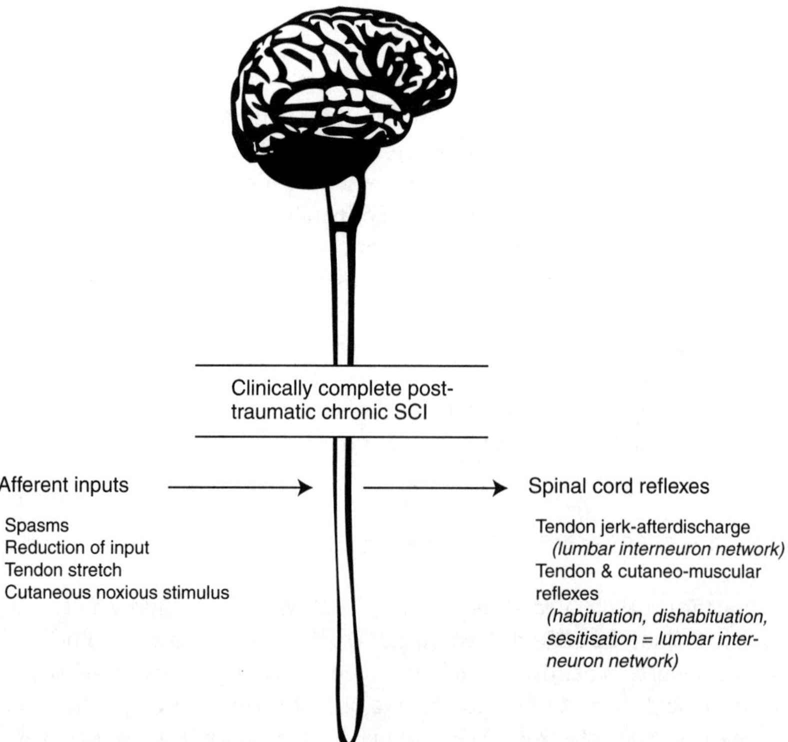

Figure 2–7 Illustration of neurological principles for evaluation of motor control after spinal cord injury. The sketch shows standardized approaches to afferent input and systematic analyses of spinal reflex output of single and repetitive responses, and their temporal and spatial distribution within different muscle groups of the lower limbs. These neurological and neurophysiological approaches provide additional characteristics of spinal reflex responses and the early and later components of their interactions within different muscle groups.

recovery of volitional motor activity. Ultimately, recovery of motor control below the level of the lesion reaches a plateau and a sustained level of altered motor control. By using the available neurophysiological methods for the assessment of motor control below chronic and established SCI, it is possible to apply in human studies methods for recording the functional characteristics of spinal reflex activity and the interaction between brain and spinal cord in SCI in clinically complete or incomplete spinal cord lesions. In this way it is possible to study neurophysiologically the *neurocontrol of spinal reflex activity*, and record its features under residual brain influence and motor control. The neurobiological scientific background, which underlies the human studies of neurocontrol evident below the level of the lesion, is derived from experimental pathophysiology of SCI in animals and their indirect translation to the human (Jankowska & Hammar, 2002; Gorassini et al., 2004; Nielsen et al., 2007; Heckman et al., 2009).

In this section, an outline of the neurophysiological background behind the protocols we use to assess motor control in the clinical practice of restorative neurology will be given. The aim is to document the effect of brain motor control on the lumbar cord network below the level of the injury, and/or the modification of reflex or volitional output under the influence of residual brain control.

3.1. Spasticity and Spasms

When the spinal cord is deprived of supraspinal control, there is a correspondingly large increase in activity of the spinal motor neurons. This is manifested as spasms in the form of prolonged, uncontrolled, excessive contractions of skeletal muscles and as pathological responses to all form of stimulation: tactile, noxious, and proprioceptive. This excessive activity interferes with basic reflexes organized at segmental levels of the spinal cord. As this activity continues, it takes an abnormally long time for one movement to be replaced by another. Motor responses become limited in their variety of stereotyped movements, and local signs of response are lost.

Multi-channel surface electrode polyelectromyography (sPEMG) is a relatively simple and noninvasive neurophysiological tool used to study features of spasticity and to explore the evidence for the contribution of clinically non-obvious suprasegmental neurocontrol. SPEMG records of motor unit activity reveal features of covert or not fully appreciated residual brain control, which has been modified by the SCI. By placing pairs of electrodes over the main muscle groups of the lower limb flexors and extensors while eliciting peripheral or central maneuvers of spinal reflex activity, it is possible to record the presence of the subject's idiosyncratic or dysynergistic responses. Reduced inflow to the spinal cord reduces the excessive activity of motoneurons and thus the features of spasticity (Dimitrijevic & Nathan, 1967a). A decrease of spinal cord hyperexcitability may reveal the basic elements of reciprocal innervation (Dimitrijevic & Nathan, 1967b), such as changes in withdrawal reflexes (Dimitrijevic & Nathan, 1968; 1970; 1971), habituation and dishabituation; that is, sensitization, of tendon reflexes (Dimitrijevic & Nathan, 1973).

SPEMG recording of *spasms* in spastic paraplegia or in paraparesis during spontaneous, reflex, volitionally induced spasms or after efforts made to perform motor tasks, has led to the recognition of various features of spasticity, as it occurs in patients with complete and incomplete spinal cord lesions. In spasticity, all or most of the muscles of the lower limbs fire together. This occurs spontaneously and/or as a response to stimulation, and, in paraparesis, as a part of purposeful movement. Antagonist and synergistic muscles continue to fire throughout the whole extent of a movement, usually increasing and decreasing their activity simultaneously with that of the agonist. An example of this activity in all the muscles sampled, including both limbs flexors and extensors, is illustrated in Figure 2–8.

3.2. Individual Stereotype Responses

Another feature of sPEMG is the *individual stereotype response* of motor unit activity recorded in spastic paraplegics. Although organized spinal cord reflex responses are expected to be common to all subjects with a similar profile of SCI deficits, they are, however, replaced or overlaid by the subject's individual response. Certain muscles or muscle groups tend to be activated on all occasions regardless of whether normal coordination indicates that they should take part in the movement or that they should be suppressed and inhibited. When there is a muscle group, which is easily activated, every sort of stimulation tends to bring it into activity. However the built-in-reflex response is not completely lost, for elements of the built-in response and the individual response are both present and detectable.

3.3. Central State of the Spinal Cord

Reduction of the local inflow of impulses to the spinal cord causes a widespread reduction in the activity of motor units. This reduction in inflow is effective in

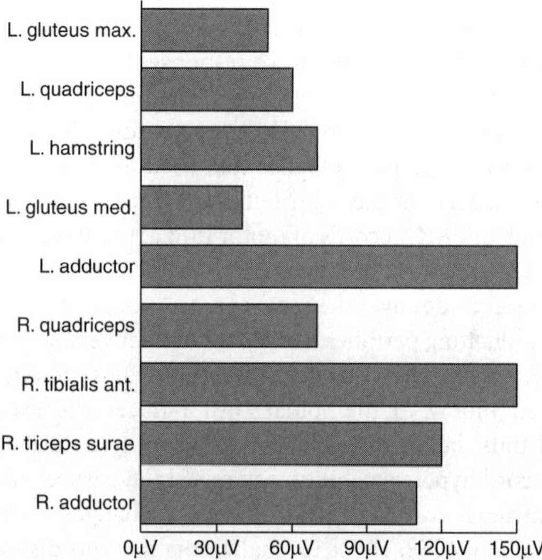

Figure 2–8 Mean values of sPEMG recorded motor unit activity from lower-limb muscle groups during an involuntary spasm. Substantial simultaneous motor unit activity in antagonistic muscle groups is present without any evidence of reciprocal inhibition, and contralateral muscle groups are activated (adapted from Figure 1 in Dimitrijevic & Nathan, 1967a).

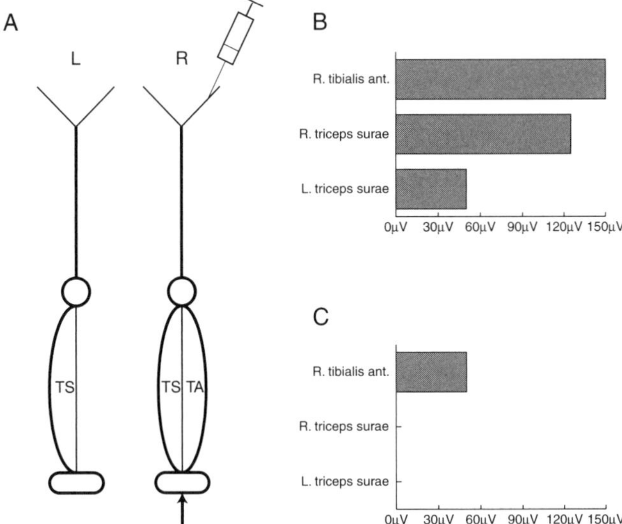

Figure 2–9 Sketch illustrating effect of a reduction of afferent input in a spastic SCI patient induced by a procaine block of the right femoral nerve (*A*), and motor unit activition elicited by plantar stimulation before (*B*) and after (*C*) nerve block. Significant reduction of motor unit activity in the ipsilateral limb as well as complete absence of activity in the contralateral limb can be observed in *C* (adapted from Figure 12 in Dimitrijevic & Nathan, 1967a).

reducing motor activity even when this activity is increased by other means such as local stimulation or stimulation from higher levels of the neuraxis. Figure 2–9 illustrates sPEMG recording of motor unit activity in spastic paraplegic subjects elicited by nociceptive stimulation of the right plantar surface, and evoked activity in ipsi- and contralateraltibialis anterior and ipsilateral triceps surae. However, after anesthetic block of the right femoral nerve and therefore reduced afferent input from the right quadriceps, only ipsilateral tibialis anterior motor units respond to sole stimulation, to the same strength. Ipsi- and contralateral triceps surae muscles do not respond after the central state of spinal cord excitability is reduced by nerve block.

3.4. Tendon Jerk after Discharge

The sPEMG recording of the stretch reflexes of the lower limbs in spastic paraplegics and paraparetics and their analysis demonstrates larger responses than in subjects with intact CNS functions. There is a synchronous discharge of motor units immediately after the tap on the tendon, followed by less synchronized, later, and longer-lasting motor unit afterdischarges. The muscle is activated during the first 100 ms following the tap on a tendon according to the normal patterns of reciprocal innervation. After the first 100 ms contractions, that is, spasms are due to the afterdischarge of motor units of the tapped muscle and of many other muscles. Distribution of this afterdischarge follows no pattern of reciprocal innervation. The manner by which the afterdischarge spreads to other muscles of the lower limbs shows that the afterdischarge is proportional to the amount of local input to the spinal cord. If the tendon jerk is reduced by any means, the afterdischarge is also reduced. As most features of spasticity are due to the afterdischarge, a reduction in the local input to the cord removes many of the features of spasticity.

Features of the tendon jerk-induced afterdischarge are schematically shown in Figure 2–10. Tendon jerk sPEMG displayed with a time base of 10 ms per division shows an Achilles tendon jerk response with a constant latency of 30 ms. When the time base is adjusted to 50 ms/division, there are clear but less synchronized and delayed motor unit discharges that follow the early, more constant response, with a variable latency of 100 ms to 200 ms. When the antagonistic muscle group is also

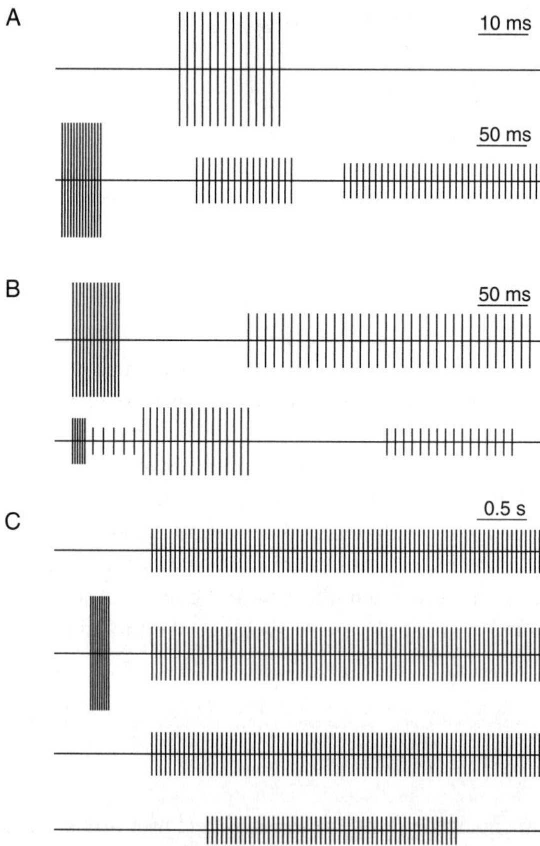

Figure 2–10 Sketch illustrating sEMG recordings of Achilles tendon jerk responses recorded with 10 ms and 50 ms per division (*A*). Two traces (*B*) are motor unit recordings in quadriceps and antagonistic hamstring muscles during the hamstring jerk. SPEMG recordings of ipsilateral muscles during the knee jerk (*C*). Sketch illustrates the afterdischarge folowing the Achilles jerk in the lower trace of (*A*) with the 50 ms per division time base; (*B*) reciprocal inhibition in antagonistic hamstring during quadriceps jerk; and (*C*) multisegmental afterdischarge in all ipsilateral thigh and leg muscles after knee jerk (adapted from Dimitrijevic & Nathan, 1967b).

recorded as is the case in Figure 2–10 B in which the patellar tendon is tapped, the hamstring muscle, can also be seen to respond with a phasic contraction, synchronized with the response in the quadriceps followed by later afterdischarges and less synchronized EMG activity. Further, when the recording period is extended to one second and other ipsilateral and contralateral muscle groups are added, even tapping the dorsal surface of the ankle or metatarsal bone heads can elicit simultaneous early phasic response, within the first 50 ms, followed by a burst of simultaneous late and prolonged afterdischarges in ipsilateral thigh, leg, and contralateral thigh muscles (Figure 2–10 C). This is a reproducible constant and repetitive finding in all subjects with spastic paraplegia and paresis, and is modified by ongoing motor activity. Afterdischarges can be elicited by tendon taps in all recorded ipsilateral and contralateral muscle groups, following phasic tendon-tap responses or with the appearance and spreading of afterdischarge motor unit activity to any muscles. Thus, in addition to the tendon reflex responses which are the result of the excessive, unregulated sensitivity of spinal neural circuitry to input from stretch receptors in the muscle and tendon, reflex responses can be result from input conducted through the bony skeleton. In this event, synchronized short and constant latency responses will appear in many muscle groups without reciprocal relationships, or when delivered during ongoing background activity, they may appear as central spreading of suppression of activity in the antagonistic muscle groups. Therefore, in a spastic SCI subject, reflex hammer taps to tendon or bone can elicit short and constant latency, phasic synchronized responses without reciprocal antagonistic interaction and radiation is both peripheral and central. However, in both cases afterdischarge motor unit activity can be triggered simultaneously in any muscle groups of the lower limbs. Thus, SCI often leaves spinal interneuronal circuitry hyper-responsive to inputs from muscle and tendon receptors and even bone leading to differing degrees to a centrally mediated distribution and spread of short-latency reflex responses and longer latency afterdischarging simultaneously to other muscles both ipsi- and contralateral to the source of input. The significance of this finding that there is a low threshold for eliciting phasic stretch reflexes in spastic paraplegia due to chronic spinal cord injury is that it provides electrophysiological evidence that spinal polysynaptic segmental and plurisegmental circuitry is hyperactive and, thus contributes to spasticity.

3.5. Cutaneo-Muscular Reflex Organization

The next step in neurophysiological exploration of the features of spasticity by sPEMG is the analysis of reflex activity evoked by noxious cutaneous stimulation (Dimitrijevic & Nathan, 1968). A system of cutaneo-muscular reflexes organized at the level of the spinal cord has been reported in the decerebrate cat and in the human with intact CNS function (Hagbarth, 1960). When the cord is deprived of supraspinal control, the finely adjusted system of cutaneo-muscular organization described by Hagbarth and colleagues is not seen (Figure 2–11). The main reason for the absence of this cutaneo-muscular system is disinhibition of the flexion reflex. Different regions of the skin give different responses. In the spinal cord subject deprived of supraspinal control, responses to noxious cutaneous stimulation are abnormally prolonged, and there is commonly a late response following the early response. With spasticity, noxious cutaneous stimulation may activate most of the

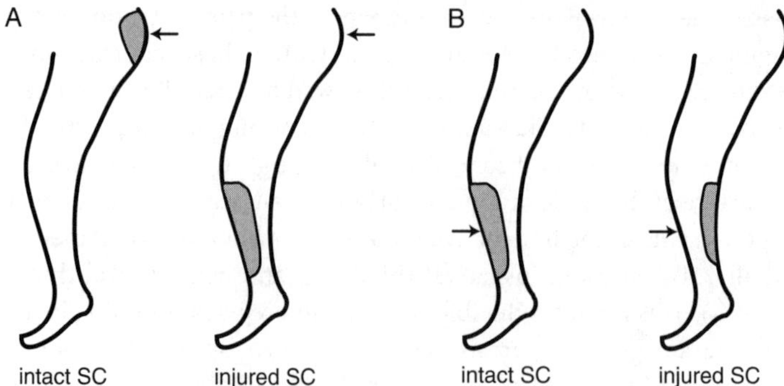

Figure 2–11 Noxious stimulus applied over gluteus maximus (*A*) and tibialis anterior (*B*). It shows that in subjects with intact CNS, the muscle below the muscle underlying the stimulation site responds, but this organized response is disrupted after SCI. Arrows represent the site of stimulation, and shaded areas, the muscle responding (adapted from Hagbarth, 1960; Dimitrijevic & Nathan, 1968).

muscles of the limb stimulated and some of the opposite limb. The result is mostly flexion of the limb stimulated, often accompanied by flexion of the opposite limb as well. Noxious cutaneous stimulation may evoke individual idiosyncratic responses. The response obtained is determined by the intensity of stimulation, by the presence or absence of motor unit activity at the time of stimulation, by the position of the limb and the phase of movement of the limb, depending on whether it is moving or being moved.

Variability in the spread, amplitude, and duration of the muscular response to identical electrical noxious stimuli is found when studying cutaneo-muscular, withdrawal reflexes of the lower limbs in spastic SCI subjects with a clinically complete spinal cord lesion. Therefore, studies of changes of the flexion reflex with repetitive cutaneous stimulation in the spinal cord injured human contribute to the neurophysiological descriptions and underlying control mechanisms of the features of spasticity. When recording reflex responses to cutaneous stimulation by sPEMG from the lower limb muscle groups by electrically induced noxious stimulation in spastic paraplegics, the time taken for the excitability to return to its previous level after a single stimulation is related to the stimulus intensity and to the number of preceding stimuli. When regularly repeated stimuli to the skin are given in a series, the spinal cord organizes a response that changes in amount and in radiation. These changes follow a certain pattern, of which the following phases are recognized: buildup, fluctuation, diminution, and cessation (see Figure 2–12).

It is not certain that there will always a phase of cessation of the response when the stimulation is intense. This phase may not be reached even after 30 minutes of stimulation. Moreover, withdrawal reflexes often have two components, an early and a later one, similar to the already illustrated afterdischarges in response to tendon jerks, and in the phase of cessation of response, the second component of the flexor reflex ceases to respond before the first one.

The duration of the phase depends on stimulus rate and intensity. With a repeated stimulus of slight intensity, each phase is of short duration. With a repeated stimulus

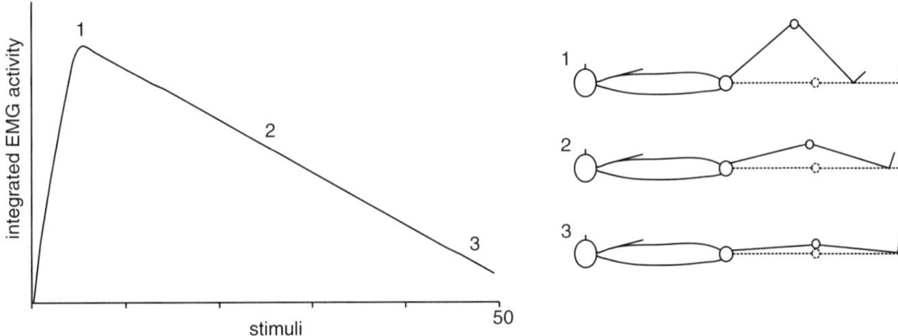

Figure 2–12 Sketch illustrating sequential integrated EMG resonses from the tibialis anterior muscle during repetitive noxious stimulation delivered to the plantar surface representing the progressively declining amplitude of this flexor muscle response (on the left side, the decreasing responses are illustrated; adapted from Dimitrijevic & Nathan, 1970).

of strongly noxious character, there may be no buildup phase, the phase of fluctuation and diminution being very long, and under the condition of testing, no phase of unresponsiveness occurs. Thus, habituation is more marked for stimuli of low rather than of high intensity.

Repetitive stimulation causes both excitatory and inhibitory processes within the local region of spinal cord. Furthermore, the first muscle to respond is the last muscle to continue to respond, and the last muscle is the first to fall out. There are also other reasons to believe that cessation of the response is not due to failure of transmitter substance anywhere in the reflex pathway. Habituation to repeated cutaneous stimuli occurs within the interneuronal pathways, somewhere near the afferent limb of the reflex. Repetitive stimulation causes, in addition to habituation, a decrease in the excitability of the whole spinal cord. This decrease follows a different time-course from habituation. This process has been called *tiring*.

Motor units brought to a phase of unresponsiveness by regular repetitive stimulation are reactivated by an increase in stimulus intensity and by an increase or decrease in stimulus rate, but they are not reactivated by a decrease in stimulus intensity. When stimulation is added or substituted at a second site, habituation occurs more quickly than it would have had there been no habituation occurring at the previous site. All dishabituating effects are less marked from contralateral than from ipsilateral stimulation.

3.6. Repetitive Tendon Jerks

Repetitive excitation of tendon reflexes of the lower limb in chronic SCI may also elicit habituation, dishabituation, or sensitization of the above-described noxious flexion reflexes. However, tendon reflexes are more likely to show sensitization. Thus the above-described polysynaptic cutaneo-muscular flexion reflex in spastic paraplegics also occurs in the case of the monosynaptic tendon reflex (Dimitrijevic & Nathan, 1973).

4. RESIDUAL BRAIN INFLUENCE AND MOTOR CONTROL BELOW THE INJURY

The absence of volitional movements and perception of sensation for touch, vibration, pain, and temperature are the clinical criteria for the syndrome of clinically complete spinal cord injury. However, when to those criteria are added the analysis of lumbar spinal cord reflex activity, simultaneously recorded electromyographically from all lumbar segmental common final pathways, and their interaction in time and space is characterized, the concept that the lesion is a complete transection of the spinal cord can be challenged. This conclusion, reached by the findings of these additional human neurophysiological assessments, is supported by postmortem findings in SCI. Therefore, by studying volitionally induced modification of spinal reflex responses below the level of the lesion, a definite supraspinal input passing through the injury zone may be identified. This concept is supported by studies on brain influence on rudimentary control below the spinal cord injury. This conclusion is reached by recording the neurophysiological characteristics of spinal cord reflexes to determine if and how they can be modified by supraspinal maneuvers.

By means of the bedside neurological examination, it is possible to ascertain deficits in motor and sensory functions in SCI patients. However, the presence of subclinical manifestations of brain influence on paralyzed muscles may substantially alter the clinical findings. This discrepancy between clinical and subclinical neurological status should be recognized in developing goals for clinical programs in restorative neurology. In order to document the nature and extent of such residual and subclinical suprasegmental brain influence, we recorded surface PEMG from multiple muscle groups, studying patterns of motor unit activity in response to a variety of stimuli, including tendon taps and tendon vibration (Dimitrijevic et al., 1977), and by voluntary suppression of plantar withdrawal reflexes (Cioni et al., 1986). SPEMG changes may also be induced by activating motor units of muscles below the lesion through reinforcement maneuvers performed above the lesion (Dimitrijevic et al., 1984). Analyses of data, derived from the brain motor-control assessment (BMCA) procedures we have developed, also provides evidence of subclinical brain influence in clinically complete spinal cord injury subjects (Sherwood et al., 1992) (see Chapter 8 in this volume). We shall review these findings and describe their frequency of occurrence and their characteristics in the following chapter sections.

4.1. Presence of Exaggerated Tendon Jerks in Spastic SCI

After post-traumatic spastic SCI, we shall expect clinically and electrophysiologically recorded stretch reflexes to be of constant latency and of exaggerated amplitude, reflecting the excessive excitability of spinal cord motoneurons responding to presynaptic inputs and the decrease of pre- and postsynaptic inhibition. However, in a study of patellar and Achilles tendon jerks in a group of 38 chronic wheelchair-bound, post-traumatic cervical and thoracic clinically complete and incomplete SCI subjects suffering from spasticity, sPEMG was used to record tendon jerk responses elicited by a handheld electrodynamic hammer (Trontelj et al., 1968); and we found

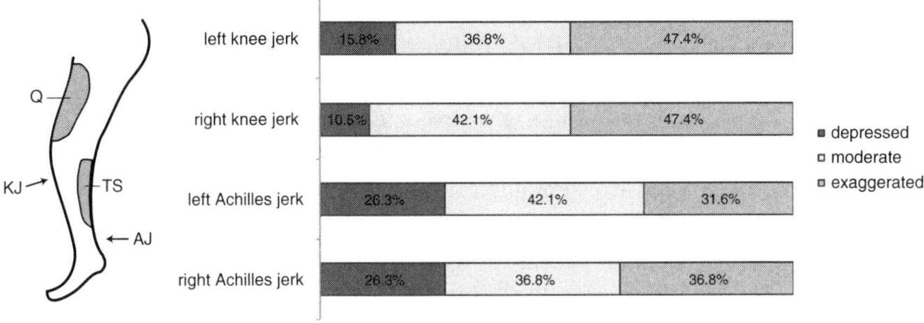

Figure 2–13 Summary of a surface EMG study of 38 chronic, wheelchair bound, spastic persons with SCI. Recorded tendon jerk responses from both quadriceps and triceps surae muscles elicited by a handheld electrodynamic (constant force and controlled rate) hammer, just above threshold for response. Ten average responses from each response have been categorized to: clinically depressed (average amplitude of 0.2 mV); moderate (average amplitude of 1.0 mV); exaggerated (average amplitude of 2.0 mV).

that spastic SCI subjects showed both exaggerated and depressed amplitude responses to the stimulus. The summary results of ten repetitive constant-strength taps to the tendon delivered at a repetitive rate of 0.5 Hz with the responses averaged to their mean value in sitting subjects is shown in Figure 2–13.

As shown in Figure 2–13, in spastic SCI subjects, tendon jerks are not only exaggerated, but in the same individual they can also be of low amplitude. This finding does not change significantly in follow-up recordings. We have shown this in five subjects of the 38 studied, by repeated measurements under an identical measurement protocol from which sPEMG amplitudes of tendon jerk responses were analyzed. Thus, when measured electrophysiologically in spastic SCI subjects, tendon reflexes may be moderate, exaggerated, or suppressed. We should point out that, in the spastic SCI subjects studied, other independent neurological conditions such as peripheral nerve damage that would impair volley conduction within the monosynaptic reflex arch were excluded. An alternative explanation for the presence of low-amplitude tendon jerks together with exaggerated reflexes can be a hypothetical modification of the central state of spinal cord excitability by residual suprasegmental influence being sufficient to modify spinal reflex behavior but not to enable volitional movement in clinically complete SCI syndromes. This hypothetical mechanism can be supported by a small population of axons with intact anatomical and functional connectivity that survive and cross through the injury zone. Moreover, there is a great deal of supportive anatomical morphological evidence for this hypothesis derived from neuropathological studies of spinal cord injuries in patients with the clinically complete lesion syndrome.

In previous publications (1999; 2004), Kakulas reported that, in the majority who have received their spinal injury from motor vehicle or diving accidents, there was continuity of spinal cord white matter; that is, conducting nerve fiber tissue at the level of the lesion observed postmortem, despite the severity of the injury and displacement of the vertebral column. Of 352 cases with vertebral injuries who were "dead on arrival" at the hospital, the spinal cord was found to be intact at the level of the lesion in 138. Generally these patients survived less than one hour after injury. Of 125 "acute survivors" with vertebral fractures (surviving for less than six months post-injury), the spinal cord was transected in only 17. Of 87 chronic cases (survivors of more than six months), 24 were neurologically incomplete, 31 were anatomically "discomplete" (see below) showing structural continuity of white matter across the injured segments, and 22 were anatomically fully complete having transected their spinal cord. The clinical status of the remaining 10 was unknown.

Thus a very clear correlation exists between the neurophysiological observations of supraspinal influences in clinically "complete" patients, well described above, and the findings in a large postmortem series. As stated, this observation offers fruitful ground for the restorative neurologist to augment and enhance residual functions of the CNS. Preserved axons traversing the lesion may be stimulated by various techniques, such as by electrical currents, in order to improve residual voluntary motor control.

To further this objective, a clinico-pathological assessment was made to discover just how much white matter is required to allow volitional control and/or retain sensation below the level of the lesion. In long-term survivors, the spinal cord lesion in SCI consists of multilocular glial lined cysts traversed by vascular bundles, regenerated nerve roots, and a variable amount of preserved white matter representing residual pathways. In 11 clinically complete patients, no residual white matter traversing the lesion was found in eight subjects, while three showed some preservation of white matter tracts. Therefore, these three may be regarded as being "anatomically discomplete." In these three discomplete patients, the area of preserved white matter was 1.09 sq mm, 1.12 sq mm, and 3.89 sq mm, respectively. In 10 clinically incomplete patients, the amount of white matter traversing the level of the lesion ranged from 1.17 sq mm to 13.89 sq mm. Thus, it is evident that there is no strict correlation between the amount of preserved white matter and the clinical status of the patient. For instance, in one of the clinically complete cases, the amount of white matter was 3.89 sq mm, and in four of the clinically incomplete patients, there was 1.94 sq mm, 3.17 sq mm, 1.94 sq mm, and 1.73 sq mm, respectively.

Axonal counts were also undertaken to establish the minimum number required for volition and sensation. Normal controls had an average of 41,472 nerve fibers in the lateral corticospinal tracts at T4 (all were cervical injuries); the smallest number found in a patient with slight motor control below the lesion was 3,173 axons. This patient had retained dorsal and plantar flexion of the right foot.

The lowest number counted in the posterior columns in a sensory incomplete patient was 117,359. This person had preserved light touch and vibration sense in the right arm and pinprick sensation perianally. Normal controls had an average of 452,480 axons in the posterior columns (Kakulas, 1999; 2004).

Returning to our neurophysiological assessments, when the excitability of spinal motoneurons is tested by tendon jerks in subjects with severe spasticity, they may be exaggerated with hyperexcitable motoneurons, or they may be reduced with motoneurons of lesser excitability. A possible spinal cord central mechanism to explain this finding is a residual supraspinal input passing through the spinal cord injury zone, reaching to influence spinal cord reflexes below the level of the lesion. In order to examine this hypothesis, we shall call on the evidence for neurophysiological subclinical brain influence on spinal cord reflexes in SCI people with the clinical syndrome of complete spinal cord injury.

4.2. The Characteristics of the Vibratory Tonic Reflex in the Clinically Complete SCI Syndrome

Vibrating a muscle tendon with a manually attached vibrator (vibration frequency 80 Hz and unload excursion of 2–3 mm) will elicit a progressively increasing tonic vibratory reflex (TVR) in the stimulated muscles in persons with intact nervous system functions (Sherwood et al., 1993). This TVR can be voluntarily facilitated and suppressed (Dimitrijevic et al., 1977). We have reported on the features of the vibratory reflexes (VR) (see Figure 2–14), beginning with no response as shown in Figure 2–14A1, followed by increasing duration of VR responses during stimulation (Figure 2–14A2–A5; Dimitrijevic et al., 1989). Responses in these subjects were smaller than those in the non-injured population, and occurred with increased thresholds compared to those without SCI. The differing features of response of vibrated paralyzed muscle groups arising from volitional control of motor-unit activity we interpret as the expression of different populations of partially active axons mediating bulbospinal influence through the injury zones in clinically complete subjects. This interpretation is supported by the fact that the TVR is abolished in the experimental cat model with a transected spinal cord (Matthews, 1966). Dependence of the TVR on the reticular formation has been demonstrated in the cat by transecting the spinal cord and stimulation of brain stem through the injury zone (Gilles et al., 1971).

Figure 2–14A4 shows the recorded features of a VR when reflex activity ceases, and it was possible to restore the activity by the reinforcement maneuver; and also shows a case featuring a continuous VR response (Figure 2–14A5) where it was possible to control the response by turning the vibration stimulus on and off. In addition, when a VR is continuously present as with the vibrated tendon of the muscle group B1, it can generate an isolated response in the vibrated muscle group only, spread to activate all ipsilateral muscle groups of one lower limb, or even to both ipsilateral and contralateral limbs. This is a constant and repetitive finding, depending on the severity of spasticity. We interpret this finding not as mechanical transmission (Lance & De Gail, 1965) but as neural mediation, being a central and not a peripheral mechanism. We have also demonstrated that such facilitation and suppression can spread across several segments via the interconnecting network of the propriospinal interneuron system (Faganel & Dimitrijevic, 1982).

4.3. Volitional Suppression of Withdrawal Flexor Plantar Reflex

After describing that residual translesional facilitation of spinal cord reflexes below the level of clinically complete spinal cord injury (Dimitrijevic et al., 1984), we sought to determine if it was possible to demonstrate evidence for suprasegmental suppression of the withdrawal flexor reflex. By recording EMG activity from leg muscles, we studied changes in segmental excitability of the plantar reflex elicited by cutaneous stimulation of the foot plantar surface. In 50 paralyzed spinal cord injury patients, we examined the ability to volitionally suppress the plantar reflex on three repeated trials after baseline records were established. The patients who had no voluntary EMG activity in the monitored muscles were able to volitionally suppress the plantar reflex response by 45% in tibialis anterior, hamstring, and triceps surae muscles, and to suppress the quadriceps response by 72%, which was reduced more than any other

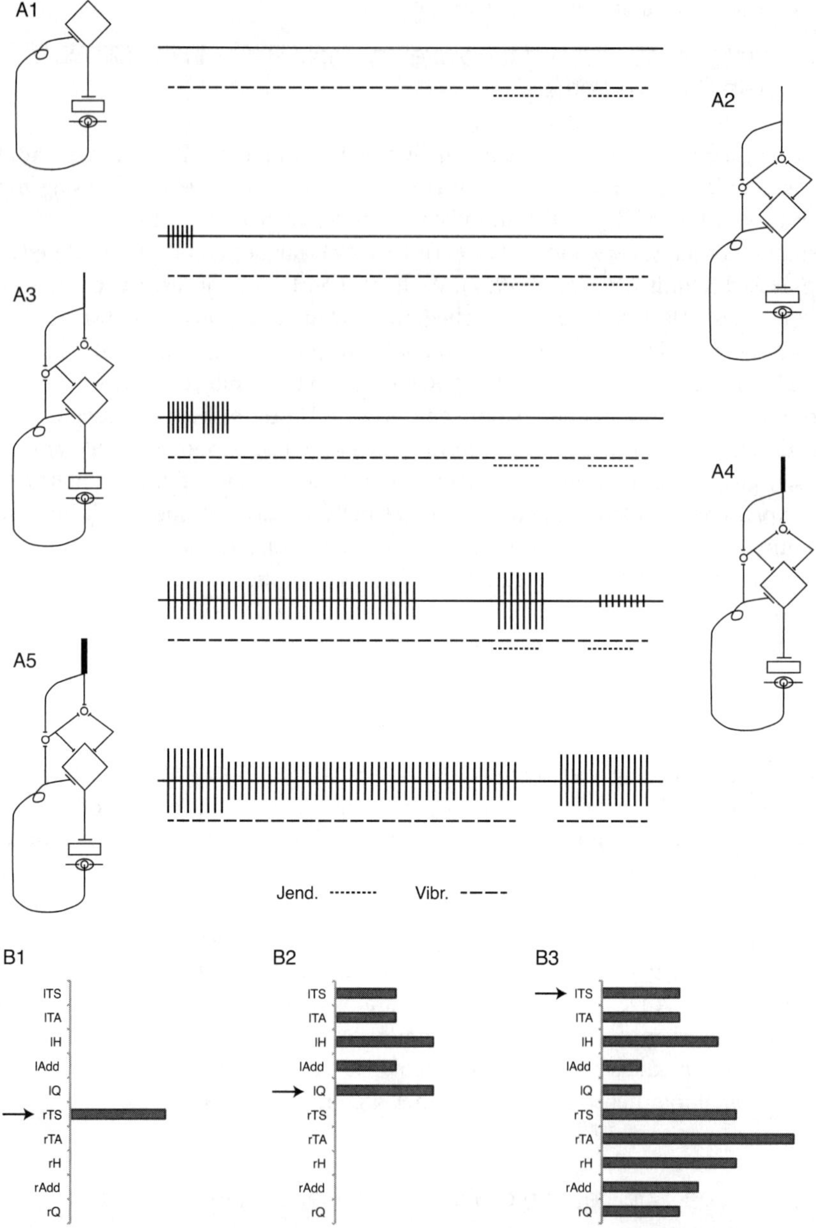

Figure 2–14 Schematic drawing of actual vibratory reflex responses induced in five different spinal cord injured subjects (*A*1–*A*5). All of them were clinically complete. Note the progressive increase from *none* in *A*1 to *a sustained response* in *A*5. Diagram of neuronal circuits illustrates the progressive increase in suprasegmental influence from larger populations of descending axons. Diamonds represent motoneurons; the circles, interneurons; the rectangles, muscles; and the lines, connections. These sketches explain that the sustained vibratory reflex response depends on residual brain segmental input, which does not contribute to any volitional motor unit activity. Sketches *B*1 through *B*3 show graphical illustrations of vibratory tonic reflex responses in three different clinically complete SCI subjects after stimulation of a single muscle, with responses recorded in only one muscle (*B*1), in all ipsilateral muscles (*B*2), and in all bilateral muscles (*B*3) (adapted from Dimitrijevic et al., 1989).

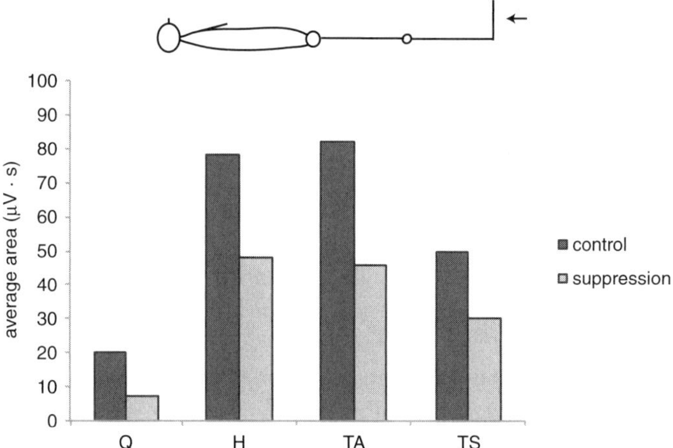

Figure 2–15 Integrated EMG activity during plantar withdrawal flexor reflex in ipsilateral quadriceps, hamstring, tibialis anterior, and triceps surae muscle groups. Without any instructions (control) and asking them to volitionally supress their reflex responses (gray).

muscle group (Peterson, 1984; Cioni et al., 1986). Summaries of these results are illustrated in Figure 2–15.

In the studied group of 50 patients, 73 of 100 tibialis anterior muscle groups showed suppression of more than 20% compared with control response. We mentioned that this suppression was not due to habituation of the plantar flexor reflex, since there was no significant difference in the response due to the sequential order within the baseline or conditioned series. On reexamination of six subjects, the findings were consistent over a period of two years. We concluded that supraspinal suppression of segmental activity does occur in otherwise completely paralyzed spinal cord injury patients. We recommend that in the neurophysiological evaluation of clinically complete patients, assessment of the degree of preservation of suprasegmental neurocontrol of segmental activity below the lesion should be included.

The findings described indicate that the injured portion of the spinal cord in some way is able to mediate suppression of the plantar withdrawal reflex movement, thus demonstrating rudimentary suppression of the test responses in these paralyzed patients. The axonal fibers mediating this suppression are probably a residual portion of the reticulospinal tract, which survived the injury, and are lying within the preserved white matter traversing the lesion as reported above in anatomical studies. We conclude that after a spinal cord injury, the residual functioning axons conduct only a small portion of the motor commands from the brain to the distal segments of the cord.

We have demonstrated that motor units potentials (MUP) elicited by vibration of muscle tendons may be recorded readily from multiple muscle groups. The MUPs are in evidence even in the absence of movement, thus demonstrating the organization of motor control in such paralyzed subjects. Patterns of such activity are different in non-injured compared to SCI subjects, and reflect the degree to which spinal motor organization is influenced by brain control, regardless of whether the brain control is able to produce voluntary movement or not.

4.4. Suprasegmentally Induced Motor Unit Activity in Paralyzed Muscles of Patients with Established Spinal Cord Injury

In attempts to demonstrate the presence of functional descending fibers in subjects with clinically inferred spinal cord transection, electromyographically recorded paralyzed muscle responses to the Jendrassik and other reinforcement maneuvers were undertaken. We have found that Jendrassik and other reinforcement maneuvers can elicit a gross flexor or extensor movement in paralyzed legs—a related effect of suprasegmentally induced facilitation of ongoing vibratory reflex activity. These observations suggest that residual structures in the injured portion of the spinal cord are able to transmit brain influence to the segments below the lesion. To examine this feature of the suprasegmentally induced activity, we investigated the phenomenon in a total of 58 SCI patients with clinically complete paralysis. None of these patients exhibited electromyographic activity in response to a volitional effort made to move their legs, but they showed preserved segmental reflexes of the lumbosacral spinal cord (Dimitrijevic et al., 1983).

Typical findings are shown in Figure 2–16. This sketch illustrates the effect of a reinforcement maneuver response (RMR) in multichannel recordings during first and second attempts of forceful volitional neck flexion. The RMR takes two forms. Firstly, the R1 response consists of single low-amplitude motor units that begin to fire approximately of 0.5 seconds after the neck flexion effort begins. On the third attempt in figure 2–16, the R1 responses are followed by large-amplitude and further delayed R2 with generalized activation of motor units in all recorded muscle groups of both lower limbs.

When R1 was followed by R2, the muscles showing the shortest onset time in R1 are the first to activate to begin the R2. The R2 was larger than the R1, usually involved all recorded leg muscles, and spread bilaterally. The R2 could occur following an

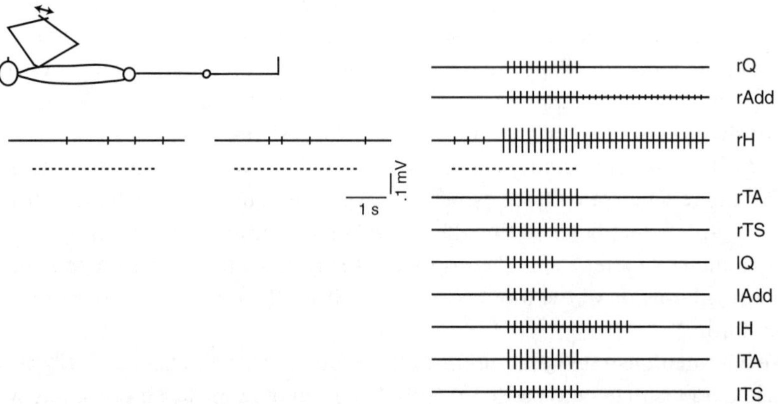

Figure 2–16 Schematic drawing of the effect of the Jendrassik reinforcement maneuver during three subsequent attempts. In the first and second (*from left to right*) attempts, only delayed activation of single motor units is recorded. In the third recording, after the early single motor-unit responses, there is a later bilateral activation of motor unit activity in all recorded muscles (adapted from Dimitrijevic et al., 1984).

R1 or appear without it. The R2 onset time, as shown on the sketch, is much longer and somewhat more variable than that of R1. When the R2 did occur more than once in a given subject, was consistent in the sequence and pattern of muscle activation across repeated trials. If there were changes in the pattern, they seemed to reflect an overall or generalized change in excitability. In separate recordings from six subjects, only one subject failed to show reproducible results over a span of more than four years.

These responses suggest the presence of preserved descending facilitatory influence on isolated populations of motor units (R1), or on segmental interneuron pools (R2). Such findings indicate the presence of functioning fibers traversing the injured portions to initiate subclinical motor unit activity or suprasegmentally induced gross movement through reinforcement maneuvers, but without influence on or control over the amplitude or duration of the response.

5. MODIFICATION OF VOLITIONAL MOTOR TASK OUTPUT BELOW LEVEL OF INCOMPLETE SCI

There can be a variety of features of motor unit activity during a volitional motor task, depending on the severity of diffuse, incomplete SCI (Sherwood et al., 1996). Dorsal and plantar flexion of the ankle is shown in the next illustration, drawn from an actual sPEMG recording. Typical findings recorded by sPEMG from lower-limb muscle groups during the subject's attempts to perform a movement illustrate this response, while four subjects with different degrees of severity of SCI performed volitionally controlled dorsal and plantar flexion of right ankle.

Figure 2–17 illustrates four different and distinct features of the motor unit activity:

- Subject A can performed ankle movement, and there was a well-developed pattern of reciprocity between tibialis anterior and triceps surae and some low-amplitude co-activation of thigh antagonistic muscles.
- Subject B's performance of ankle movement is present but of decreased amplitude and force, and motor unit activity in the tibialis anterior showed large amplitude, sharp onset and cessation; at the same time, however, co-activation of adductors and lesser-degree hamstrings activation were followed by well-developed activity of the triceps surae and suppression of activity of the previously co-activated muscle group.
- Subject C illustrates a subject whose clinical movement was absent, but electromyographic recording showed the presence of activation in the tibialis anterior and an absence of reciprocity or pattern of co-activation between triceps surae.
- Subject D is a similar but mirror-image pattern, wherein activation of the triceps surae motor units was present only during plantar flexion of the ankle, but was absent in both triceps surae and tibialis anterior during dorsal flexion of the ankle, without any co-activation or clinical movement.

Those illustrative features of motor unit activity during performance or attempts to perform the motor task of ankle movement by subjects with clinically absent

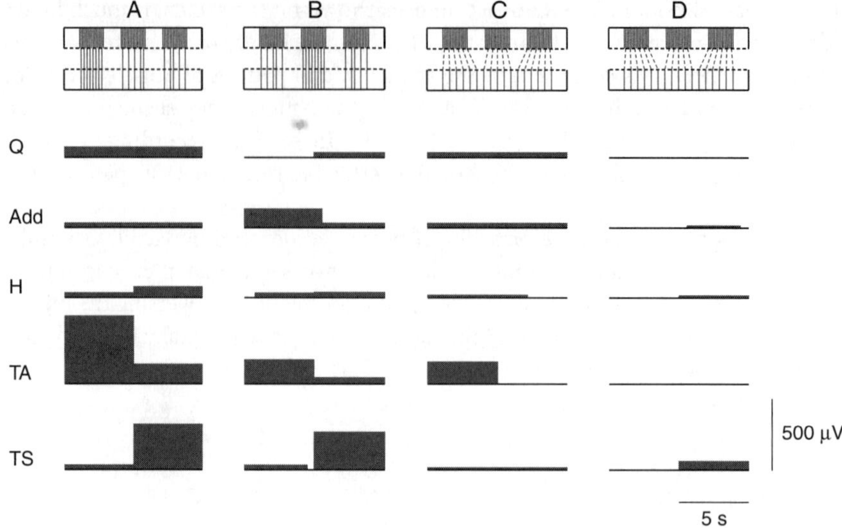

Figure 2–17 Graphic representation of integrated EMG activity during volitional ankle dorsal and plantar flexion motor tasks in four SCI subjects with increasing severity of lesion from *A* to *D*. Above EMG amplitude plots are drawings that reflect the dependence of the amount and nature of EMG response during motor task from the degree of preserved residual volitional control (adapted from Dimitrijevic, 1984).

movement are repetitive and are a reproducible finding in follow-up sessions under an unchanged environment, position, and recording technique paradigm.

Figure 2–17 summarizes a sPEMG recording of motor unit features during the volitional motor task of ankle movement in four different subjects with different degrees of paresis and paralysis. It shows that modified residual connectivity of long descending tracts to the spinal network can establish different patterns of coupling within the network below the level of lesion and, as a result, may elicit well-defined and consistent motor unit activity features, defined by sPEMG distributed in time and space during actually performed motor tasks, during partially completed motor tasks, or even when the attempted motor task is clinically absent.

In order to demonstrate another example of motor unit patterns, we shall illustrate PEMG recordings in a chronic, incomplete post-traumatic thoracic (T-8) SCI. In Figure 2–18, recordings of motor unit features in a single subject during the performance of different volitional motor tasks are illustrated.

Here we see that in A, the subject is executing a single ankle-joint movement, dorsal and plantar flexion. Movement is clinically present, and there is some reciprocity of the motor unit activity between tibialis anterior and triceps surae, with co-activation of thigh muscles with distinct features during the two segments of this ankle volitional motor task. In B, the subject is making an attempt to execute the multi-joint volitional motor task of flexion and extension of the whole lower limb. The features of motor unit output are strikingly different and of much larger output, involving the leg and thigh muscle groups. However, the same subject is, in C, performing a reinforcement maneuver by forceful neck flexion against resistance. This generalized increase in excitability above the level of lesion activates low amplitude

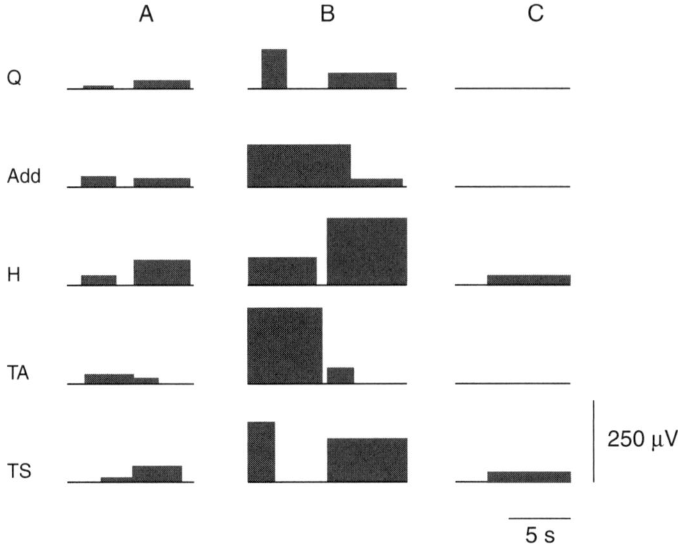

Figure 2–18 Graphical presentation of integrated EMG recordings in a single subject during three different motor tasks. (*A*) Volitional ankle dorsal and plantar flexion, (*B*) volitional whole lower limb flexion and extension, and (*C*) reinforcement maneuver (neck flexion against resistence) (adapted from Dimitrijevic, 1984).

sPEMG activity with longer delay than during the volitional motor task, and significantly lower motor unit amplitudes are seen only in hamstrings and triceps surae muscle. Thus three different motor tasks in the same subject can elicit three different features of motor unit activity.

Figures 2–17 and 2–18 suggest that motor output can be different during the same motor task in subjects with different degrees of supraspinal innervation. However, performance of different motor tasks will have different outputs in the same subject.

6. NEUROCONTROL OF HUMAN LOCOMOTION

There are two important aspects to the study of the neurocontrol of human locomotion. The first is to monitor spinal motor-nuclei output from their corresponding muscle groups during the performance of locomotor activity. The second is stimulation of spinal cord posterior roots and externally controlled afferent input to lumbar network pattern generators (Minassian et al., 2007).

6.1. Gait after Spinal Cord Injury

As a result of SCI, gait in humans is altered, but often possible without or with assistive devices. Instead of developing a broad range of speed, the ambulatory SCI subject is often only capable of a very slow gait. Intervening factors are the degree of spasticity present and the alteration of muscle activation patterns, that lead to weakness and impaired control of weight support and transfer during ambulation (Yakura et al., 1990; Waters et al., 1992). A study of the neurocontrol of gait in patients with upper motor neuron lesions (Dimitrijevic & Lenman, 1980) included 38 subjects with traumatic SCI and three with brain stem lesions, all 18 or more months after injury, with neurophysiological evidence of a stationary condition. The purpose of the study was, first, to measure how far stepping movements can be initiated in chronic SCI, and, second, to determine to what extent such stepping movements are dependent on contributions from supraspinal input. We studied motor unit activity using sPEMG with the patient supine, standing, and walking, and their segmental reflexes were examined according to the above-described principles for assessment of residual motor control below SCI. We concluded in this study that segmental reflexes with and without supraspinal influence at the level of discomplete SCI are not sufficient to generate stepping movements during attempted gait, unless brain stem influences—control—are also present. This brain stem influence can suppress hyperexcitability of spinal reflex activity and initiate patterned and alternating phases of excitation and suppression.

In a study of volitional control of motor units in SCI (Dimitrijevic et al., 1997), we obtained results from 91 chronic SCI patients and 15 neurologically healthy individuals. All SCI subjects suffered from non-penetrating SCI between C2 and T10, and 49 of 91 were ambulatory. Integrated EMG activity during gait is shown as the repetitive pattern of bursts of discharges followed by silent periods. Two examples of typical integrated EMG activity during gait of ambulatory SCI subjects are given in Figure 2–19. In Subject A, the EMG activity reveals the reciprocal relationship between the activity of antagonistic muscle groups. In Subject B, ambulation is much slower, with longer durations of the stance and swing phases and much lower frequencies of repetitive bursts of EMG activity. There is also a significant reduction of EMG output in the quadriceps, tibialis anterior, and triceps surae when compared with Subject A. At the same time, a reciprocal pattern of EMG activity between the tibialis anterior and the triceps surae muscles is partially preserved during swing.

In a study of locomotor patterns after SCI (McKay et al., 1993) of 16 ambulatory subjects, three of them were functional ambulators, as walkers with faster stepping (average stride times 1.2 sec.) without any supportive devices, and 13 subjects manifested various levels of functional ambulation with a slower rate of steps (average stride times 4 sec.) with assistive devices, from unilateral canes to bilateral braces. In the parallel recording of the same 16 ambulatory SCI subjects, there was a close relationship between volitionally induced flexor/extensor patterns in the supine position and during gait performance (McKay et al., 1993).

All three studies of neurocontrol of gait after spinal cord injury mentioned here (Dimitrijevic & Lenman, 1980; Dimitrijevic et al., 1997; McKay et al., 1993) and their consistent, repetitive features of motor control during single-joint and multi-joint volitional motor tasks are supportive of the hypothesis that this control is the result of newly established functional connections between spinal and supraspinal structures involved in motor control after injury. This proposal is supported by finding that the quality of gait performance depends on the extent of neurocontrol functional organization as a result of residual suprasegmental interactions with the spinal cord network.

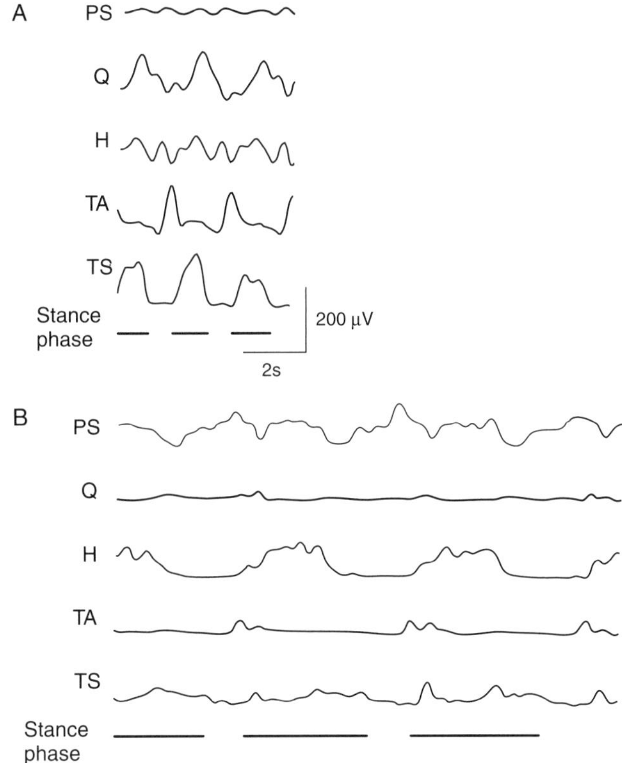

Figure 2–19 Integrated EMG pattern of two ambulatory SCI individuals. Subject A walks faster than Subject B, but motor unit activity in Subject B was significantly less than in Subject A (adapted from Dimitrijevic et al., 1997).

6.2. Spinal Cord CPG; Spinal Cord Stimulation

There is another approach to eliciting stepping movements from the isolated lumbosacral cord, which differs from the activation of patterned, sensory, phasic input from the lower limbs associated with load-bearing stepping and elicited locomotor-like EMG activity and stepping movement. This approach involves electrical stimulation of the spinal cord with sustained, un-patterned electrical stimuli of externally controlled frequency, amplitude, and duration. We also conducted a study of the locomotor capabilities of the lumbosacral cord induced by epidural spinal cord stimulation in six subjects with complete, long-standing SCI and found that non-patterned electrical stimulation of the posterior structures of the lumbar cord induced patterned, locomotor-like motor output (Dimitrijevic et al., 1998). An increase in the frequency of the stimulating train corresponded to an increase in the frequency of rhythmic activity, whereas an increase in the strength of the stimulus resulted in a decrease in rhythmic activity. This observation led us to the conclusion that when the integrity of segmental input-output is preserved, the mechanisms within the lumbosacral cord network, which determines the temporal pattern of rhythmic generation and shapes motor output, is able to initiate and maintain locomotor-like activity in response to non-patterned, segmental stimulation of a particular site of the lumbosacral cord.

References

American Spinal Injury Association. *International Standards for Neurological Classification of Spinal Cord Injury, rev. 2002.* Chicago, IL: American Spinal Injury Association, 2002.

Cioni, B., Dimitrijevic, M. R., McKay, B., Sherwood, A.M. "Voluntary supraspinal suppression of spinal reflex activity in paralyzed muscles of spinal cord injury patients." *Experimental Neurology* 93 (1986): 573–583.

Dimitrijevic, M. M., Dimitrijevic, M. R., Sherwood, A. M., van der Linden C. "Clinical neurophysiological techniques in the assessment of spasticity." In *Physical Medicine And Rehabilitation: State of the Art Reviews, vol. 3*, nr. 2, edited by R. Davis, G. V. Kondraske, W. W. Tourtellotte, K. Syndulko, 64–83. Philadelphia, PA: Hanley & Belfus, 1989.

Dimitrijevic, M. R. "Withdrawal reflexes. New developments in electromyography and clinical neurophysiology." In *Progress in Clinical Neurophysiology, vol. 3,* edited by J. E. Desmeth, 744–750. Basel, Switzerland: Karger, 1973.

Dimitrijevic, M. R. "Neurocontrol of chronic upper motor neuron syndromes." In *Electromyography in CNS Disorders: Central EMG*, edited by B. T. Shahani. Boston, MA: Butterworth, 1984.

Dimitrijevic, M. R. "Neurophysiology in spinal cord injury." *Paraplegia* 25 (1987): 205–208.

Dimitrijevic, M. R. "Clinical assessment of spasticity." In *Neurosurgery for Spasticity*, edited by M. Sindou, R. Abbott, Y. Keravel, 33–37. New York: Springer, 1991.

Dimitrijevic, M. R. "Development of neurophysiological aspects of the spinal cord during the past ten years." *Paraplegia* 30 (1992): 92–95.

Dimitrijevic, M. R., Dimitrijevic, M. M., Faganel, J., Sherwood, A. M. "Suprasegmentally induced motor unit activity in paralyzed muscles of patients with established spinal cord injury." *Annals of Neurology* 16 (1984): 216–221.

Dimitrijevic, M. R., Faganel, J. "Motor control in he spinal cord." In *Recent Achievements in Restorative Neurology: Upper Motor Neuron Functions and Dysfunctions,* edited by J. C. Eccles, M. R. Dimitrijevic, 150–162. Basel, Switzerland: Karger, 1985.

Dimitrijevic, M. R., Gerasimenko, Y., Pinter, M. M. "Evidence for a spinal central pattern generator in humans." *Annals of the New York Academy of Sciences* 860 (1998): 360–376.

Dimitrijevic, M. R., Faganel, J., Lehmkuhl, L. D., Sherwood, A. M. "Motor control in man after partial or complete spinal cord injury." In *Motor Control Mechanisms in Health and in Disease. Advances in Neurology, vol. 39*, edited by J. E. Desmedt, 915–926. New York: Raven, 1983.

Dimitrijevic, M. R., Lenman, J. A. R. "Neural control of gait inpatients with upper motor neuron lesions." In Spasticity: Disordered Motor Control, edited by R. G. Feldman, R. R. Young, W. P. Koella, 101–114. Chicago: Year Book Medical Publishers, 1980.

Dimitrijevic, M. R., Lissens, M. A., McKay, W. B. "Characteristics and extent of motor activity recovery after spinal cord injury." In *Advances in Neural Regeneration Research,* edited by F. J. Seil, 391–405. New York: Wiley-Liss, 1990.

Dimitrijevic, M. R., McKay, W. B., Sherwood, A. M. "Motor control physiology below spinal cord injury: Residual volitional control of motor units in paretic and paralyzed muscles." In *Advances in Neurology, vol. 72: Neuronal Regeneration, Reorganization and Repair*, edited by F. J. Seil, 335–345. Philadelphia, PA: Lippincott-Raven, 1997.

Dimitrijevic, M. R., Nathan, P. W. "Studies of spasticity in man. 1. Some features of spasticity." *Brain* 90 (1967a): 1–30.

Dimitrijevic, M. R., Nathan, P. W. "Studies of spasticity in man. 2. Analysis of stretch reflexes in spasticity." *Brain* 90 (1967b): 333–358.

Dimitrijevic, M. R., Nathan, P. W. "Studies of spasticity in man. 3. Analysis of reflex activity evoked by noxious cutaneous stimulation." *Brain* 91 (1968): 349–368.

Dimitrijevic, M. R., Nathan, P. W. "Studies of spasticity in man. 4. Changes in flexion reflex with repetitive cutaneous stimulation in spinal man." *Brain* 93 (1970): 743–768.

Dimitrijevic, M. R., Nathan, P. W. "Studies of spasticity in man. 5. Dishabituation of the flexion reflex in spinal man." *Brain* 94 (1971): 77–90.

Dimitrijevic, M. R., Nathan, P. W. "Studies of spasticity in man. 6. Habituation, dishabituation and sensitization of tendon reflexes in spinal man." *Brain* 96 (1973): 337–354.

Dimitrijevic, M. R., Spencer, W. A., Trontelj, J. V., Dimitrijevic, M. M. "Reflex effects of vibration in patients with spinal cord lesions." *Neurology* 27 (1977): 1078–1086.

Eidelberg, E. "Spinal cord syndromes." In *Handbook of the Spinal Cord: Vol. 4, Congenital Disorders and Trauma; Vol. 5, Infections and Cancer*, edited by R. A. Davidoff, 1–17. New York: Marcel Dekker, Inc.,1987.

Faganel, J., Dimitrijevic, M. R. "Study of propriospinal interneurone system in man: Cutaneous exeroceptive conditioning of stretch reflexes." *Journal of Neurological Science* 56 (1982): 155–172.

Gilles, J. D., Burke, D. J., Lance, J. W. "Supraspinal control of tonic vibration reflex." *Journal of Neurophysiology* 34 (1971): 302–309.

Gorassini, M. A., Knash, M. E., Harvey, P. J., Bennett, D. J., Yang, J. F. "Role of motoneurons in the generation of muscle spasms after spinal cord injury." *Brain* 127 (2004): 2247–2258.

Guttmann, L. "Symptomatology." In *Spinal Cord Injuries: Comprehensive Management and Research*, edited by L. Guttman, 260–279. London: Oxford University Press,1976.

Hagbarth, K. E. "Spinal withdrawal reflexes in the human lower limbs." *Journal of Neurology, Neurosurgery & Psychiatry* 23 (1960): 222–227.

Heckman, C. J., Mottram, C., Quinlan, K., Theiss, R., Schuster, J. "Motoneuron excitability: The importance of neuromodulatory inputs." *Clinical Neurophysiology* 120 (2009): 2040–2054.

Jankowska, E. and Hammar, I. "Spinal interneurones; how can studies in animals contribute to the understanding of spinal interneuronal systems in man?" *Brain Res Rev.* 40 (2002):19–28.

Kakulas, B. A. "A review of the neuropathology of human spinal cord injury with emphasis on special features." *J Spinal Cord Medicine* 22 (1999): 119–124.

Kakulas, B. A. "Neuropathology: The foundation for new treatments in spinal cord injury." *Spinal Cord* 42 (2004): 549–563.

Lance, J. W., De Gail, P. "Spread of phasic muscle reflexes in normal and spastic subjects." *Journal of Neurology, Neurosurgery & Psychiatry* 28 (1965): 328–334.

Lundberg, A. (1967) "The supraspinal control of transmission in spinal reflex pathways." *Electroencephalography and Clinical Neurophysiology* 25 (1967): 35–46.

Matthews, P. B. C. "The reflex excitation of the soleus muscle of the decerebrate cat caused by vibration applied to its tendon." *Journal of Physiology (Lond.)* 184 (1966): 450–472.

McKay, W. B., Verhagen, M. L., Dimitrijevic, M. M., Sherwood, A. M., Dimitrijevic, M. R. "Locomotor pattern in humans with impaired spinal cord functions." In *Motor Control Disorders, Physical Medicine and Rehabilitation Clinics of North America, Vol. 4*, edited by G. H. Kraft, B. Shahani, 707–730. Philadelphia, PA: W.B. Saunders Co., 1993.

Minassian, K., Persy, I., Rattay, F., Pinter, M. M., Kern, H., Dimitrijevic, M. R. "Human lumbar cord circuitries can be activated by extrinsic tonic input to generate locomotor-like activity." *Human Movement Science* 26 (2007): 275–295.

Nielsen, J. B., Crone, C., Hultborn, H. "The spinal pathophysiology of spasticity—from a basic science point of view." *Acta Physiologica* 189 (2007): 171–180.

Peterson, B. W. "The reticulospinal system and its role in the control of movement." In *Brain Stem Control of Spinal Cord Function*, edited by C. D. Barnes, 28–86. New York: Academic Press, 1984.

Sherwood, A. M., Dimitrijevic, M. R., Bacia, T., McKay, W. B. "Characteristics of the vibratory reflex in humans with reduced suprasegmental influence due to spinal cord injury." *Restorative Neurology and Neuroscience* 5 (1993): 119–129.

Sherwood, A. M., Dimitrijevic, M. R., McKay, B. "Evidence of subclinical brain influence in clinically complete spinal cord injury: Discomplete SCI." *Journal of the Neurological Sciences* 110 (1992): 90–98.

Sherwood, A. M., McKay, W. B., Dimitrijevic, M. R. "Surface EMG." *Muscle & Nerve* 19 (1992): 966–979.

Sherwood, A. M., McKay, W. B., Dimitrijevic, M. R. "Motor control after spinal cord injury: assessment using surface EMG." *Muscle Nerve.* 19 (1996): 966–79.

Steeves, J. D., Lammertse, D., Curt, A., Fawcett, J. W., Tuszynski, M. H., Ditunno, J. F. et al. "Guidelines for the conduct of clinical trials for spinal cord injury (SCI) as developed by the ICCP panel: Clinical trial outcome measures." *Spinal Cord* 45 (2007): 206–221.

Trontelj, J. K., Dimitrijevic, M. R., Prevec, T. "A mechanical stimulator for eliciting tendon reflexes and somatosensory cerebral responses in man." Symposium on Electronics in Medicine (1968): Ljubljana, Slovenia.

Waters, R. L., Yakura, J. S., Adkins, R. D. "Gait performance after spinal cord injury." *Clinical Orthopedics* 288 (1992): 87–96.

Yakura, J. S., Waters, R. L., Adkins, R. H. "Changes in ambulation parameters in spinal cord injury individuals following rehabilitation." *Paraplegia* 28 (1990): 364–370.

3

Restorative Neurology of Motor Control after Spinal Cord Injury

Clinical Practice

KEITH TANSEY, META M. DIMITRIJEVIC, WINFRIED MAYR, MANFRED BIJAK, AND MILAN R. DIMITRIJEVIC

CONTENTS

1. Introduction
2. Environment and Clinical Setup for Assessment of Motor Performance
3. Restorative Neurology Interventions
   3.1. Physiotherapy
   3.2. Neuromuscular Stimulation and Functional Electrical Stimulation
   3.3. Clinical Program for Fitting a Foot-Drop Stimulator
   3.4. The Program for Electrical Stimulation for Therapeutically and Mobility-Oriented Recovery after Spinal Cord Injury
   3.5. Neuromuscular Stimulation (Trophic State of the Muscle)
   3.6. Nerve and Neuromuscular Electrical Stimulation and Modification of Muscle Hypertonia
   3.7. Neuromuscular Stimulation for the Modification of Patterns of Movement
   3.8. Functional Electrical Stimulation for Impaired Functional Movement of the Single Muscle Group
   3.9. Externally Electrically Induced Modification of Altered Neurocontrol
   3.10. Recommendation
4. Spinal Cord Stimulation for Control of Spasticity and Movement Augmentation
5. Spinal Cord Stimulation and Movement Elicitation
6. Intrathecal Baclofen Pumps
7. Spasticity Treatment with Botulinum Toxin
8. General Conclusion
References

1. INTRODUCTION

Motor control in people with chronic, post-traumatic spinal cord injury can be so severely affected that they are not able to perform any volitional muscle activation. With decreasing severity of motor pathway damage, they will have the ability to perform gross multi-joint movements. Less severe lesions will allow performance of more precise single-joint movements, and ultimately, the ability to generate any kind of well-coordinated motor task. There are also people with SCI who can only generate minute traces of movements within affected regions of the body. Another clinically relevant, characteristic feature of chronic SCI is the inability to stand or walk, even when certain other motor tasks can be performed. There are also those who are able to move from the sitting to the standing position and others who can proceed to walking. Thus, the chronic phase of SCI includes a very broad range of motor capabilities and impairments.

In view of the variety of underlying mechanisms responsible for this chronic impairment of motor control, restorative neurology is faced with specific treatment issues. Therefore, a particular physiotherapy maneuver, such as the electrical stimulation of large peripheral nerve afferents or of the spinal cord through implanted or surface electrodes, can induce very different effects in people with similar SCI clinical-scale-score values. Thus, in the practice of restorative neurology, it is important to be aware not only that the site, strength, and duration of any intervention are important, but also that the surviving or residual nervous system function plays a significant role in the outcome of treatment. Therefore, when we apply restorative neurological procedures, it is important to first neurophysiologically assess and document the residual function and base the intervention protocol on those findings. Moreover, we should also assess the effect of the applied intervention by regularly monitoring changes to residual function and take these findings into consideration when adjusting the intervention protocol. If there is no residual activity, we can simply substitute missing activation of muscles and nerves in order to prevent the effects of disuse. However, if there are some residual functions present, then restorative procedures will need to be selected and applied in a way that specifically facilitates and enhances existing motor performance.

The possibility that residual motor control can be preserved to different degrees explains why we do not have a rigid clinical protocol for particular, clinically defined, motor deficits. Furthermore, restorative neurological clinical practice requires a multidisciplinary team that includes physicians, human neurophysiologists, therapists, and biomedical engineers. In this chapter, we shall discuss how established procedures using physiotherapy, neuromuscular and peripheral nerve stimulation, and spinal cord stimulation can be used as restorative procedures. Moreover, we shall describe how the same restorative neurological procedures can be used to assess motor control. We shall also present the intrathecal application of Baclofen and intramuscular injection of botulinum toxin (Botox®) as examples of interventions that do not take advantage of residual motor control but rather suppress it. Briefly, we shall describe how clinical restorative neurological treatment can best be practiced in medical centers where multidiscipline programs exist. Whether such programs are cost-effective is determined by local cost structures, but, to date, our experience is that they can be very cost-effective if they are performed in an appropriate environment. Its biggest advantage is that much of this program can be carried out in the home after proper assessment, instruction, and training have been completed.

2. ENVIRONMENT AND CLINICAL SETUP FOR ASSESSMENT OF MOTOR PERFORMANCE

Potential candidates entering a restorative neurology program should already have been clinically assessed and graded using the International Standard for Neurological Classification of Spinal Cord Injury examination (Marino et al., 2003) and their overall health condition reviewed. Before a treatment program is initiated, the candidate's spasticity and residual motor control should also be assessed using neurophysiological principles and methods described in Chapters 2 and 8. Based on the findings of these examinations, an appropriate intervention can be selected, and a protocol for applying it can be designed that will augment residual motor control. Finally, the effects of the selected intervention will then need to be evaluated through repeated assessments.

The individuals should be examined in a pleasant and comfortable environment. Assessment is best conducted, as already discussed in Chapter 2, in the supine, sitting, and, when possible, standing positions. Furthermore, the subject's attention span and endurance should be taken into account, as their cooperation is essential. Therefore, motor-control assessment sessions should never be longer than one hour. Also, subjects ought to be given sufficient periods of rest whenever needed. When assessing responsiveness to motor tasks, conditioning effects of externally controlled afferent input using stretch, cutaneous touch, or electrical stimulation may be added to raise excitability when needed. Findings should be documented in a clear and simple way when describing volitional motor task performance. Simple scores for the findings can be applied: 0 for *absent*; 1 for *trace*; 2 for *incomplete* (only initial performance); 3 for *complete performance with radiation to other muscle groups*; 4 for *complete performance without radiation to other muscle groups*; 5 for *normal control*. These can then be summarized to obtain a final score across a group of volitional tasks. Naturally, combining scoring and descriptions of the performance of different motor tasks can provide a more comprehensive documentation. Standardized volitional motor tasks, including single and multi-joint tasks, are relatively easy to describe, and the extent to which these different tasks can be executed should be characterized over multiple, usually three, repetitions within an exam session. This approach allows us to answer the question of whether or not the brain can reliably generate a given simple motor task, such as a single-joint and multi-joint movement, in the face of SCI. These two motor tasks are directed by two different neural-control mechanisms. Therefore, by assessing two different motor tasks, we can determine the degree of brain-derived motor control, whether or not it is capable of isolating a motor act. Furthermore, when that motor task is performed, we can assess whether it is organized to selectively or non-selectively activate synergistic and/or antagonistic muscle groups.

After assessing their residual motor activity in the supine position, additional assessments of motor control in those able to stand or walk, with or without support, should be carried out. While several methods could be used, we assess standing with eyes opened, and then with them closed for at least one minute and up to three minutes, depending on the ability of the patient to stand safely. Standing with eyes open allows the use of visual input to aid in maintaining equilibrium, while closing the eyes requires the patient's control to be based only on vestibular and proprioceptive input. After quiet standing, we ask them to lean forward and backward from a neutral position to assess dynamic control of equilibrium. For gait assessments, we test a subject's ability to change from sitting in a chair to walking three steps forward and then return to a sitting position in the chair. The total time it takes to perform sitting, standing, stepping forward, and returning to sitting provides a measure of performance skill. In subjects with greater gait capacity, measurement of maximal gait speed along a 10-meter path or gait distance accomplished in 6 minutes are common tests for determining gait capability.

The findings from this examination process and neurophysiological assessment results (Chapter 8) are then used to develop a clinical treatment plan designed to selectively augment existing residual motor function. This planning process should involve the patient's attending physician and the treatment team and have the patient's agreement. We also recommend that the neurophysiological Brain Motor Control Assessment be performed during execution of the treatment plan to confirm that effects support the goals and that it be repeated at the time of discharge. Furthermore, patients are asked to record their observations in a diary for use by the treatment team to evaluate the appropriateness of the plan and goals during the treatment process. Thus, every patent is treated on a single-case basis with interventions selected and applied to augment that particular patient's profile of residual motor control.

3. RESTORATIVE NEUROLOGY INTERVENTIONS

3.1. Physiotherapy

Chronic spinal cord injury changes important aspects of neuromuscular function: (1) joint mobility becomes restricted, and non-neural changes increase muscle stiffness; (2) increased muscle tone develops due to inappropriate motor control; and (3) volitional control of motor tasks is limited or absent.

Maintenance and/or restoration of muscle length and muscle compliance are essential for people with muscle weakness. Limited volitional movement and a restriction in the full range of motion at the joints due to changes in periarticular connective tissue and joint connective tissue are common treatment targets in many with chronic SCI. Techniques commonly used by physical therapists to alleviate these problems include active and passive stretching, a standing regimen, casting, the use of orthoses, optimized sitting posture in a wheelchair, and manual massage of muscles. These treatments can be effective, but at the same time, we should be aware of their limitations. These are time-consuming issues, and it is not clear how long these treatment protocols should be applied.

Increased muscle tone can be decreased by regular, repetitive, sustained stretching of antagonistic muscle groups, and suppression of reflex muscle hypertonia can be achieved by 10 to 20 repetitions of full range-of-motion stretching. Suppression of reflex muscle tone can last beyond cessation of stretching treatments. An alternative method for decreasing the severity of spasticity, or muscle reflex hypertonia, is to train the subject in a physical therapy program to learn how to relax hypertonic muscles. This procedure should be performed in a quiet and comfortable environment and position for the subject. The subject is asked to induce spasticity in a definite body region or part of the limbs and then to follow this by relaxing. With some training in one or more sessions, the SCI spastic subject can often master the ability to initiate and suppress spasticity. It is important to point out that this ability may be affected by anti-spasticity medications, which can eliminate this residual capability of the brain below the level of the spinal cord lesion. Unfortunately there are few additional specific physiotherapeutic techniques for permanently decreasing spasticity.

There are two different approaches used for training motor control in individuals with spinal cord injury. First, making use of facilitation—movement enhancement by afferent augmentation techniques (Rood, 1947), and second, motor relearning by practicing task-specific activities and strength training (Brunström, 1970; Bobath, 1978). Verbal instructions are used to direct correct movement performance, and auditory and visual cuing is also used. Sometimes those two techniques are combined with sensory facilitation provided by tactile input and/or muscle stretch.

In spinal cord injured individuals with the ability to stand, physiotherapeutic approaches can incorporate training of balance and posture after initial fixation of unstable body segments. Treadmill training, body-weight-supported treadmill training (BWSTT) and over-ground walking have similar average outcomes (Dobkin et al., 2006). However, Wolpaw (2006) concluded that BWSTT will help develop new treatment methods. Furthermore, Wolpaw (2007) reviewed spinal cord plasticity in acquisition and maintenance of motor skills and pointed out that, throughout normal life, activity-dependent plasticity occurs in the spinal cord at numerous sites as well as within the brain due to a variety of mechanisms. There are several new possibilities for intervention that combine over-ground gait training and robotic training with and without electrical stimulation (Field-Fote et al., 2005). Another approach is to use reflex conditioning (Chen et al., 2010). Recently added to these are neurophysiological methods to enhance neurocontrol of locomotion through transcutaneous stimulation of lumbar posterior roots (see Chapter 10). In the past few years there has been significant development of robotic devices, which can provide prescribed movements under the supervision of physical therapists (Jezernik et al., 2003).

In conclusion, physiotherapeutic interventions can prevent diminished secondary tissue changes that result from the effects of disuse due to impaired movement, and those interventions can support the relearning of movements.

3.2. Neuromuscular Stimulation and Functional Electrical Stimulation

Electrical stimulation—the depolarization of nerve cells to elicit action potentials—can be applied to peripheral sensory or motor nerves to evoke contractions from muscles otherwise affected by impaired motor control due to upper motor neuron dysfunction. Neuromuscular stimulation (NMS) includes all applications whereby muscle responses are elicited by stimulation of the supplying motor nerve; functional electrical stimulation (FES) is the more general generic term for all applications targeting the activation or restoration of functions by electrical stimulation; that is, efferent and afferent nerve, neuromuscular, and muscle stimulation. NMS and FES can be used in people with SCI to build muscle bulk and to externally control patterned movements or even to restore motor control in weak and nonfunctional muscle groups. In reality, to apply these methods properly and to accomplish therapeutic goals is a rather demanding job that requires knowledge of the functional anatomy of muscles and nerves, kinesiology, motor control, and biomedical engineering for the electrical stimulators and their operation.

Electrical stimulation of muscle groups at their lowest-threshold intensity for eliciting muscle contraction, using a train of stimuli delivered to the muscle motor point, or for eliciting functional movements by sustained electrical stimulation of those muscles' corresponding nerves, are methods that have been used for some time to build the trophic condition of paralyzed muscles. Over the past decades, electrical stimulation of peripheral nerves to elicit functional movement brought about the development of commercially available devices. Simple applications also exist for ambulatory spinal cord injured individuals, in the form of the foot-drop stimulator to enhance gait by providing dorsal foot-flexion during swing.

Liberson and colleagues (1961) did the pioneering work of functional electrical therapy, later renamed FES, for the correction of upper-motor-neuron dysfunction. He described in his autobiography how critical for his work was his neurophysiological education, gained from leading Russian neuroscientists, and the opportunity to work with distinguished French neuroscientists in the field of electrical stimulation (Liberson, 1999). An additional contributing factor was the technological development of transistorized stimulators that made possible portable stimulators for functional electrical stimulation.

On his discovery of the peroneal FES in 1961, Liberson wrote in his autobiography:

> With the help of Dr. Franklin Offner, a manufacturer of EEG equipment, I was able to demonstrate my idea on limited scale. I took for a model the drop foot of a hemiplegic patient. I placed a switch in the shoe. Each time the patient would lift his leg from the floor a current would be initiated and would stimulate the tibialis anticus and peroneal muscles. The tibialis anticus elicits dorsiflexion of the foot and its shoe. Thus a closed loop was created and an automatic correction of the hemiplegic gait was achieved (Liberson, 1999).

Before Liberson discovered "FES for correction of the drop foot," he worked in the laboratory of Nikolai Wedensky (1852–1922), a Russian neurophysiologist. Lapicque (1866–1952) introduced him to electrodiagnosis while working in Salpêtrière, Paris. Liberson's educational and research path and his medical practice, supported by technological electronic developments, clearly illustrates the development of "yesterday's" FES toward new solutions for medical problems by integrating contemporary neurophysiology and technology. Liberson consequently developed other systems for the improvement of locomotion, an electromechanical brace for the stimulation of soleus and gluteus maximus activity in 1966, and "reflex walking" in paraplegic patients in 1973 (Liberson, 1999).

It is worth mentioning that Liberson published his *Functional Electrotherapy* . . . in 1961, and today, some 50 years later, there are several foot-drop stimulators that are commercially available; for example, from Innovative Neurotronics, Inc; the Walk-Aide system; from Finetech-Medical, the StimuStep system; from Bioness, the L300; and from Otto Bock, the ActiGait. These systems for peroneal nerve stimulation and drop-foot correction are appropriate FES approaches for ambulatory individuals with SCI who have recovered antigravity, extensor functions of the trunk and lower limbs but have weaker flexor muscle groups (Gracanin & Marincek, 1969). Peroneal nerve stimulation can enhance swing phase during gait and correct drop foot. Naturally, in order for the subject to maximally benefit from the drop-foot system, it is important that they be properly fitted with the device and trained to use the system.

The muscles of SCI patients, both those in wheelchairs and those who are ambulatory, become weaker and more fatigable, with poor endurance, increased muscle tone, and other consequences of chronic upper-motor-neuron dysfunctions. NMS and FES approaches can have a therapeutic effect on paralyzed muscles and enhance mobility. In this case we are developing a clinical protocol for therapeutic enhancement to improve the function of muscles, mobility, and self-care (Ragnarsson, 2008). Furthermore, FES can reverse wasting, improve strength, enhance cardiovascular fitness, and improve other impaired motor functions (Stein et al., 2002; Creasey et al., 2004). Thus we should divide supportive clinical programs in two different types: those for fitting patients with commercial systems for drop foot; and electrical stimulation for therapy and mobility after spinal cord injury (Stein et al., 2002).

3.3. Clinical Program for Fitting a Foot-Drop Stimulator

A specially trained physician or physical therapist, who is familiar with prescribing stimulators such as commercial FES foot-drop stimulators, should conduct this training protocol. The physician would examine the patient's cardiovascular fitness and their skeletal, circulatory, and preserved peroneal nerve lower-motor-neuron condition before beginning stimulation. The patient must be informed about the method and protocol for learning how to use a foot-drop stimulator. Beginning while a hospital inpatient, they would be taught how to apply the foot-drop stimulator during daily sessions with the therapist. After discharge, a few outpatient sessions should be scheduled to assess their progress and address any problems that may arise. Furthermore, patients should participate for several weeks in a home program combined with at least one to two outpatient sessions during which the patient is guided toward optimal use of the device. In short, the protocol is that application be provided by a physician or therapist who is familiar with the device and the patient's characteristics and who is able to provide instruction for any adjustment of the foot-drop stimulator to residual neurocontrol of gait. Biomedical engineering support is not expected to be necessary in routine treatment, but in case it is needed, the manufacturer should provide it.

3.4. The Program for Electrical Stimulation for Therapeutically and Mobility-Oriented Recovery after Spinal Cord Injury

We shall explain to the patient the operation of the stimulation unit, and then, whenever possible, apply it first to a site where we expect normal sensation to provide an opportunity for the subject to experience the tingling sensation evoked by a train of stimuli, and to show the subject progressively the effect of different stimulus parameters and thresholds. The thresholds are of sensation and just below sensation, definite and comfortable sensation, evoked movement, and sensory tolerance.

All of these thresholds can be changed through repeated stimulation. Patients can accommodate to these externally induced sensations, raising the threshold for sensation. Motor thresholds can be decreased by stimulus parameters and the duration of application. We take care to avoid application of NMS or FES within areas where altered or decreased thresholds for electrical stimulation, hyperesthesia, or hyperalgesia are experienced. After such a training session, we are ready to proceed with the evaluation of the functional responses and examine the neuromuscular physiological condition and the effects that such electrical stimulation has on the initiation, external control, and modification of movement.

The second step consists of an evaluation procedure to determine the muscle's ability to respond to repetitive percutaneous stimuli with visible or palpable muscle twitches. If we measure the length of time a muscle responds with muscle twitches, we can learn about the endurance and fatigability of the muscle's contraction and force-production capabilities. Afterwards, depending on the patient's condition and our tentative goals, we should examine the response to the stimulation of cutaneous nerves for modulation of muscle tone and modification of volitional movements, as well as, when necessary, determining what will be the effects of stimulation of a mixed nerve or motor point on functional movements.

In short, we should not start a treatment program of NMS or FES until we test the effects of the planned stimulation to prove that we can obtain the expected results from electrical stimulation of the nerve structures that are available, or until those results can be obtained with stimulation parameters that are within the patient's range of comfort. We should also carry out examinations of the physiological properties of the neuromuscular system and responses of altered motor control to stimulation parameters at different sites and with the use of different sizes of electrodes. Such clinical evaluations should be repeated over several sessions.

After an evaluation is completed, we will be ready to start developing clinical goals, and NMS and FES protocols to meet those goals, that can improve conditioning, augment existing function, and/or train the patient for task performance. None of these protocols excludes the others, and their sequence or application will depend on the findings of the evaluations carried out during the course of treatment (Dimitrijevic & Dimitrijevic, 2002).

3.5. Neuromuscular Stimulation (Trophic State of the Muscle)

Upper-motor-neuron dysfunction, either partial or complete, will result in progressive disuse atrophy of the affected muscles and alter their capacity to produce adequate force and resist fatigue. Muscle bulk decreases, and when muscle contractions are induced via electrical stimulation, the de-conditioned muscle may only make a few contractions before developed force begins to progressively diminish. Thus it is essential to develop a rigorous daily NMS program to recondition muscles before beginning externally controlled electrical stimulation for the generation of functional muscle force.

After muscle force has been restored, we add a program of physical therapy with the subject performing active movements so that we can increase the endurance of their whole body in addition to that of the stimulated muscles.

3.6. Nerve and Neuromuscular Electrical Stimulation and Modification of Muscle Hypertonia

Muscle hypertonia is another common result of chronic upper-motor-neuron dysfunction. When it is not too severe, and its distribution is restricted to only several muscle groups, stimulation of appropriate cutaneous nerves or spastic muscle groups can be applied to effectively diminish increased muscle tone (Bajd et al., 1985; Dimitrijevic & Dimitrijevic, 2002).

A train of stimuli (20 Hz–50 Hz) adjusted to an intensity that is below the threshold of sensation is appropriate for the control of spasticity. In a case where the patient has no sensation, we can substitute the missing sensory threshold by stimulation strength below the threshold of minimal motor response. Stimulation should be applied for 30 minutes, twice a day. It is important to take care of the skin and to build skin tolerance for long-lasting electrical stimulation. Once skin tolerance is developed, and if muscle hypertonia is persistent, it is possible to stimulate one or several cutaneous nerves of the skin above the spastic muscle groups for several hours and several times per day.

Overall, electrical nerve and neuromuscular stimulation for the modification of muscle hypertonia has the advantage of being simple to apply, but proper placement of the electrodes can be difficult. Common stimulation targets are cutaneous nerves of the sural, saphenus, and lateral cutaneous femoral nerves and the cutaneous branches of the radialis, musculocutaneous, ulnaris, radialis, and axillaris nerves. Another requirement is that the strength of the train of stimuli must be carefully tuned to achieve the desired effect. This procedure is useful in patients in whom spontaneous recovery will ultimately diminish spasticity.

3.7. Neuromuscular Stimulation for the Modification of Patterns of Movement

Another feature of upper-motor-neuron dysfunction is the presence of multi-joint patterned flexion-extension movements that can occur when fine coordinated control is needed to perform a desired motor task. A predominant extensor thrust pattern with a weakened flexor pattern is well known to occur in some patients with SCI. This causes a circumduction movement during the swing phase of gait, leading to slow gait and requiring the use of crutches or other support devices. In these patients, it is first necessary to use the muscle-conditioning procedure described above, and when muscle resistance and endurance is recovered, to proceed simultaneously with electrical stimulation and volitional movement (Vodovnik et al., 1984).

There is always a need for multi-site stimulation because motor deficits are always present in several muscle groups. Moreover, no general recipe for how and when to stimulate different muscle groups exists due to the diversity of residual function in persons with SCI. Thus, in ambulatory spinal cord injured subjects, rarely do the motor patterns for both limbs match those of other SCI patients, even when they have similar spinal cord injury levels. Therefore, we have found that it is beneficial to use multi-site stimulation in the laboratory environment to assess the responsiveness of the motor pattern, and then to prescribe one- or two-channel stimulators for daily training and use at home.

3.8. Functional Electrical Stimulation for Impaired Functional Movement of the Single Muscle Group

Foot and wrist drop are rarely the only motor deficits in patients with chronic spinal cord injury. However, these conditions are likely to respond positively to the application of FES to substitute for the loss of control over a single muscle group within the residual volitional control of the other muscle groups. This approach is also very effective for correcting greater deficits and improving motor activity.

However, while working with upper-motor-neuron foot or wrist drop, we have found that, on eliciting functional movement of single muscle groups, the presence of subclinical impairment of the other leg and thigh or arm muscle groups becomes more noticeable. Therefore, even when applying FES to one muscle group, it is imperative to incorporate exercise and gait training to correct motor activity in the other muscle groups.

3.9. Externally Electrically Induced Modification of Altered Neurocontrol

The application of this external electrical control in patients with paralyzed extremities has given rise to two basic questions. First, how effective is this approach in overcoming motor neuron dysfunction? Second, is it possible to accomplish long-term modification of motor control even without electrical stimulation?

The answer to these questions depends on the degree of impairment, the pattern of upper motor neuron dysfunction, and the location of the lesion (spinal cord, brain stem, or brain). In ambulatory SCI patients, observations have been reported that find, after longer periods of NMS or FES, a patient can achieve new motor activity (Figure 3–1) that may persist without any further stimulation (Dimitrijevic et al., 1988a; Bajd et al, 1999; Boucher & Pepin, 1989; Dimitrijevic et al., 1990).

The electrically and externally induced modification of altered neurocontrol in this population of patients requires that stimulation be tailored according to the patient's residual motor control. Therefore, it is essential to have a multi-site stimulation system with a variety of controls for the amplitude and duration of the trains of stimuli from different channels. The patient's understanding of this approach and commitment to the relatively modest functional outcome is also a factor to be considered. Locomotor recovery enhancement through sensori-motor stimulation has also been reviewed from the neuroscientific point of view, by Muir and Steeves (1997) and from the clinical point of view by Gorman (2000). An example of the effect of FES is shown in Figure 3–2. Figure 3–2A shows a gait recording in a spinal cord injured person 60 months after injury. Figure 3–2B shows the gait pattern, without stimulation, of the same person as in Figure 3–2, after a period of two months of training with peroneal FES to assist ankle dorsiflexion. This FES-assisted training led to an improved dorsiflexion and overall regulation of the activation of other muscles during ambulation without stimulation.

3.10. Recommendation

Clinical practice using NMS and FES in SCI people can be very successful if we respect the following rules: Treat individual persons with specific motor disorders;

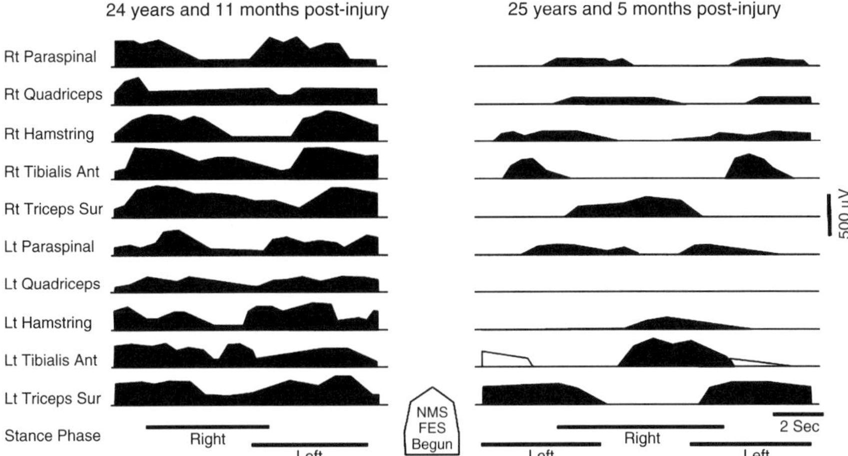

Figure 3–1 Brain Motor Control Assessment (BMCA) recording from a person with an incomplete ambulatory post-traumatic T7 spinal cord injury (SCI) during gait carried out 24 and 25 years after the onset of the injury, illustrating a significant change in the neurocontrol pattern after NMS and FES programs were carried out (from Dimitrijevic et al., 1990).

have the support of biomedical engineering to maintain the operation of the stimulator and to have appropriate systems for outpatient and home programs; apply the treatment program only after conducting a clinical assessment of motor function (see Chapter 2) and a clinical neurophysiological assessment (see Chapter 8). In order to illustrate how FES programs can be very different in similar categories of SCI patients, we shall use two publications by the same group of biomedical engineers who applied FES in people with incomplete SCI. In the first case, FES in the lower extremities of incomplete spinal cord injured individuals was used (Bajd et al., 1999). They have found that there are two possible applications of FES in incomplete SCI patients. The first is short-term therapeutic treatment in the clinical environment. The second application is the permanent orthotic use of an FES rehabilitation system. In the second case, they applied sensory-supported FES control in gait training to the L3/4 dermatome during treadmill walking (Cikajlo et al., 2005). They proved that stimulation was effective in diminishing extensor tone occurring after loading of the paralyzed limb during the stance phase of walking, which resulted in improved flexion of the leg during swing phase.

Thus, motor syndromes in persons with SCI can comprise a variety of impairments, including increased muscle tone, decreased muscle force, altered coordination between different joints, and impairments in the implementation of motor tasks. However, neuromuscular stimulation and functional electrical stimulation can be effective in improving altered function, from trophic muscle support up to enhanced movement control. Furthermore, a muscle and nerve stimulation program should be comprehensive and adjusted for the particular motor-control conditions of each patient. Finally, after achieving the intended improvement goal, the treatment plan should be adjusted to focus on maintaining this state.

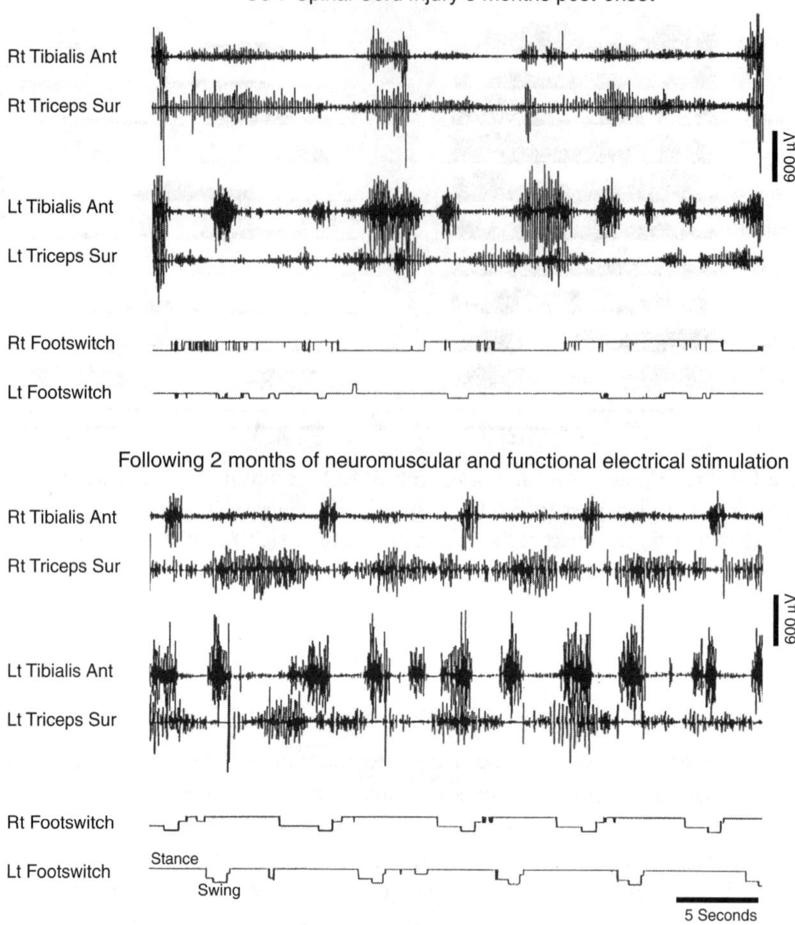

Figure 3–2 Electromyogram recorded with surface electrodes over right (*R*) and left (*L*) dorsal (*TA*) and plantar (*TS*) ankle flexor muscles during gait. Gait cycles were recorded with foot-contact switches (*FSW*) placed over the heel and ball of the foot. Recordings performed under identical conditions before application of neuromuscular and functional electrical stimulation (*A*) and two months after the start of the treatment (*B*) reveal a significant change in the pattern of electromyographic activity and neurocontrol, as well as performance (swing and stance phases; from Dimitrijevic, 1990).

It is important to ensure that the physical therapist conducting treatment and the restorative neurology program has received additional training in electrical stimulation and in the motor control of spinal cord injured people and works in an environment with biomedical engineering resources and a physician with human neurophysiology expertise. In conclusion, NMS and FES are effective modalities to improve trophic functions, increase fatigue resistance, decrease spasticity, and enhance volitional movement, but the degree of improvement depends on the residual motor control found below the spinal cord injury.

4. SPINAL CORD STIMULATION FOR CONTROL OF SPASTICITY AND MOVEMENT AUGMENTATION

If a successful NMS and FES restorative neurology program for chronic SCI individuals depends on the expertise of the physician and the physical therapist and on biomedical engineering support, then spinal cord stimulation (SCS) of the posterior structures of the lumbar spinal cord cannot be practiced unless that intervention is coordinated in a multi-professional environment that includes a neurosurgeon the attending SCI physician, a clinical neurophysiologist, a biomedical engineer, a well-oriented anesthesiologist, and an informed nursing staff, all of whom know how to care for a person with SCI after the surgical placement of epidural electrodes and an implanted stimulator. Spinal cord stimulation is a neurophysiological intervention tool that, to be properly implemented, should only be applied after an assessment of spinal cord function has been performed, with the ability to neurophysiologically monitor the effects of spinal cord stimulation during the procedure as well as afterwards. When such criteria are fulfilled, SCS can be effective as a treatment for the control of spasticity, the augmentation of residual motor control, and the activation of motor functions not present before its application.

An example of SCS-induced improvement of motor-task performance is shown in Figure 3–3.

Overall, SCS is a dynamic neurophysiological procedure that can be effective if all technical requirements can be met. Otherwise it is a method with many technical challenges, especially if conducted by a single neurosurgeon without neurophysiological or biomedical engineering support.

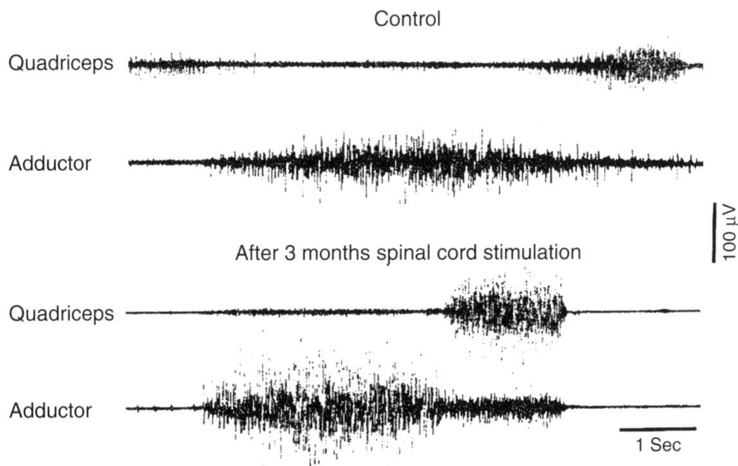

Figure 3–3 Electromyographic response to volitional movement of the leg before and after three months of spinal cord stimulation in an MS patient. Adductor activity appears during flexion and decreases during extension. The quadriceps is activated only during extension. A comparison of control responses and responses after three months of spinal cord stimulation shows the improved control in the sudden onset and cessation of motor unit activity (from Dimitrijevic & Sherwood, 1980).

Richardson and McLone (1978) succeeded in suppressing spasticity and flexor spasms in six patients with clinically complete, chronic thoracic spinal cord lesions by applying SCS with the electrode placed caudal to the lesion. Siegfried and colleagues (1980), who treated 15 chronic SCI patients by placing the electrode above the lesion, failed to confirm this finding. In an effort to clarify the precise impact of the site of stimulation, Dimitrijevic and coworkers (1986a, 1986b) used SCS in 58 chronic SCI patients and found, by clinical evaluation in all and by neurophysiological observation in 15, that spasticity is more effectively controlled when the epidural electrode was placed below, rather than above, the spinal lesion. This finding was confirmed by Barolat and his team (1995), who, based on a total of 48 patients, concluded that SCS applied caudal to the level of the lesion was an effective and safe method to control SCI-related spasms.

The 1990s saw interest in this approach decline, mainly due to technical problems and the realization that SCS as a method to control spasticity was less effective in patients with severe spasms of the lower limbs (Dimitrijevic et al., 1986b; Barolat et al., 1995; Pinter et al., 2000). In our earlier work on motor control in human SCI, we described the complex neurocontrol mechanisms of the lumbar cord below the level of injury and described residual supraspinal input in clinically motor-complete SCI (Dimitrijevic, 1988b; Dimitrijevic et al., 1997).

Thus our studies have revealed that SCS induced a generalized (diffuse) suppression, which suggests that the adopted approach of spinal cord stimulation enhanced the activity of an inhibitory plurisegmental network situated within the lumbar cord (Dimitrijevic et al., 1972).

It has been shown repeatedly, that mild forms of spasticity can be effectively controlled by stimulating through electrodes placed caudal to the level of the spinal cord lesion (Dimitrijevic et al., 1986a; Gybels & Van Roost, 1985; Illis, 1992; Barolat et al., 1995). Why this approach has failed in cases of severe spasticity becomes clear when we realize how heavily the anti-spastic effect of SCS depends on the site of stimulation. Rather than just placing the electrode below the level of the lesion, it is essential that the stimulation site target the dorsal roots of the upper lumbar cord segment. As a possible explanation for this difference, we suggest that the previously adopted approach can only activate nonspecific inhibitory mechanisms within the dorsal column–brain stem–spinal loop (Saade et al., 1984), whereas our own approach succeeds in activating a specific inhibitory mechanism accessed through dorsal root inputs within the lumbar spinal cord. Because the remarkable anti-spastic effect of targeting the dorsal roots of the upper lumbar cord segment was absent when the stimulus was applied to the neighboring lower thoracic or lower lumbar segment, we suggest that there exists a network within the lumbar cord that can be activated by exciting the posterior structures of the L2 segment. The same specific dependence on the site of stimulation is noted when stimulation is applied to elicit activity of a spinal pattern generator for locomotion in chronic paraplegic patients (Dimitrijevic et al., 1998).

Thus, there apparently exist two different sites of stimulation, one of which is suitable only for SCI patients with mild spasticity and incomplete lesions. In their situation, stimulation below the level of the lesion may be a perfectly serviceable approach, but in patients with severe spasticity in the lower limbs, it is essential to selectively stimulate upper lumbar dorsal roots. A detailed description of how to locate the correct site of upper lumbar stimulation is provided by Murg and colleagues (2000).

All other stimulation parameters are variable. Frequencies and amplitudes must be adapted on a case-by-case basis, regardless of whether the electrode is operated in unipolar or bipolar mode. We have found a trend that the more severely affected patients required either higher amplitudes or higher frequencies of stimulation. The range of effective frequencies of stimulation is 50 Hz–100 Hz.

Looking to the future, there is a need to develop new epidural electrodes specifically designed for the stimulation of lumbar cord dorsal roots. This design would involve an extended reach to cover multiple sites not only in the vertical but also in the horizontal plane. The results of our studies offer testimony to the fact that we are gradually learning how to restore normal function of the spinal cord by identifying specific sites for stimulation to achieve specific and predictable results.

Finally, we should address the question of how long the induced effects of SCS can last. The first answer to this question is that SCS can have different effects, suppression of spasms as well as augmentation of the control of spasms and some minimal movement, to improve functional movements. These effects will depend on the setup of the stimulator's frequency, polarity, and strength, and be influenced by whether the SCI subjects can learn how to set up those stimulator parameters to suppress as well as to elicit their spasticity. This effect is present and repeatable and should last unless there are problems with electrode migration. Proper care of extensive mobility of the lumbar spine can minimize potential danger for electrode migration. Moreover, there is also the possibility of resetting which electrode contacts are active and thus adjusting the optimal stimulation site. Furthermore, there is ongoing development of new designs with electrode arrays; that is, with 16 contacts, for field steering and with a long-term attachment to the dura in the posterior lumbar or thoracic region.

In conclusion, the epidural SCS method is based on external interaction with residual spinal cord functions and proves, therefore, that the nervous system is dynamic and that a variety of excitatory or inhibitory effects can be elicited, which can be incorporated to upgrade residual motor control. Thus SCS is not a treatment procedure for spasticity. On the contrary, it is an active system for interacting with the residual motor control that is manifested as spasticity. Therefore, the overall goal of SCS is not treatment of spasticity but rather the enhancement of spinal cord motor control after SCI, that is, converting pathophysiology to task appropriate functional physiology.

5. SPINAL CORD STIMULATION AND MOVEMENT ELICITATION

SCS is effective in the control of spasticity by delivering non-patterned, electrical stimulation of posterior lumbar structures with a frequency range of between 50 Hz and100 Hz. However, when the frequency is reduced to 25 Hz–35 Hz, we have been able to demonstrate that, in clinically complete, spinal cord injured subjects, it is possible to evoke patterned spinal motor output to the muscles and produce stepping-like movement of the paralyzed lower limbs (Minassian et al., 2004). SCS frequencies in the range of 5 Hz–15 Hz can initiate and maintain tonic activation of extensor muscles and produce lower limb extension (Jilge et al., 2004). In fact, within each clinically complete subject tested, SCS first induced reflex responses that tracked each impulse at lower frequencies. With increasing frequency, 5 Hz to 15 Hz, tonic, predominantly extensor-dominant activation occurred. Further frequency increase, 20 to 25 Hz, brought the stepping-like movements, and higher frequencies brought full relaxation of the muscles. Thus, the spinal cord was able to "process" the continuous input signal into output patterns that were determined by the frequency of the input and included four different characteristic forms: reflex responses; simultaneous tonic activity; reciprocating phasic activity; full electrical silence.

Computer modeling has demonstrated that large-diameter afferents within the posterior roots are directly depolarized by this epidurally delivered electrical stimulation (Rattay et al., 2000; Ladenbauer et al., 2010). These afferents project to motoneurons via monosynaptic and polysynaptic connections as well as to populations of lumbar spinal interneurones involved in motor control of the lower limbs. Non-patterned electrical stimulation at the range of 25 Hz–35 Hz activates multifunctional spinal circuits by synaptically evoked depolarization. The generation of functional motor outputs and movements of the paralyzed lower limbs hinges essentially on the application of appropriate parameters for tonic electrical stimulation. In the following illustration, the multifunctional character of elicited motor responses with different stimulation strengths and frequencies is shown (Figure 3–4).

Finally, it has been shown that in addition to the above-described observations in complete SCI subjects, in motor-incomplete SCI, epidural stimulation of the posterior structures of the lumbar cord, in addition to suppression of spasticity, can augment motor control.

6. INTRATHECAL BACLOFEN PUMPS

There are two profiles of SCI subjects, one representing people who, after SCI, are highly motivated to take all advantage of their residual motor control, capitalize on improving their volitional control over spasticity and to adapt to a degree of disability and use residual motor control. These individuals are candidates for comprehensive physiotherapy, electrical stimulation procedures, and spinal cord stimulation, and usually they are able to advance their motor control and convert their spasticity to functional movements. The other profile is of individuals who are unable to cope with therapy to enhance motor control over their spasticity and are, therefore, looking for an efficient external control of their spasticity. In such cases, intrathecal delivery of baclofen may provide the control of spasticity that they seek. Moreover, intrathecal baclofen provides relatively safe, titratable, and reversible control over spasticity. Baclofen is an agonist of the inhibitory neurotransmitter γ-aminobutyric acid (GABA) receptor (B type). It acts presynaptically to reduce motor neuron excitability by inhibiting the release of excitatory neurotransmitters (Ochs, 1999; Penn, 2009). In some cases it may be useful to combine intrathecal baclofen application for control of spasticity during the night for better sleep, and then during the day to apply SCS to augment motor output. In our experience, in some patients this can be an optimal solution for providing comfort for hypertonia during the night while preserving their ability to enhance functional activity with SCS during the day.

In conclusion, the application of intrathecal baclofen is an intervention reserved for the condition when the successful control of spasticity and enhancement of

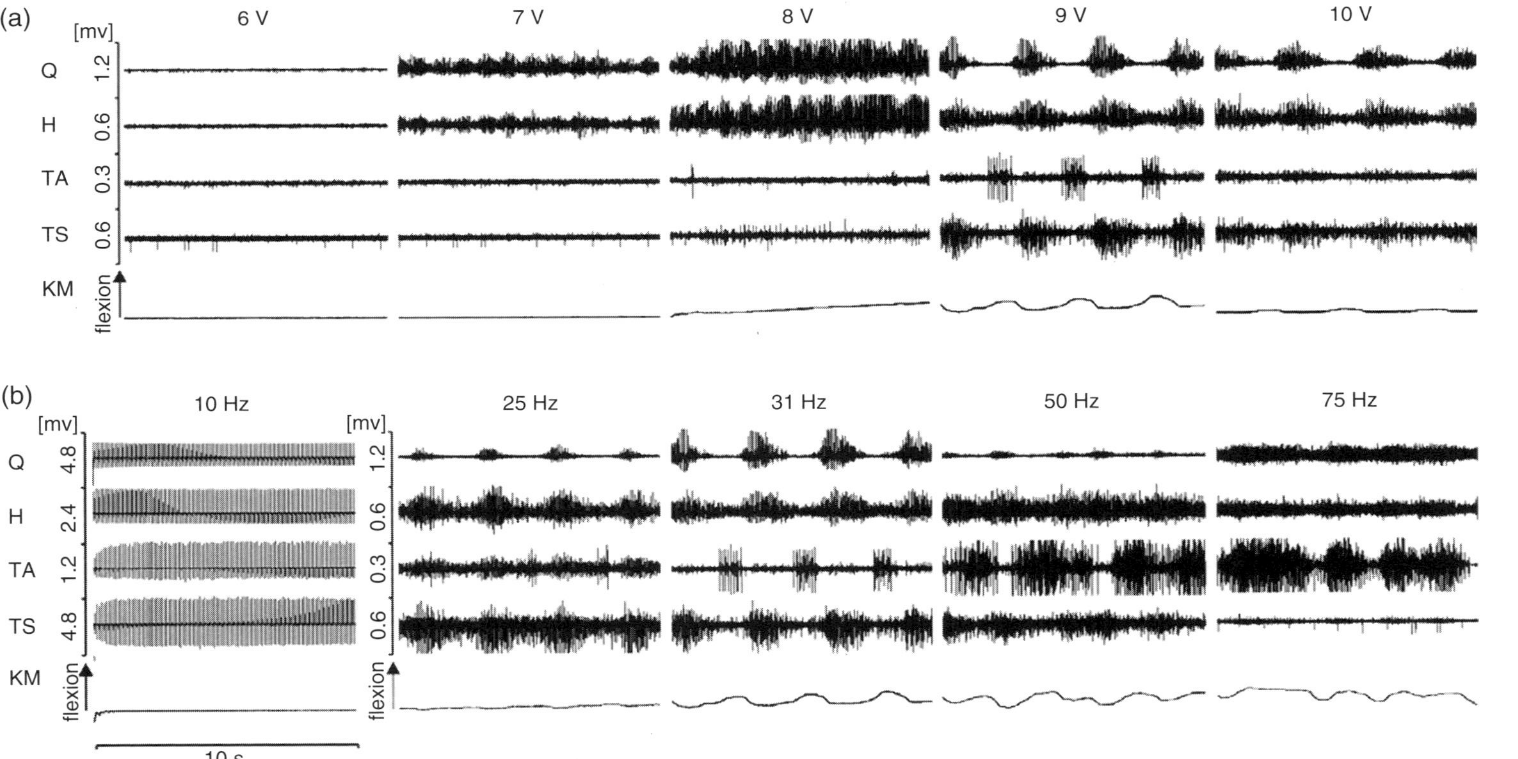

Figure 3–4 Multifunctional character of the human lumbar cord circuitry and dependence on extrinsic tonic input. This is an example presenting a variety of nonfunctional and functional motor outputs induced in a single subject with constant electrode position. (a) Constant frequency of 31 Hz and increasing the stimulus strength from 6 V–10 V. (b) Constant stimulus strength of 9 V and variation of stimulation frequencies between 10 Hz and 75 Hz. Steady rhythmic patterns appropriate to generate stepping-like movements were only induced within particular stimulation parameters (from Minassian et al., 2007).

residual motor control is otherwise not possible. Furthermore, intrathecal baclofen application can be used in such amounts that spasticity will be diminished only partially, since a certain degree of spasticity may be useful, particularly when combined with other neurophysiological augmentive procedures.

7. SPASTICITY TREATMENT WITH BOTULINUM TOXIN

Successful control of spasticity by injecting overactive muscles responsible for the clinical picture of spasticity with botulinum toxin, thereby causing muscle paralysis for several months, is, today, a widely accepted and practiced method for focal and multifocal control of spasticity (Ward, 2008). It is a potent neurotoxin that inhibits the release of neurotransmitter chemicals by disrupting the functioning of the SNARE (an acronym derived from "**SNA**P (Soluble NSF Attachment Protein) **RE**ceptor") complex required for exocytosis of synaptic vesicles (Dolly, 2003; Ward, 2008). This is a short-term means of improving patients' functioning and providing an opportunity to work actively toward a long-term management strategy. It is important, as in all the above-mentioned restorative neurological procedures, that the physician be trained in patient selection and the safe and effective application of the intervention.

8. GENERAL CONCLUSION

Motor control in chronic post-traumatic spinal cord injured individuals is the expression of residual descending function that ranges from very minimal brain influence over spinal cord reflex activity, to greater control needed to perform a variety of motor tasks in both individuals in wheelchairs and in those who can stand and ambulate. The clinical practice of restorative neurology is driven by the elucidation of clinical, and sub-clinical, neurophysiological motor control features to select and design the application of existing treatment methods. Such treatment modalities as physiotherapy, peripheral electrical stimulation, and spinal cord stimulation can be used to elicit a variety of interactions between external inputs and internal residual motor control. When practiced as part of a multidisciplinary team approach with the needed expertise to comprehensively assess the underlying mechanisms of muscle hypertonia, spasms, and disrupted volitional motor control, it is possible to enhance functional outcomes and the quality of life for people with chronic spinal cord injuries.

References

Bajd, T., Gregoric, M., Vodovnik, L., Benko, H. "Electrical stimulation in treating spasticity due to spinal cord injury." *Archives of Physical Medicine and Rehabilitation* 66 (1985): 515–517.

Bajd, T., Kralj, A., Stefancic, M., Lavrac, N. "Use of functional electrical stimulation in the lower extremities of incomplete spinal cord injured patients." *Artificial Organs* 23 (1999): 403–409.

Barolat, G., Singh-Sahni, K., Staas, W. E., Shatin, D., Ketcik, B., Allen, K. "Epidural spinal cord stimulation in the management of spasms in spinal cord injury: A prospective study." *Stereotactic and Functional Neurosurgery* 64 (1995): 153–164.

Bobath, B. *Adult Hemiplegia: Evaluation and Treatment*. London: William Heinemann Medical Books Ltd., 1978.

Boucher, J. P., Pepin, A. "Effects of patterned electrical stimulation in recent and chronic quadriplegia." In *Neuromuscular Stimulation: Basic Concepts and Clinical Implications*, edited by F. C. Rose, R. Jones, G. Vrbova, 83–91. New York: Demos, 1989.

Brunström, S. *Movement Therapy in Hemiplegia*. Philadelphia, PA: Harper and Row, 1970.

Cikajlo, I., Matjacic, Z., Bajd, T., Futami, R. "Sensory supported FES control in gait training of incomplete spinal cord injury persons." *Artificial Organs* 29 (2005): 459–461.

Chen, X. Y., Chen, Y., Wang, Y., et al. "Reflex conditioning: A new strategy for improving motor function after spinal cord injury." *Annals of the New York Academy of Sciences* 1198 (2010): E12–E21.

Creasey, G. H., Ho, C. H., Triolo, R. J., et al. "Clinical applications of electrical stimulation after spinal cord injury." *Journal of Spinal Cord Medicine* 27 (2004): 365–375.

Dimitrijevic, M. M., Dimitrijevic, M. R. "Clinical elements for the neuromuscular stimulation and functional electrical stimulation protocols in the practice of neurorehabilitation." *Artificial Organs* 26 (2002): 256–259.

Dimitrijevic, M. M., Dimitrijevic, M. R., Illis, L. S., Nakajima, K., Sharkey, P. C., Sherwood, A. M. "Spinal cord stimulation for the control of spasticity in patients with chronic spinal cord injury: I. Clinical observations." *Central Nervous System Trauma* 3 (1986a): 129–144.

Dimitrijevic, M. M., Illis, L. S., Nakajima, K., Sharkey, P. C., Sherwood, A. M. "Spinal cord stimulation for the control of spasticity in patients with chronic spinal cord injury: II. Neurophysiologic observations." *Central Nervous System Trauma* 3 (1986b): 145–152.

Dimitrijevic, M. M., Dimitrijevic, M. R., Patridge, M., Verhagen-Metman, L. "Alteration of neurocontrol in chronic ambulatory spinal cord injury patients after long-term peripheral nerve stimulation." In *Abstract Digest*, American Spinal Injury Association, 32 (1988a).

Dimitrijevic, M. R. "Residual motor functions in spinal cord injury." In *Advances in Neurology, Vol. 47: Functional Recovery in Neurological Disease*, edited by S. G. Waxman. New York: Raven Press, 1988b.

Dimitrijevic, M. R. "Neurological rehabilitation and restorative neurology of spastic syndromes." In *The Origin and Treatment of Spasticity*, edited by R. Benecke, M. Emre, R. A. Davidoff, 113–124, Lancashire, UK: The Parthenon Publishing Group, 1990.

Dimitrijevic, M. R., Faganel, J., Gregoric, M., Nathan, P. W., Trontelj, J. K. "Habituation: Effects of regular and stochastic stimulation." *Journal of Neurology, Neurosurgery and Psychiatry* 35 (1972): 234–242.

Dimitrijevic, M. R., Gerasimenko, Y., Pinter, M. M. "Evidence for a spinal central pattern generator in humans." *Annals of the New York Academy of Sciences* 860 (1998): 409–420.

Dimitrijevic, M. R., Gracanin, F., Prevec, T., Trontelj, J. "Electronic control of paralyzed extremities." *Biomedical Engineering* 3 (1968): 8–19.

Dimitrijevic, M. R., Illis, L. S., Nakajima, K., Sharkey, P. C., Sherwood, A. M. "Spinal cord stimulation for the control of spasticity in patients with chronic spinal cord injury: II. Neurophysiologic observations." *Central Nervous System Trauma* 3 (1986b): 145–152.

Dimitrijevic, M. R., McKay, W. B., Sherwood, A. M. "Motor control physiology below spinal cord injury: Residual volitional control of motor units in paretic and paralyzed muscles." In: *Neuronal Regeneration, Reorganization and Repair*, edited by F. J. Seil, 335–345. New York: Raven Press, 1997.

Dimitrijevic, M. R., Sherwood, A. M. "Spasticity: medical and surgical treatment." *Neurology* 30 (1980): 19–27.

Dobkin, B., Apple, D., Barbeau, H., et al.: Spinal Cord Injury Locomotor Trial Group. "Weight-supported treadmill vs. over-ground training for walking after acute incomplete SCI." *Neurology* 66 (2006): 484–493.

Dolly, O. "Synaptic transmission: Inhibition of neurotransmitter release by botulinum toxins." *Headache* 43 Suppl 1 (2003): S16–S24

Field-Fote, E. C., Lindley, S. D., Sherman, A. L. "Locomotor training approaches for individuals with spinal cord injury: A preliminary report of walking-related outcomes." *Journal of Neurological Physical Therapy* 29 (2005): 127–137.

Gorman, P. H. "An update on functional electrical stimulation after spinal cord injury." *Neurorehabilitation and Neural Repair* 14 (2000): 251–263.

Gybels, J., Van Roost, D. "Spinal cord stimulation for the modification of dystonic and hyperkinetic conditions: A critical review." In *Recent Achievements in Restorative Neurology*, edited by J. Eccles, M. R. Dimitrijevic, 56–70. Basel, Switzerland: Karger, 1985.

Gracanin, F., Marincek, I. "Development of new systems for functional electrical stimulation." Proceedings of the 3rd International Symposium on External control of Human Extremities: Yugoslav Committee for Electronics and Automation, Belgrade, Yugoslavia, 495–502, August 25–30, 1969.

Illis, L. S. "Spinal cord stimulation in spasticity and bladder dysfunction." In *Spinal Cord Dysfunction, Vol. 3*, edited by L. S. Illis, 294–303. New York; Tokyo: Oxford University Press, 1992.

Jezernik, S., Colombo, G., Keller, T., Frueh, H., Morari, M. Robotic orthosis lokomat: A rehabilitation and research tool. *Neuromodulation* 6 (2003): 108–115.

Jilge, B., Minassian, K., Rattay, F., et al. "Initiating extension of the lower limbs in subjects with complete spinal cord injury by epidural lumbar cord stimulation." *Experimental Brain Research* 154 (2004): 308–326.

Kralj, A. R., Bajd, T. *Functional Electrical Stimulation: Standing and Walking After Spinal Cord Injury*. Boca Raton, FL: CRC Press, 1989.

Ladenbauer, J., Minassian, K., Hofstoetter, U. S., Dimitrijevic, M. R., Rattay, F. "Stimulation of the human lumbar spinal cord with implanted and surface electrodes: A computer simulation study." *IEEE Transactions on Neural System and Rehabilitation Engineering* 18 (2010): 637–645.

Liberson, W. T. "Functional electrical stimulation." In: *Brain, Nerves, Muscles and Electricity: My Life in Science*, edited by R. Choen, 74–87. Union City, CA: Smyrna Press, 1999.

Liberson, W. T., Holmquest, M. E., Scott, D., Dow, M. "Functional electrotherapy stimulation of the peroneal nerve, synchronized with the swing phase of gait of hemi-paraplegic patients." *Archives of Physical Medicine and Rehabilitation* 42 (1961): 101–105.

Marino, R. J., Barros, T., Biering-Sorensen, F., et al.: ASIA Neurological Standards Committee. "International standards for neurological classification of spinal cord injury." *Journal of Spinal Cord Medicine*, 26 Suppl 1 (2003): S50–S56.

Minassian, K., Jilge, B., Rattay, F., et al. "Stepping-like movements in humans with complete spinal cord injury induced by epidural stimulation of the lumbar cord: Electromyographic study of compound muscle action potentials." *Spinal Cord* 42 (2004): 401–416.

Minassian, K., Persy, I., Rattay, F., Pinter, M. M., Kern, H., Dimitrijevic, M. R. "Human lumbar cord circuitries can be activated by extrinsic tonic input to generate locomotor-like activity." *Human Movement Science* 26 (2007): 275–295.

Muir, G. D., Steeves, J. D. "Sensorimotor stimulation to improve locomotor recovery after spinal cord injury." *Trends in Neuroscience* 20 (1997): 72–77.

Murg, M., Binder, H., Dimitrijevic, M. R. "Epidural electric stimulation of posterior structures of the human lumbar spinal cord: 1. Muscle twitches—a functional method to define the site of stimulation." *Spinal Cord* 38 (2000): 394–402.

Ochs, G., Naumann, C., Dimitrijevic, M. R., Sindou, M. "Intrathecal Baclofen therapy for spinal origin spasticity: Spinal cord injury, spinal cord disease, and multiple sclerosis." *Neuromodulation* 2 (1999): 108–119.

Penn, R. D. "Intrathecal drugs for spasticity." In *Textbook of Stereotactic and Functional Neurosurgery*, edited by A.M. Lozano, P. L. Gildenberg, R. R. Tasker, 1973–1981. Berlin: Springer Verlag, 2009.

Pinter, M. M., Gerstenbrand, F., Dimitrijevic, M. R. "Epidural electrical stimulation of posterior structures of the human lumbosacral cord: 3. Control of spasticity." *Spinal Cord* 38 (2000): 524–531.

Rattay, F., Minassian, K., Dimitrijevic, M. R. "Epidural electrical stimulation of posterior structures of the human lumbosacral cord: 2. Quantitative analysis by computer modeling." *Spinal Cord* 38 (2000): 473–489.

Ragnarsson, K. T. "Functional electrical stimulation after spinal cord injury: Current use, therapeutic effects and future directions." *Spinal Cord* 46 (2008): 255–274.

Richardson, R. R., McLone, D. G. "Percutaneous epidural neurostimulation for paraplegic spasticity." *Surgical Neurology* 9 (1978): 153–155.

Rood, M. S. "A program for paraplegics." *American Journal of Occupational Therapy* 1 (1947): 22–25.

Siegfried, J., Lazorthes, Y., Broggi, G. "Electrical spinal cord stimulation for spastic movement disorders." *Applied Neurophysiology* 44 (1980): 77–92.

Saade, N. E., Tabet, M. S., Atweh, S. F., Jabbur, S. J. "Modulation of segmental mechanisms by activation of a dorsal column brain stem spinal loop." *Brain Research* 310 (1984): 180–184.

Stein, R. B., Chong, S. L., James, K. B., et al. "Electrical stimulation for therapy and mobility after spinal cord injury." *Progress in Brain Research* 137 (2002): 27–34.

Vodovnik, L., Bajd, T., Kralj, A., Gracanin, F., Strojnik, P. "Functional electrical stimulation for control of locomotor systems." *CRC Critical Reviews in Bioengineering* 6 (1981): 63–131.

Vodovnik L, Bowman BR, Hufford P. "Effects of electrical stimulation on spinal spasticity." *Scand J Rehabil Med.* 16 (1984): 29–34.

Ward, A. B. "Spasticity treatment with botulinum toxins." *Journal of Neural Transmission* 115 (2008): 607–616.

Wolpaw, J. R. "Treadmill training after spinal cord injury: Good but not better." *Neurology* 66 (2006): 466–467.

Wolpaw, J. R. "Spinal cord plasticity in acquisition and maintenance of motor skills." *Acta Physiologica* 189 (2007): 155–169.

4

Neural Control of Locomotion

GERTA VRBOVÁ, URSZULA SŁAWIŃSKA, AND HENRYK MAJCZYŃSKI

CONTENTS

1. Introduction
2. Spinal Cord Network for Locomotion
3. Supraspinal Control
4. Changes in Locomotion after Spinal Cord Injury
    4.1. Changes in Locomotion after Spinal Cord Injury in Cats
        — Total spinal cord transection
        — Partial transection of the spinal cord
    4.2. Changes in Locomotion after Spinal Cord Injury in Rats
        — Total spinal cord transection
        — Partial spinal cord transection
        — Contusion and compression injuries
5. Afferent Influence
6. The Role of Different Neurotransmitters for Locomotor Movement
References

1. INTRODUCTION

Spinal cord injury (SCI) damages the structures that connect the brain to the spinal cord so that the communication between the brain and the spinal cord is interrupted and the functions controlled by the brain via the spinal cord are altered. The effects of SCI are determined by the site and extent of the damage (lesion). In patients, SCI may cause severe functional impairments, among which locomotor disability (difficulty in walking) is one of the most critical. This can have a devastating social and economic impact on those affected. In the United States alone, there are more than 10,000 cases of SCI every year. In European countries, an annual incidence of 15 to 40 traumatic SCI cases per million population are reported (combined data from SCI centers). Due to the impact of this condition on the quality of life of the affected individual, considerable effort has been directed to enhance the recovery of locomotion as well as to develop effective therapies to reduce the debilitating effects of spinal cord injury on other functions. Animal models of SCI have been extremely helpful in (1) understanding the mechanisms responsible for producing the locomotor pattern, which evokes rhythmic limb movements associated with locomotion, and (2) in developing interventions to help to repair the effects of spinal cord injury.

Nevertheless, it is still unclear how close animal models of spinal cord injury come to reproducing SCI in humans. In this review we will discuss how the location and extent of spinal cord damage influence locomotion in experimental animals, and what kind of neuroactive substances are involved in the activation of the spinal cord neural system for the control of locomotion. We will focus on locomotion and the mechanisms that control it because it is relatively well understood, and the principles that govern it may apply to the control of other neural functions of the spinal cord, which at present are less well understood. The reader will be referred to a number of reviews that show the tremendous progress that has been made over the last decade in this field (Dietz, 2003; Duysens & Van de Crommert, 1998; Edgerton et al., 2001; Jordan & Schmidt, 2002; Jordan et al., 2008; Jordan & Sławińska, 2011; Kay-Lyons, 2002; Kiehn, 2006; Majczyński & Sławińska, 2007; McCrea, 2001; Pearson, 2004; Rossignol et al., 2004; 2009).

2. SPINAL CORD NETWORK FOR LOCOMOTION

It is now generally accepted that the neural control of locomotion is organized through a central pattern generator (CPG). This consists in mammals of a network of spinal cord neurons producing signals evoking alternating activity in groups of flexor and extensor muscles, which result in leg movements and locomotion. Much of the understanding of the basic functional principles of neural circuits (networks of interneurons) within the spinal cord that are responsible for locomotion and interact with specific sensory inputs is based on information obtained from invertebrates and primitive fish (the lamprey). Much less is known about the organization of the CPG in higher vertebrates.

Our understanding of stereotyped motor responses to external stimuli produced by neural structures in the spinal cord is mainly based on observations of locomotion in cats. Brown (1911; 1912) discovered that in cats, after total transection of the spinal cord and dorsal roots, rhythmic alternating contraction of ankle flexor and extensor muscles could be elicited. This observation could only be explained by the existence of a specialized neuronal network in the spinal cord that can elicit complex movements. The pioneering studies of Sherrington (Sherrington, 1910) and Brown (Brown, 1911; 1912) indicated that the mechanisms responsible for regulating these limb movements are complex. Later observations led to the proposal that rhythmic motor activity is generated by the reciprocal inhibition of two "half-centers." One half-center produces activity in the flexor and the other in the extensor muscles (Brown, 1911; 1912). Thus, in addition to mono- and polysynaptic reflexes described by Sherrington (Sherrington, 1910), the spinal cord circuitry can generate movements of several joints. Subsequent experiments have confirmed these findings (for review, see Dietz, 2003; Duysens & Van de Crommert, 1998; Grillner & Zangger, 1975; Grillner, 1985; Jankowska et al., 1967b; Jankowska et al., 1967a; Kay-Lyons, 2002b; Pearson, 2004; Rossignol et al., 1996; Wetzel & Stuart, 1976; Whelan, 1996), and it is now established that locomotor activity is generated by the neuronal circuitry located in the spinal cord and the group of neurons responsible are referred to

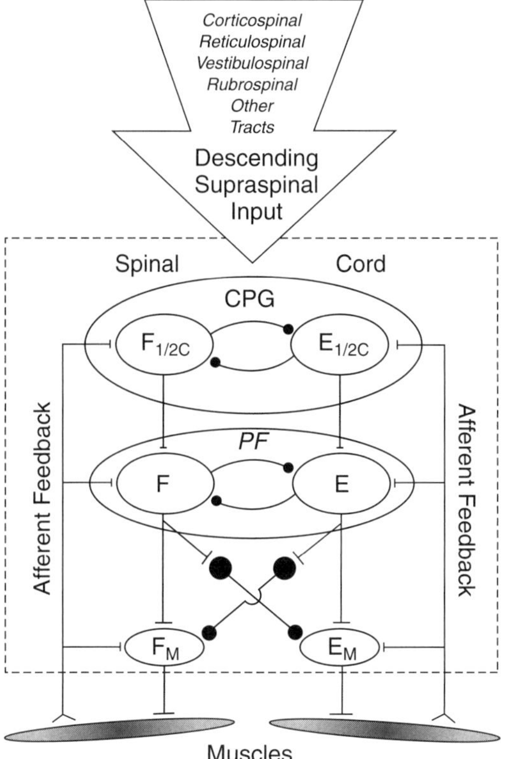

Figure 4–1 Simplified schematic diagram of spinal circuitry involved in producing locomotor patterns and peripheral and supraspinal inputs, which can modify locomotor activity at various levels . Spinal cord circuitry consists of a separate network for rhythm generation and a network for pattern formation that distributes excitation and inhibition to motoneurons. This circuitry is under the influence of descending supraspinal inputs and intraspinal connections as well as of muscle, joint, and skin afferents. *Abbreviations*: CPG – central pattern generator, $F_{1/2C}$ – flexor half center, $E_{1/2C}$ – extensor half-center, F, E – respectively flexor and extensor part of a pattern formation network, E_M – extensor motoneurons, F_M – flexor motoneurons, PF – pattern formation (adapted from Majczyński & Sławińska, 2007).

as the CPG (Grillner and Zangger, 1975; Grillner, 1985; Lundberg, 1979; Shik et al., 1969; Shik & Orlovsky, 1976). A schematic representation of the spinal cord circuitry and its inputs is illustrated in Figure 4–1, which indicates that its activity can be modulated by many afferent inputs (descending supraspinal pathways, propriospinal and ascending afferents from the periphery). Nevertheless, while limb movements are modified by sensory inputs, they do not depend on them, for rhythmic activity can be generated by the CPG even in the absence of these inputs when the descending pathways have been disrupted by total spinal cord and dorsal root transection. Total transection of the spinal cord disrupts the influence of supraspinal structures on the part of the spinal cord below the lesion containing the network responsible for generating the locomotor pattern and prevents any information from the spinal cord below the lesion from reaching the brain. Cutting the dorsal roots does not completely abolish afferent inputs, because some afferent information reaches the spinal cord through the ventral roots (Coggeshall et al., 1997; Loeb, 1976). Nevertheless, it is unlikely that ventral root afferents play a role in locomotion, because most of them originate from the visceral region (Grillner & Zangger, 1979) and stimulation of ventral roots does not evoke any obvious sensation or movement (Duysens & Van de Crommert, 1998).

The most convincing evidence for the existence of the CPG in the spinal cord of cats was provided by recordings of rhythmic patterns of locomotor activity from ventral roots of animals in which the limb movement (and therefore the "feedback" of movement) was eliminated by paralyzing the muscles or by cutting the motor nerves. Because these rhythmic patterns occurred in the absence of any movement, such neural activity was called "fictive locomotion" (for review, see Kay-Lyons, 2002). Further investigations using the "fictive locomotion" model led to a better understanding of the organization of the reflex pathways and to the identification of some of the spinal interneurons involved in locomotor-dependent reflexes and the organization of the mammalian CPG (for review, see McCrea, 2001). Recently, McCrea with his colleagues (Angel et al., 2005; Lafreniere-Roula & McCrea, 2005; Rybak et al., 2006a; Rybak et al., 2006b; Stecina et al., 2005; Yakovenko et al., 2005) proposed a model of the spinal circuitry for locomotion with a layer of interneurons between the CPG and the motoneurones. Thus, the CPG acting upon a limb can be divided into two networks: one for rhythm generation (i.e., cycle period and phase), and the other for pattern formation, by distributing excitation and inhibition to particular motoneurones, (see Figure 4–1).

3. SUPRASPINAL CONTROL

None of these findings diminishes the importance of supraspinal and sensory inputs in regulating locomotion under normal conditions. Supraspinal structures have several functions in the control of locomotion in cats (Orlovsky, 1991): (a) initiating and terminating the activity of the spinal locomotor CPGs, (b) controlling the level of their activity, (c) maintaining equilibrium in locomotion, (d) adapting paw movements to external circumstances, and (e) coordinating other performances with locomotion. The spinal circuitry is reserved only to generate the complex pattern of muscle activity needed for locomotion.

Thus the spinal network that can generate basic locomotor rhythmicity without any supraspinal or sensory input to the spinal cord in spinal animals, can also be activated in decerebrated animals by tonic descending activation from centers in the brain stem: mesencephalic locomotor region (MLR) and subthalamic locomotor region (SLR) (Orlovsky, 1969; Shik & Orlovsky, 1976). Stimulation of these regions initiates and controls locomotor movements. To maintain locomotion, many other supraspinal structures are engaged, including the sensorimotor cortex, the cerebellum, and the basal ganglia. There is now good evidence that neurones originating from several areas of the brain stem are important for initiating and maintaining locomotion (for review, see Fouad & Pearson, 2004; Jordan et al., 2008). Recently it was described that a group of serotonergic neurones located in the brain stem near the pyramidal tract (just rostral to the inferior olivary nucleus at the level of the nucleus of the VIIth cranial nerve) is also involved in initiation of locomotor movement (Liu & Jordan, 2005). The brain stem structures that are the source of the reticulo- and vestibulospinal pathways play an important role in controlling contractions of muscles necessary to support the body weight, for ensuring the lateral stability of the animal and for regulating the sequence of muscle activity during locomotion. In addition, the reticulospinal pathways can modulate the body posture to ensure stability under dynamic conditions. In comparison, the rubrospinal pathway, which is well developed in lower mammals and less so in humans, exerts excitatory effects on flexor muscles and inhibits extensor muscles. Removing the sensorimotor cortex or cutting the corticospinal tract did not influence stereotyped locomotion, whether walking uphill, downhill, or running at different speeds (Orlovsky, 1991). However, more demanding locomotor tasks, like walking over barriers, produced increased bursting activity in pyramidal tract neurones in an intact cat. Thus, it seems that the corticospinal pathway contributes to the control of basic locomotor movements required to negotiate obstacles in the environment.

The role of the cerebellum in locomotion is not completely clear. Mori and colleagues (Mori et al., 1999) observed that stimulation of the hook bundle of Russell in the midline cerebellar white matter evokes coordinated quadrupedal locomotion in the decerebrate cat. It is also known that the cerebellar cortex integrates proprioceptive, exteroceptive, visual, and vestibular afferent information originating from a wide variety of sources (Armstrong, 1988; Armstrong et al., 1997). The cerebellum receives information about the state of the CPG via the ventral spinocerebellar and spinoreticulocerebellar tracts and afferent information from the peripheral motor apparatus via the dorsal spinocerebellar tract. The cerebellum indirectly influences motoneurones through the vestibulospinal, rubrospinal, reticulospinal, and corticospinal tracts. Furthermore, removal of the cerebellum results in the deterioration of locomotor movements characterized by poor interlimb coordination, inaccurate foot placement, and impairment of balance. The basal ganglia are now also recognized as part of a larger motor-control system involving the cerebral cortex and thalamus, which is responsible for planning, initiation, execution, and termination of motor tasks, as well as motor learning (Graybiel, 1995). Both the cerebellum and the basal ganglia are thought to maintain the timing of sequential muscle activation, with the basal ganglia working over a long time-scale (Kay-Lyons, 2002).

CPG activity is modulated by a number of different neurotransmitters, employed by several pathways that originate from supraspinal structures: the serotonergic cells of raphe nucleus, the noradrenergic cells of the locus coeruleus, plus glutamatergic cells in the nucleus reticularis gigantocellularis, the pontine reticular nucleus, and possibly from other descending pathways. At least two descending projections of the monoaminergic system; i.e., serotonergic and noradrenergic; play a crucial role in the control of the excitability of the spinal circuitry. The supraspinal serotonergic descending projections are involved in initiation and control of locomotor hind limb movements (Jordan & Schmidt, 2002; Jordan et al., 2008; Liu & Jordan, 2005). There is ample evidence showing that descending serotonergic pathways make synaptic contact with motoneurones (Holstege & Kuypers, 1987; Jordan & Schmidt, 2002; Ulfhake et al., 1987) and increase their excitability (Jankowska et al., 1967a; Jankowska et al., 1967b; Jankowska et al., 1997; Jankowska et al., 1998; Jordan & Schmidt, 2002; White & Neuman, 1980; White & Neuman, 1983).

The reduced release of noradrenaline and serotonin after spinal cord injury markedly alters the locomotor functions as well as the bladder, bowl control, and sexual reflexes. Total spinal cord transection induces almost complete disappearance of monoaminergic neurotransmitters below the lesion (Faden et al., 1988), and this leads to critical changes in extensor excitability and alteration of the stretch reflexes. Administration of serotonin precursors or agonists can restore these functions (Ahlman et al., 1971; Ellaway & Trott, 1975). Systemic administration (intravenous or intraperitoneal) of monoamine agonists has produced some modifications of spinal reflexes and improvement of locomotor performance of animals that had their spinal cord transected (Barbeau & Rossignol, 1987; 1991; 1994). While systemic administration of monoaminergic drugs positively modulates many neurological functions, it has serious side effects because it affects the peripheral autonomic nervous system (Fung et al., 1990). During the last 20 years, alternative methods for applying this drug were developed. Intrathecal application of serotonin itself improves locomotor movements in spinal adult rats (Feraboli-Lohnherr et al., 1999). Moreover, the implantation of embryonic tissue from the raphe nucleus containing serotonergic neurones significantly improves hind limb stepping in spinal rats (Feraboli-Lohnherr et al., 1997; Majczyński et al., 2005b; Ribotta et al., 2000; Sławińska et al., 2000).

Interestingly, a comparison of results from rats and cats indicates that there is a species difference between the actions of the same drug; the same drugs may act differently in separate species and in different animal models. Clonidine can initiate locomotion in acute spinal cats and improve ongoing locomotor movements in chronic spinal cats (Barbeau & Rossignol, 1991), but it is ineffective in acute and chronic spinal rats (Fouad & Pearson, 2004). In contrast, serotonin is effective in initiating locomotor activity in spinal rats (Feraboli-Lohnherr et al., 1999) but ineffective in spinal cats (Barbeau & Rossignol, 1991). Recent data indicate that, at least in rats, both serotonergic and noradrenergic systems play an important role in locomotion, because blocking receptors to these transmitters with specific antagonists abolishes locomotion in intact animals (Majczyński et al., 2005a; Majczyński et al., 2006).

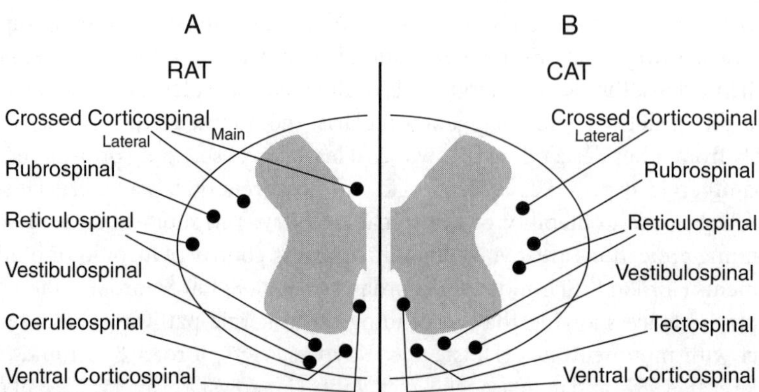

Figure 4–2 Descending tracts in the spinal cord of (*A*) rat and (*B*) cat. Note that in rat, unlike in cat, the corticospinal tract runs mainly in the dorsal spinal cord, with only a small number of fibers located in the ventral part of the spinal cord (adapted from Majczyński & Sławińska, 2007).

The supraspinal structures influence motor activity through descending pathways that can be grouped into two principal systems according to their medial or lateral location in the spinal cord (Drew et al., 2002). A medial system includes the reticulo- and vestibulospinal pathways, while the lateral system comprises the cortico- and rubrospinal pathways (Figure 4–2). The former has a relatively diffuse action on flexor and extensor muscles (Mori, 1987; Mori et al., 1992), while the latter is responsible for fine control and voluntary modification of locomotion (Beloozerova & Sirota, 1993; Kuypers, 1963).

4. CHANGES IN LOCOMOTION AFTER SPINAL CORD INJURY

In the spinal cord, each descending, ascending, or intrinsic neural system is topographically organized and has functional specificity (Figure 4–2). Thus injuries to different sites of the cord and their extents can cause different degrees of deterioration of locomotion. The effect of the site and extent of lesions at the low thoracic level on the impairment of locomotion in cats and rats will be discussed.

4.1. Changes in Locomotion after Spinal Cord Injury in Cats

As mentioned earlier, several investigations have demonstrated the substantial contribution of the spinal cord to both the generation and control of vertebrate locomotion (for review, see Grillner & Zangger, 1975; Grillner, 1985; Rossignol et al., 2002b; Schmidt & Jordan, 2000). In awake cats, locomotion has been mainly studied by examining either overground movement or that on a treadmill. In both conditions, intact cats demonstrate well-defined patterns of coordination of forelimb-forelimb, hind limb-hind limb, and forelimb-hind limb steps. Walking is a complicated motor act that requires in quadrupedal animals coordinated movements of four limbs; it involves the activity of many skeletal muscles and coordinated movement of several joints. This complex behavior is controlled by the integrated activity of descending and peripheral afferent inputs that act upon the neural spinal cord circuitry. In spite of the complex nature of the control of locomotion, cats can regain hind limb locomotor movements after a large lesion or even after a complete transection of the spinal cord (De Leon et al., 1998a; 1998b; Edgerton et al., 2001; Rossignol et al., 2001; 2002a; 2002b). This is possible because of the remarkable ability of the spinal cord to reorganize locomotor functions within the structures of the CNS below the lesion that are still connected to the muscles, indicating the existence of some plasticity in the mechanisms controlling locomotion. Many recent studies have provided evidence that after a lesion, the spinal cord network is gradually modified, and in this way the ability to express more or less appropriate locomotion is eventually regained.

Total spinal cord transection

The cat seems to be particularly privileged in its capacity to regain locomotor movements after spinal cord injury at the low thoracic level. The recovery of hind limb locomotion in cats after total spinal cord transection may occur as early as a few days as well as a few weeks after the lesion (Rossignol et al., 2002a; 2004). This phenomenon, however, is only observed when the cats' hind limbs are placed on a treadmill while the forelimbs stand on a stationary platform, and not during spontaneous overground locomotion. Only a few days after injury, when the animal is placed on the treadmill, strong manual stimulation of the perineum or the base of the tail elicits small alternating rhythmic movements of the otherwise flaccid hind limbs. Such stimulation evokes more or less rhythmic flexion movements, mainly at the hips, while very little knee and ankle flexion is observed. At this stage of recovery, the animals are unable to support the weight of their hindquarters. After a relatively quick progression (10 to 21 days), the cats reach a plateau in locomotor performance with plantar contact of the paw when supported over a treadmill and can generate adequate muscle force to support their hindquarters (Belanger et al., 1996; Rossignol et al., 2002a). Thus, two to three weeks after a complete transection of the spinal cord at T13, cats can recover almost authentic hind limb locomotor movements on a treadmill making plantigrade contact, and can support the weight of their hindquarters (Barbeau & Rossignol, 1987; Belanger et al., 1996; Rossignol et al., 2004). Moreover, spinal cats can then adapt their hind limb steps to the varying speed of the treadmill and are able to avoid obstacles (Forssberg et al., 1975). However, there are some obvious deficits in hind limb locomotor movements of spinal cats, such as a lack of voluntary control, an absence of sustained coordination between the fore- and the hind limbs during quadrupedal locomotion, and an almost total absence of balance control. Typical locomotor deficits include dragging the foot in the initial part of the swing phase of the step cycle, irregularities in the stepping frequency, exaggerated adduction of the hind limbs, and sometimes, incomplete weight support (Belanger et al., 1996). Although spinal cats can walk on a treadmill, they are unable to perform any hind limb overground locomotor movements in their home cages—they move around using forelimbs only. It seems that the specific defects observed in cats after total spinal cord transection can be attributed to the loss of normal control provided by the descending pathways from the cortex, brain stem, and propriospinal system (Brustein & Rossignol, 1998; Jiang & Drew, 1996; Rossignol et al., 1999).

Partial transection of the spinal cord

Investigations carried out using animal models with total spinal cord transections indicate the existence of spinal mechanisms controlling hind limb locomotor movement, related to the interneuronal circuitry that can produce a basic pattern of rhythmic activity. As described above, the activity of this circuitry is under the control of many descending pathways that can be divided into two principal spinal systems: medial, including the reticulo- and vestibulospinal pathways, and lateral, including the cortico- and reticulospinal pathways (Figure 4–2). A number of investigations on the recovery of cat overground quadrupedal locomotion after partial thoracic spinal cord lesions at different sites and extents have provided information concerning the role of various supraspinal structures in the regulation of hind limb locomotion (e.g., Afelt, 1974; Eidelberg & Yu, 1981; English, 1980; Górska et al., 1990; Górska et al., 1993b; Górska et al., 1993a; Górska et al., 1993c; Górska et al., 1996; Rossignol et al., 1999). It has to be noted that, in contrast to the results of investigations of animals with total spinal cord transection, the findings concerning cats with partial lesions are less consistent. For example, Górska and coworkers (Bem et al., 1995; Górska et al., 1990; Górska et al., 1993b; Górska et al., 1993c) reported that in general there are three different forms of impairment of fore–hind limb coordination after partial thoracic spinal cord lesions of different extent: (1) lesions sparing the dorsolateral or the ventral funiculus on one side preserve the equality of the step cycle duration between the fore- and hind limbs but change the coupling between the movements of these limbs compared to intact animals, so a tendency toward pacing-like locomotion is obtained; (2) more extensive lesions involving the ventral quadrants of the spinal cord and major parts of the dorsolateral funiculi as well as lesions sparing ventrolateral and ventral funiculi result in a small difference between step cycle durations of forelimbs and hind limbs (being shorter in forelimbs and longer in hind limbs) associated with episodes of substantial dissociation of fore- and hind limb step cycle duration; (3) lesions destroying almost the whole spinal cord sparing only small parts of the dorsolateral funiculus and/or parts of dorsal columns, as well as lesions sparing the ventral funiculus result in permanent impairment of front–hind limb coordination; that is, there is a permanent difference between the duration of the step cycle of the fore- and hind limbs, which leads to lack of synchronization (desynchronization) between forelimb and hind limb movements. The main conclusion from these results is that in addition to the ventral funiculi, the dorsolateral ones also play an important role in the preservation of the equal rhythm of the front and hind limbs.

The results of earlier studies based on lesions sparing small patches of spinal cord tissue (Afelt, 1974; Eidelberg, 1981; Eidelberg et al., 1981) imply that the ventral and ventrolateral pathways are crucial for quadrupedal locomotion. Signals conveying information about the body's balance in particular appear to play an important role. The observed desynchronization between front and hind limbs might be a consequence of possible deficits in the control of equilibrium in animals in which lumbar enlargement neurones were deprived of the vestibulospinal pathway (Bem et al., 1995; Brustein & Rossignol, 1998). However, in contrast to the findings of the aforementioned studies, there is now growing evidence that, despite extensive lesions in the ventral and lateral quadrants that eliminate the vestibulospinal and severely damage the reticulospinal pathways, recovery of voluntary locomotion is possible in the long term (Bem et al., 1995; Brustein & Rossignol, 1998; Górska et al., 1993b; Górska et al., 1996). We may conclude that even after a massive lesion to the ventral and ventrolateral quadrants, severing the vestibulospinal pathway, the recovery of quadrupedal locomotion is possible and is related to structures in the dorsolateral funiculus such as the corticospinal pathway. Moreover, these results suggest that dorsolateral funiculi play a major role in preserving the equality of rhythms in the fore- and hind limbs, while lesions to the ventral quadrants influence the coupling between limbs. Other investigators (Jiang & Drew, 1996) have reported that complete interruption of both the cortico- and rubrospinal pathways at the thoracic level produced long-term deficits in overground locomotion, including paw-dragging, while smaller lesions produced similar deficits only initially, from which the cats recovered relatively quickly (Drew et al., 2002). Even several months after injury, cats with the largest lesions affecting the dorsolateral funiculi were unable to modify their gait when obstacles were attached to a treadmill belt. According to Drew and colleagues (Drew et al., 2002), damage to the cortico- and rubrospinal input to motoneurones controlling distal muscles as well as muscles acting around the hip and knee might be responsible for such deficits. In addition, the propriospinal pathways in the dorsal columns may participate in interlimb coordination (English, 1980; English & Lennard, 1982; English, 1985; English et al., 1985). However, lesions of dorsal columns at low thoracic levels alone did not evoke any deficits in fore–hind limb coordination (Górska et al., 1996); it is also possible that mechanical coupling via the trunk is responsible for this coordination. The trunk muscles are likely to play an important role because any pulling or pushing action from one limb to another is transmitted via the trunk, resulting in a change in the position of the body in relation to the limb in contact with the ground (Rossignol et al., 1993). Thus, it is likely that long descending and ascending propriospinal pathways interconnecting the spinal enlargements plays a crucial role.

The results of numerous studies concerning the role of the lateral system (for review, see Drew et al., 2002) imply that, although the corticospinal tract is not essential for the production of the basic locomotor rhythm in cats, it does contribute to the regulation of locomotion, particularly in situations where there is a requirement for precise control of paw placement or limb trajectory. This means that the medial, reticulo- and vestibulospinal pathways are unable to fully compensate for damage to the lateral pathways (Drew et al., 2002).

These results illustrate the great variability in the different types of functional impairments, which might stem from either the lack of functional specification of various descending or ascending pathways or from a considerable variability in the extent of the spinal lesions and of afferent input destruction in different experiments. Brustein and Rossignol (1998) suggested that inconsistency in partial spinal lesion studies might be related to limitations in the method of light microscopy used for estimating the surviving axons. In highly necrotic and deformed tissue, more axons could survive than estimated from the observed lesion size, which could explain recovery.

The results obtained from studies on cats have increased our understanding of the behavioral and pathophysiological effects of spinal cord injury. Although these findings cannot be directly transferred to explaining the consequences of SCI in humans, this knowledge is helpful in the development of new treatments (therapeutic interventions) for promoting the recovery of locomotion in patients.

4.2. Changes in Locomotion after Spinal Cord Injury in Rats

Rodents and especially rats are currently the most popular animal model of SCI. Despite physiological and functional differences between rodents and humans, the rat model can assist in understanding the mechanisms of locomotor impairment and processes of recovery after CNS trauma and has been vital in the development of many new techniques for encouraging recovery after spinal cord injury, which may be applied to patients.

Total spinal cord transection

In adult rats, complete transection of the spinal cord at the low thoracic level (T8–T10) abolishes hind limb locomotor movements (Feraboli-Lohnherr et al., 1997; Majczyński et al., 2005b; Sławińska et al., 2000). These spinal rats move around using only their forelimbs, while the caudal part of the trunk, the hindquarters, and the hind limbs drag behind them. The activity of hind limb muscles recorded during locomotor-like movement induced by tail pinching in spinal rats suspended over the treadmill indicated substantial abnormalities in burst duration and timing of

EMG activity. In spinal rats, unlike in intact ones, the activity between flexor and extensor muscle very often overlap, and simultaneous contractions of homologous muscles in the right and left hind limbs are obtained. When sitting motionless, spinal rats keep their hind limbs extended passively behind their body.

Partial spinal cord transection

Following partial lesions of the spinal cord at the low thoracic level, rats can regain quadrupedal walking after a period of recovery, although with obvious deficits that depend on the number of the remaining intact fibers (Górska et al., 2007). The question as to which supraspinal structures are crucial and the amount of spared fibers sufficient for the recovery of the support of hindquarters and for maintaining hind limb locomotor movements has been addressed by numerous studies over the last decade. In general it has been shown that, in rats (as in cats; see the previous section), the spinal white matter in the ventral and ventrolateral parts seems to be more important than that contained in the dorsal part of the spinal cord (Grill et al., 1997a; Loy et al., 2002a; Loy et al., 2002b; Schucht et al., 2002). Dorsal hemisection at the low thoracic level (T7), which interrupted several motor pathways, including the corticospinal, rubrospinal, coeruleospinal, and some raphespinal, vestibulospinal, and propriospinal tracts, did not affect overground locomotion when rats were tested one month after surgery (Grill et al., 1997). Similar results were obtained in rats after dorsal hemisection when tested three months after surgery (Metz et al., 2000b); out of 71 operated rats, most attained high locomotor ability and only 17 recovered partial body weight support (13–14 out of 21 scores in BBB (Basso, Beatie, and Bresnahan) scale evaluating locomotor functions (Basso et al., 1995)). More severe impairment of locomotion was observed in rats following dorsal hemisection at T9 (Hamers et al., 2001). Soon after surgery, the rats showed only occasional weight-supported plantar stepping by the hind limbs (BBB score of 10), but they recovered significantly within 28 days, reaching a score 13 on the BBB scale (frequent fore–hind limb coordination).

Similar experiments were performed on rats with dorsal lesions at the T8 spinal cord level (Kaegi et al., 2002). The day after surgery, rats with the severest lesions could not walk, while those with mild injury showed hind limb plantar stepping with body weight support. Despite the fact that some of the rats had less than 30% of the spared white matter at the site of the lesion, all regained hind limb locomotor movements within three days, and a gradual improvement in locomotor movement quality was observed up to the end of the experiment (14 days after surgery). Analysis showed a strong correlation between the quality of hind limb locomotor movements and the amount of white matter spared. The EMG activity of two hind limb muscles, the tibialis anterior and vastus lateralis, recorded during the recovery period indicated substantial abnormalities in parameters such as the amplitude and duration of activity, the activity overlap between flexor and extensor muscles, and coupling between the activities of the same muscles in the right and left hind limbs. Most of these measures returned to control levels after 14 days, but a prolonged flexor burst and an overlap between the activity of the flexor and extensor muscles persisted.

The strong correlation between the locomotor performance, the amount of spared white matter, and the significant role of the ventrolateral funiculi in the recovery of locomotion in rats was also revealed by You and colleagues (You et al., 2003). They showed that sparing less than 5% of the white matter in the ventrolateral part of the spinal cord at T9 level was enough to allow eventual restoration of hind limb locomotor movements. Moreover, it has been demonstrated that bilateral demyelination of ventrolateral funiculus (VLF) or ventral column (VC) alone had little impact on spontaneous overground locomotion, while joint lesion of VLF and VC or a more extensive lesion induced severe deficits in hind limb locomotor movements (Loy et al., 2002a). The pathways that are likely to be severed by this type of lesion include the coeruleospinal, spinocerebellar, raphespinal, reticulospinal, and vestibulospinal tracts. In the same experimental model it was shown that combined lesion of the myelinated fibers in the dorsal column (DC) and in the dorsal corticospinal tract (CST) and in VLF caused mild locomotor deficits, while lesion of these fibers in both the dorsolateral funiculus (DLF) and VLF produce more severe locomotor impairment (Loy et al., 2002b). Descending fibers that are likely to be damaged in part by VLF + DLF lesions include those in the corticospinal, rubrospinal, reticulospinal, vestibulospinal, coeruleospinal, raphespinal, and propriospinal tracts. Separate destruction of most of these tracts does not cause deterioration of locomotion. These results raise the question of the significance of these individual pathways in controlling locomotion. Nevertheless, because neither dorsal hemisection, VLF lesion, nor VC lesion alone produced major locomotor deficits, it was concluded that a tract present in all of these parts of the spinal cord is likely to be responsible for the initiation of locomotion. Loy and coworkers (Loy et al., 2002b) proposed that the reticulospinal tract, which projects in the rat ventral columns, VLF, lateral columns, and DLF, fulfills this function.

The work of Schucht and coworkers supports this possibility (Schucht et al., 2002). In rats with dorsal or ventral lesions at low thoracic level (T8), the relationship between the spared spinal cord white matter and the effect on locomotion was examined. The results demonstrated the importance of fibers descending in the ventrolateral funiculus and the insignificance of fibers in the dorsal funiculus for overground locomotion. Sparing the entire dorsal funiculus was insufficient for hind limb locomotion, but if in addition a small amount of white matter in the ventral or lateral funiculus was left intact, recovery of locomotor movements took place. In both dorsal and ventral lesions, there was a high level of correlation between the amount of spared white matter and the quality of locomotor movements. However, ventral parts of the spinal cord have a stronger influence on "open-field" locomotion because the correlation between the amount of spared white matter and the quality of locomotor movements for the dorsal lesions was higher than for the ventral. In addition, after extensive dorsal lesions, rats recovered to perform rhythmic hind limb movements without body weight support, while after ventral lesions, rats did not show any hind limb movement. These results indicate the significant role of fibers in the dorsolateral, lateral, and ventrolateral funiculi for control of locomotion. Descending pathways within these funiculi include vestibulospinal fibers, serotonergic fibers from the raphe nucleus, noradrenergic fibers from the locus coeruleus, and glutamatergic fibers mainly from the nucleus reticularis gigantocerularis and the pontine reticular nucleus. These reticulospinal glutamatergic axons seem to be the most important for the initiation of locomotion, and a small residual number of this tract reaching the lower spinal cord appears to be sufficient to initiate locomotor movements.

Although the BBB scale (Basso et al., 1995) allows us to quantify a wide range of locomotor deficits following various types of CNS or PNS lesions, we need more precise tools to evaluate changes in the locomotor pattern following spinal cord lesion (Ballermann et al., 2006; Majczyński et al., 2007). In a study in which the dorsal part of the spinal cord at T8 was sectioned, rats reached a plateau in their locomotor performance after eight to 22 days, depending on the severity of the lesion. The quality of locomotor performance was strongly correlated with the amount of spared white matter (Ballermann et al., 2006). Moreover, subtle changes in locomotor movements were observed in the EMG activity and trajectory of hind limb movements, even in rats that had recovered apparently normal locomotion. The most important changes were an increase in hind limb extension during the stance phase, leading to a more upright position; an increase in the EMG amplitude of the triceps brachii (a forelimb extensor), indicating compensation of the deficit in hind limb propulsion; and an increase in the temporal separation between activity of the tibialis anterior and vastus lateralis muscles. These findings indicate that, following recovery from spinal cord damage, the pattern of locomotor movement does not return to that seen in intact animals, and new strategies develop in the lesioned spinal cord. The BBB score cannot describe these subtle changes of movement.

Small, defined lesions restricted to the corticospinal tract at the T8 level produced similar effects to those of the rubrospinal tract (RST). Rats showed plantar walking with weight support and frequent but inconsistent fore-hind limb coordination, corresponding to a BBB score of 13 (Muir & Whishaw, 1999; 2000). However, the time-scale of recovery from these two types of lesion was significantly different. Animals with a CST lesion reached a plateau of locomotor recovery within one week, whereas those with an RST lesion recovered to the same level of locomotor performance after seven weeks. This result shows the relative unimportance of the corticospinal tract in the control of locomotion in rats. Rats with a dorsal hemisection were most severely impaired and reached a plateau of locomotor performance two weeks after surgery, with a score of 11 on the BBB scale (plantar stepping with no fore-hind limb coordination). A unilateral pyramidal tract section evoked less severe locomotor impairment (Metz et al., 1998). On the first day after surgery, toe-dragging and external rotation of the hind limb contralateral to the lesion as well as trunk instability were observed. Rats recovered rapidly during the first postoperative week, but by day 28, some discrete movement impairment, like hypermetria and trunk instability, persisted.

Contusion and compression injuries

In addition to surgical methods of spinal cord injury that produce more or less specific lesions of particular ascending and descending connections, it is important to use methods that will mimic lesions seen in human SCI patients. Contusion and compression injuries of the spinal cord studied in rodents are more reproducible than transection of the spinal cord and more akin to the majority of SCI seen in humans. The disadvantage of these methods is that selective disruption of particular spinal cord tracts is unlikely. Contusion and compression usually cause a central cavity surrounded by an outer rim of spared white matter (Metz et al., 2000a). The amount of tissue that is spared depends on the energy of the impact or the extent of the pressure applied. At small contusion severities, the pathological changes are mainly confined to the central gray matter, but with increasing severity the damage progresses outward (Kloos et al., 2005). In small lesions of this type, dorsal fiber tracts, including the corticospinal and propriospinal tracts, are usually disrupted; while in larger lesions, the dorsal, lateral, and ventral tracts are severely damaged. Dorsal white matter is usually more affected by contusion and compression lesions than the ventral white matter. Moreover, large-diameter axons are more vulnerable than small-diameter axons.

In most experiments in which the spinal cord was damaged by contusion and compression at the low thoracic level (T8-T10), there is a strong correlation between the percentage of spared white matter and the locomotor performance, and in general, the relationship between them is linear (Basso et al., 1995; Basso et al., 1996; Bresnahan et al., 1987; Cao et al., 2005; Collazos-Castro et al., 2006; Gruner et al., 1996; Kloos et al., 2005). Contrary to these results, in another study in which locomotion in the open field was studied, the relationship between locomotor ability and the spared white matter area were best fitted by second-order polynominal regression plots (Gruner et al., 1996). Also, a large-scale study revealed that a progressive increase in lesion severity did not produce proportionate changes in the degree of locomotor impairment (Kloos et al., 2005), and the relationship between them was a curvilinear, fourth-order polynominal regression. Similar results concerning the percentage of spared white matter and the hind limb locomotor ability of rats were reported by Kloos and colleagues (Kloos et al., 2005).

The investigation of contusion injuries has also confirmed the importance of ventral, ventrolateral, and lateral funiculi in the recovery of locomotion. In the study of Cao and coworkers (Cao et al., 2005), the most pronounced alterations in locomotor performance were seen when the lateral and ventral funiculi were injured, and the degree of locomotor ability as measured by the BBB score was dependent on the amount of white matter spared. These authors claimed that the likeliest candidate for promoting locomotor recovery is the reticulospinal tract, diffusely distributed in the ventral and lateral funiculi. Kloos and colleagues (Kloos et al., 2005) also suggested that the reticulospinal tract is dominant in mediating the recovery of locomotion after spinal cord injury at the low thoracic level, especially when the impairment is severer. They claimed that in mild lesions, which evoke small changes of locomotor movement like loss of fore–hind limb coordination, centrally located corticospinal and propriospinal tracts are the most likely to be extensively damaged. Moreover, the small alterations in locomotion, such as precise paw position, after very small injuries may be due to damage to large-diameter axons, which are more vulnerable to injury than small-diameter axons. Among these, the large axons belonging to the reticulospinal pathway seem to play a significant role in the observed rudimentary locomotor impairment.

The role of propriospinal tracts, which are involved in transmitting information between the cervical and lumbar enlargements and from supraspinal locomotor centers to the lumbar CPG, in the recovery of motor function after thoracic spinal cord injury, was highlighted by Cao and coworkers (Cao et al., 2005). These tracts may not be essential for locomotion in intact rats, but in the injured spinal cord they might at least partly compensate for impaired supraspinal projection to the lumbar spinal cord.

5. AFFERENT INFLUENCE

Although limb movements do not depend entirely on sensory inputs, it is well known that the afferent feedback influences the neural network responsible for producing the locomotor pattern in order to adapt movements to changes of the internal and external environment (Kay-Lyons, 2002). According to Pearson (Pearson, 1993) there are three main functions of afferent influences on the CPG: (1) to augment CPG activity, especially during the excitation of weight-bearing muscles, like limb extensor muscles active in the stance phase; (2) to control the timing of the motor output to ensure that the muscle drive is appropriate for the biomechanical state of the moving body with regard to its position, direction of movement, and force; and (3) to control the phase transition to avoid the switching of gait phases until a suitable biomechanical state of the limbs and body has been achieved.

Augmentation of the CPG activity was demonstrated in experiments in which stretching the Achilles tendon increased both the amplitude and duration of EMG bursts in the ankle extensor and decreased EMG bursts in flexor muscles in a "pre-mammillary cat" (a cat with a brain transection made rostrally to the superior colliculus and continued rostroventrally to the rostral tip of the mammillary bodies; for review of preparation, see Whelan, 1996b) walking on a treadmill (Duysens & Pearson, 1980). Also electrical stimulation of extensor Group I afferents in the same preparation prolonged the extensor EMG burst (Whelan et al., 1995). It is not clear which afferents are responsible for this reinforcement of the EMG burst: Group Ib, from the Golgi tendon organs, or Group Ia, from muscle spindles. However, most experiments support the hypothesis that, during the stance phase, the signal from Group Ib afferents inhibits the flexor half-center of the CPG (Duysens & Pearson, 1980). A second function of the influence of afferents on the CPG is related to low-threshold cutaneous afferents innervating the foot. Stimulation of the cutaneous nerve supplying the dorsum of the foot enhances extensor activity during the stance phase and flexor activity during the swing phase (Guertin et al., 1995; LaBella et al., 1992). This input to the CPG can inhibit motor centers producing flexion during the stance phase, so during this phase they act in a manner similar to that of Group I afferents. Several experiments demonstrated that afferent signals from the hip influence the termination of the stance and initiation of the swing phase of that limb (for review, see Grillner, 1985). This phase transition is associated with the angle of the leg extension at the hip joint (Grillner & Rossignol, 1978). Two categories of receptors might be involved: those from the hip joint and those from hip muscles. The results of experiments studying fictive locomotion (Kriellaars et al., 1994) and the walking of decerebrate cats on a treadmill indicate that signals from position-related Ia afferents of flexor muscles influence the transition from the stance to the swing phase. Thus, feedback from muscle and skin afferents as well as from other senses influence the timing of major phase transitions in the motor pattern, and is required for the adaptation of motor patterns in response to alterations of the environment (for detailed review, see Pearson, 2004).

More recently, observations obtained in humans after spinal cord injury by Dimitrijevic and his colleagues (Dimitrijevic et al., 2005; Jilge et al., 2004; Kern et al., 2005; Minassian et al., 2004; 2007), showing that epidural and transcutaneous stimulation of the dorsal roots of the severed cord can elicit movement of paralyzed limbs, inspired experiments in animals. In animals, epidural stimulation can be more easily combined with pharmacological interventions, a more precise localization of the most effective site of stimulation for a particular movement can be established, and precise patterns of stimulation on various motor performances can be tested (Guevremont et al., 2006; Lemay & Grill 2004; Mushahwar et al., 2007). In spinal cats it is possible to induce locomotion with an adequately positioned single electrode (dorsal superficial part of the spinal cord at L6–L7 level), but only when cats are well trained, or when clonidine is administered prior to stimulation. Single-electrode stimulation is very promising for rehabilitation, especially because locomotion can be evoked at low current intensities (Barthelemy et al., 2006; 2007). Although much information has already been obtained from these animal experiments, it is going to be difficult to transfer this knowledge to the human situation.

6. THE ROLE OF DIFFERENT NEUROTRANSMITTERS FOR LOCOMOTOR MOVEMENT

Development of pharmacological therapies for the control of locomotion in patients with spinal cord injury or disease requires an understanding of the mode of action of substances involved in the control of the spinal cord neural network for control of locomotion. For example, studies using the *in vitro* preparation of the lamprey, frog embryo, and newborn rat indicate that excitatory amino acids are involved in the initiation of locomotion (Douglas et al., 1993; Grillner, 1985). For investigating the role of other neurotransmitters for control of locomotion, the preparation of the decerebrated cat was used for many years, because either spontaneous episodes of locomotor movement occur in these animals, or they can be easily induced by electrical stimulation of the mesencephalic locomotor region in the midbrain, the subthalamic locomotor region in the hypothalamus; that is, areas that activate the spinal locomotor neural circuits and mediate the locomotion evoked from higher motor centers (Shik & Orlovsky 1976; Jordan 1991; 1998; Whelan 1996). In addition, in conscious animal experiments, intrathecal intraspinal local drug application was used (Giroux et al., 2001; 2003; Majczyński et al., 2005a; 2006).

As described in Section 6 of this chapter, the activity of this CPG circuitry responsible for generating locomotor movements is controlled by descending inputs from supraspinal structures and the afferent information from the periphery, and these are mediated by specific transmitters. The locomotor movement of hind limbs elicited by the CPG circuitry when it is completely separated from supraspinal and afferent inputs can therefore be modified by application of transmitters or modification or receptors of these transmitters on neurones of the CPG or those that control their activity. The influence of monoamines and serotoninergic drugs and their antagonists has been mostly studied. To give just one example, local application of monoamines modulates the transmission between primary afferents and premotor interneurones. This has a particularly strong impact on reflex actions, because these interneurones directly excite or inhibit motoneurones (Jankowska et al., 2000). Clonidine, an agonist of noradrenergic alpha-2 receptors can initiate locomotion in acute spinal cats (Barbeau et al., 1993; Forssberg & Grillner, 1973).

It has long been known that in spinal cats treated with L-dopa (L-dihydroxyphenylanine), a precursor of dopamine and norepinephrine, electrical stimulation of small diameter cutaneous and muscle afferents (FRA–flexor reflex afferents) can evoke long lasting bursts of activity in ipsilateral flexor motoneurones (Jankowska et al., 1967a; Jankowska et al., 1967b). If contralateral afferents were stimulated bursts of activity in extensor motoneurones were observed. This activity was similar to motoneurone activity observed during locomotion. Transmission between primary afferents and motoneurones was also influenced by L-dopa administration in spinal cats (Anden et al., 1966). The importance of the noradrenergic system for locomotion was also confirmed in a study in which L-dopa, in the presence of naliamid (the monoamine oxidase inhibitor), triggered "fictive" locomotion in cats soon after spinalization (Forssberg & Grillner, 1973). Also clonidine, (an alpha-2–adrenergic agonist), evoked treadmill locomotion in acutely spinalized cats. The same agonist improved locomotor performance in spinal cats that recovered some locomotion (Giroux et al., 2001). Moreover, intrathecally delivered yohimbine, an antagonist of adrenergic alpha-2 receptors, caused serious locomotor difficulties in intact cats (Giroux et al., 2001) and blocked spontaneous hind limb locomotion in decerebrated cats tested on a treadmill (Leblond & Rossignol, 2003). Among other monoaminergic systems, only the serotonergic one seem to play a role in recovery of hind limb locomotion. Although injections of serotonin (5-hydroxytryptophan, 5-HT) precursor failed to initiate locomotion in acute spinal cats, the 5-HT2 receptor agonist, quipazine, could modulate retrained locomotor movements by increasing the amplitude and duration of EMG bursts in hind limb flexors and extensors (Barbeau & Rossignol, 1991).

In spinal rats, the serotonergic system seems to play a more important role than the noradrenergic one in the recovery of hind limb locomotor activity. It has been shown that activation of 5-HT2 receptors restores the extensor tone and stretch reflex excitability in the spinal cat (Miller et al., 1996) and increases polysynaptic reflex transmission and motoneurone excitability in the rat (Nagano et al., 1988). Other studies have revealed that the serotonergic system, and especially 5-HT2 receptors, play an important role in the control of locomotor activity in spinal rats. It was demonstrated that a single administration of 5-HT or quipazine, a 5-HT2 agonist, improved locomotor-like movements in spinal rats (Feraboli-Lohnherr et al., 1999). In addition, chronic treatment with quipazine, delivered continuously to the spinal cord below the transection, induced partial restoration of hind limb motor functions (Antri et al., 2002), and daily injections of 5-HT1A/7 agonists ameliorated locomotion to a similar extent as did a 5-HT2 agonist (Antri et al., 2003). Also, grafting embryonic raphe nuclei containing serotonergic cells into the adult rat spinal cord below the level of transection was shown to improve hind limb locomotor-like movements (Feraboli-Lohnherr et al., 1997; Majczyński et al., 2005b; Ribotta et al., 2000; Sławińska et al., 2000). The essential role of serotonergic grafts in the recovery of locomotor movements was confirmed in experiments in which the intra peritoneal (i. p.) administration of a low dose (1 mg/kg) of cyproheptadine, a 5-HT2 receptor agonist, dramatically altered hind limb locomotor-like movements in spinal rats that had grafted embryonic raphe nuclei (Majczyński et al., 2005b). Moreover, cyproheptadine, delivered intrathecally at the midlumbar region, transiently blocked locomotion in intact rats (Majczyński et al., 2005a).

In vitro studies of neonatal rat spinal cord preparations have also confirmed the important role of the serotonergic system in the initiation and regulation of a locomotor-like pattern of flexor and extensor nerve activity. There is evidence that serotonin-sensitive locomotor network components are distributed throughout the spinal cord. Moreover, the different serotonin receptor subtypes having different rostrocaudal distribution can contribute to control of locomotion in different ways (for review, see Schmidt & Jordan 2000). Serotonin or 5-HT2 agonists could evoke locomotor-like activity more reliably than other substances, and 5-HT2 receptor antagonists blocked this activity (Cazalets et al., 1990a; Cazalets et al., 1992;

Cowley & Schmidt 1994; 1995 Maclean et al., 1998). It has been also shown that the serotonergic system may act, not only through 5-HT2 receptors, but via some other receptors, especially by 5-HT7. For example, in a neonatal rat spinal cord preparation, 5-HT7 receptor antagonists influenced the locomotor rhythm by acting directly on neurones of the central pattern generator, whereas 5-HT2 antagonists affected locomotion by reducing the motoneurone output (Jordan & Schmidt, 2002; Liu & Jordan, 2005). Although the functions of the serotonergic system seem to be crucial for locomotion in the rat, the relative involvement of other monoaminergic systems remains an open question. It was demonstrated that in neonatal rat 1 day after midthoracic spinal cord transection, the rhythmic alternating pattern of flexor–extensor muscle activity obtained after L-dopa was remarkably similar to that recorded from intact animals (Navarrete, et al., 2002). Moreover, in the *in vitro* neonatal rat spinal cord preparation, brain stem–evoked fictive locomotion could be blocked, not only by 5-HT receptor antagonists, but also by noradrenergic and dopaminergic antagonists (Zaporozhets et al., 2003). This is in agreement with another study showing that yohimbine, an alpha-2 noradrenergic antagonist, could transiently impair overground locomotion in intact rats (Majczyński et al., 2006).

Recently, increasing attention has been paid to the role of other transmitter systems, especially to glutaminergic and cholinergic ones, which are present in the spinal cord below the lesion. The glutamatergic system plays a substantial role in the initiation of locomotor movements in cats (Chau et al., 2002; Douglas et al., 1993) and rats (Cazalets et al., 1992; Cazalets et al., 1995; Cowley & Schmidt, 1995; Kiehn et al., 1999; Kjaerulff & Kiehn, 1996). It seems that spontaneous spinal locomotion observed in chronic spinal cats depends on excitatory amino acids (Giroux et al., 2003) or acetylcholine (Rossignol et al., 2005, Jordan, - personal communication).

The significance of the glutamatergic system was confirmed in experiments in which excitation of NMDA (N-methyl-D-aspartate) receptors by EAAs (excitatory amino acids) (Cazalets et al., 1992) or NMDA (Maclean et al., 1998a; Cazalets et al., 1990b; Kudo & Yamada, 1987) evoked locomotor activity in neonatal rat spinal cord preparation. In decerebrate cats, intrathecal administration of NMDA elicited hind limb fictive locomotion (Douglas et al., 1993). Although NMDA failed to evoked treadmill locomotion in acute spinal cats (two to five days after spinalization), it substantially improved locomotor performance when cats started to show rhythmic hind limb movements (Chau et al., 2002). In late spinal cats, NMDA evoked more regular locomotion. Intrathecal delivery of 2-amino-5-phosphonovaleric acid (AP-5), an NMDA receptor antagonist, caused a deterioration of hind limb locomotion with bilateral foot-drag and poor weight support, while the same dose of AP-5 completely blocked locomotion in spinal cats. This may suggest that locomotion in intact cats is controlled by different systems than in spinal animals (Giroux et al., 2003).

All of these recent findings show potential application for the development of new rehabilitation methods for human patients.

References

Afelt, Z. “Functional significance of ventral descending tracts of the spinal cord in the cat.” *Acta Neurobiologiae Experimentalis* (Warsaw) 34 (1974): 393–407.

Ahlman, H., Grillner, S., Udo, M. "The effect of 5-HTP on the static fusimotor activity and the tonic stretch reflex of an extensor muscle." *Brain Research* 27 (1971): 393–396.

Anden, N. E., Jukes, M. G., Lundberg, A., Vyklicky, L. "The effect of Dopa on the spinal cord. 1. Influence on transmission from primary afferents." *Acta Physiologica Scandinavica* 67 (1966): 373–386.

Angel, M. J., Jankowska, E., McCrea, D. A. "Candidate interneurones mediating Group I disynaptic EPSPs in extensor motoneurones during fictive locomotion in the cat." *Journal of Physiology* 563 (2005): 597–610.

Antri, M., Mouffle, C., Orsal, D., Barthe, J. Y. "5-HT1A receptors are involved in short- and long-term processes responsible for 5-HT-induced locomotor function recovery in chronic spinal rat." *European Journal of Neuroscience* 18 (2003): 1963–1972.

Antri, M., Orsal, D., Barthe, J. Y. "Locomotor recovery in the chronic spinal rat: Effects of long-term treatment with a 5-HT2 agonist." *European Journal of Neuroscience* 16 (2002): 467–476.

Armstrong, D. M. "The supraspinal control of mammalian locomotion." *Journal of Physiology* 405 (1988): 1–37.

Armstrong, D. M., Apps, R., Marple-Horvat, D. E. "Aspects of cerebellar function in relation to locomotor movements." *Progress in Brain Research* 114 (1997): 401–421.

Ballermann, M., Tse, A. D., Misiaszek, J. E., Fouad, K. "Adaptations in the walking pattern of spinal cord injured rats." *Journal of Neurotrauma* 23 (2006): 897–907.

Barbeau, H., Chau, C., Rossignol, S. "Noradrenergic agonists and locomotor training affect locomotor recovery after cord transection in adult cats." *Brain Research Bulletin* 30 (1993): 387–393.

Barbeau, H., Rossignol, S. "Recovery of locomotion after chronic spinalization in the adult cat." *Brain Research* 412 (1987): 84–95.

Barbeau, H., Rossignol, S. "Initiation and modulation of the locomotor pattern in the adult chronic spinal cat by noradrenergic, serotonergic and dopaminergic drugs." *Brain Research* 546 (1991): 250–260.

Barbeau, H., Rossignol, S. "Enhancement of locomotor recovery following spinal cord injury." *Current Opinions in Neurology* 7 (1994): 517–524.

Barthélemy, D., Leblond, H., Provencher, J., Rossignol, S. "Non-locomotor and locomotor hindlimb responses evoked by electrical microstimulation of the lumbar cord in spinalized cats." *Journal of Neurophysiology* 96 (2006): 3273–3292.

Barthélemy, D., Leblond, H., Rossignol, S. "Characteristics and mechanisms of locomotion induced by intraspinal microstimulation and dorsal root stimulation in spinal cats." *Journal of Neurophysiology* 97(3) (2007): 1986–2000.

Basso, D. M., Beattie, M. S., Bresnahan, J. C. "A sensitive and reliable locomotor rating scale for open field testing in rats." *Journal of Neurotrauma* 12 (1995): 1–21.

Basso, D. M., Beattie, M. S., Bresnahan, J. C. "Graded histological and locomotor outcomes after spinal cord contusion using the NYU weight-drop device versus transection." *Experimental Neurology* 139 (1996): 244–256.

Belanger, M., Drew, T., Provencher, J., Rossignol, S. "A comparison of treadmill locomotion in adult cats before and after spinal transection." *Journal of Neurophysiology* 76 (1996): 471–491.

Beloozerova, I. N., Sirota, M. G. "The role of the motor cortex in the control of accuracy of locomotor movements in the cat." *Journal of Physiology* 461 (1993): 1–25.

Bem, T., Górska, T., Majczyński, H., Zmyslowski, W. "Different patterns of fore–hind limb coordination during overground locomotion in cats with ventral and lateral spinal lesions." *Experimental Brain Research* 104 (1995): 70–80.

Bresnahan, J. C., Beattie, M. S., Todd, F. D., Noyes, D. H. "A behavioral and anatomical analysis of spinal cord injury produced by a feedback-controlled impaction device." *Experimental Neurology* 95 (1987): 548–570.

Brown, T. G. "The intrinsic factors in the act of progression in mammal." *Proceedings of the Royal Society B* 84 (1911): 308–319.

Brown, T. G. "The factors in rhythmic activity of the nervous system." *Proceedings of the Royal Society B* 85 (1912): 278–289.

Brustein, E., Rossignol, S. "Recovery of locomotion after ventral and ventrolateral spinal lesions in the cat. I. Deficits and adaptive mechanisms." *Journal of Neurophysiology* 80 (1998): 1245–1267.

Cao, Q., Zhang, Y. P., Iannotti, C., et al. "Functional and electrophysiological changes after graded traumatic spinal cord injury in adult rat." *Experimental Neurology* 191 Suppl 1 (2005): S3–S16.

Cazalets, J. R., Borde, M., Clarac, F. "Localization and organization of the central pattern generator for hind limb locomotion in newborn rat." *Journal of Neuroscience* 15 (1995): 4943–4951.

Cazalets, J. R., Grillner, P., Menard, I., Cremieux, J., Clarac, F. "Two types of motor rhythm induced by NMDA and amines in an in vitro spinal cord preparation of neonatal rat." *Neuroscience Letters* 111 (1990): 116–121.

Cazalets, J. R., Sqalli-Houssaini, Y., Clarac, F. "Activation of the central pattern generators for locomotion by serotonin and excitatory amino acids in neonatal rat." *Journal of Physiology* 455 (1992): 187–204.

Chau, C., Giroux, N., Barbeau, H., Jordan, L., Rossignol, S. "Effects of intrathecal glutamatergic drugs on locomotion I. NMDA in short-term spinal cats." *Journal of Neurophysiology* 88 (2002): 3032–3045.

Coggeshall, R. E., Lekan, H. A., Doubell, T. P., Allchorne, A., Woolf, C. J. "Central changes in primary afferent fibers following peripheral nerve lesions." *Neuroscience* 77 (1997): 1115–1122.

Collazos-Castro, J. E., Lopez-Dolado, E., Nieto-Sampedro, M. "Locomotor deficits and adaptive mechanisms after thoracic spinal cord contusion in the adult rat." *Journal of Neurotrauma* 23 (2006): 1–17.

Cowley, K. C.; Schmidt, B. J. "A comparison of motor patterns induced by N-methyl-D-aspartate, acetylcholine and serotonin in the in vitro neonatal rat spinal cord." *Neuroscience Letters* 171 (1994): 147–150.

Cowley, K. C., Schmidt, B. J. "Effects of inhibitory amino acid antagonists on reciprocal inhibitory interactions during rhythmic motor activity in the in vitro neonatal rat spinal cord." *Journal of Neurophysiology* 74 (1995): 1109–1117.

De Leon, R. D., Hodgson, J. A., Roy, R. R., Edgerton, V. R. "Full weight-bearing hind limb standing following stand training in the adult spinal cat." *Journal of Neurophysiology* 80 (1998a): 83–91.

De Leon, R. D., Hodgson, J. A., Roy, R. R., Edgerton, V. R. "Locomotor capacity attributable to step training versus spontaneous recovery after spinalization in adult cats." *Journal of Neurophysiology* 79 (1998b): 1329–1340.

Dietz, V. "Spinal cord pattern generators for locomotion." *Clinical Neurophysiology* 114 (2003): 1379–1389.

Dimitrijevic, M. R., Persy, I., Forstner, C., Kern, H., Dimitrijevic, M. M. "Motor control in the human spinal cord." *Artifitial Organs* 29(3) (2005): 216–219.

Douglas, J. R., Noga, B. R., Dai, X., Jordan, L. M. "The effects of intrathecal administration of excitatory amino acid agonists and antagonists on the initiation of locomotion in the adult cat." *Journal of Neurophysiology* 13 (1993): 990–1000.

Drew, T., Jiang, W., Widajewicz, W. "Contributions of the motor cortex to the control of the hind limbs during locomotion in the cat." *Brain Research Brain Research Review* 40 (2002): 178–191.

Duysens, J., Pearson, K. G. "Inhibition of flexor burst generation by loading ankle extensor muscles in walking cats." *Brain Research* 187 (1980): 321–332.

Duysens, J., Van de Crommert, H. W. "Neural control of locomotion: The central pattern generator from cats to humans." *Gait & Posture* 7 (1998): 131–141.

Edgerton, V. R., Leon, R. D., Harkema, S. J., et al. "Retraining the injured spinal cord." *Journal of Physiology* 533 (2001): 15–22.

Eidelberg, E. "Consequences of spinal cord lesions upon motor function, with special reference to locomotor activity." *Progress in Neurobiology* 17 (1981): 185–202.

Eidelberg, E., Story, J. L., Walden, J. G., Meyer, B. L. "Anatomical correlates of return of locomotor function after partial spinal cord lesions in cats." *Experimental Brain Research* 42 (1981): 81–88.

Eidelberg, E., Yu, J. "Effects of corticospinal lesions upon treadmill locomotion by cats." *Experimental Brain Research* 43 (1981): 101–103.

Ellaway, P. H., Trott, J. R. "The mode of action of 5-hydroxytryptophan in facilitating a stretch reflex in the spinal cat." *Experimental Brain Research* 22 (1975): 145–162.

English, A. W. "Interlimb coordination during stepping in the cat: effects of dorsal column section." *Journal of Neurophysiology* 44 (1980): 270–279.

English, A. W. "Interlimb coordination during stepping in the cat: the role of the dorsal spinocerebellar tract." *Experimental Neurology* 87 (1985): 96–108.

English, A. W., Lennard, P. R. "Interlimb coordination during stepping in the cat: In-phase stepping and gait transitions." *Brain Research* 245 (1982): 353–364.

English, A. W., Tigges, J., Lennard, P. R. "Anatomical organization of long ascending propriospinal neurons in the cat spinal cord." *Journal of Comparative Neurology* 240 (1985): 349–358.

Faden, A. I., Gannon, A., Basbaum, A. I. "Use of serotonin immunocytochemistry as a marker of injury severity after experimental spinal trauma in rats." *Brain Research* 450 (1988): 94–100.

Feraboli-Lohnherr, D., Barthe, J. Y., Orsal, D. "Serotonin-induced activation of the network for locomotion in adult spinal rats." *Journal of Neuroscience Research* 55 (1999): 87–98.

Feraboli-Lohnherr, D., Orsal, D., Yakovleff, A., Ribotta, M., Privat, A. "Recovery of locomotor activity in the adult chronic spinal rat after sublesional transplantation of embryonic nervous cells: Specific role of serotonergic neurons." *Experimental Brain Research* 113 (1997): 443–454.

Forssberg, H., Grillner, S. "The locomotion of the acute spinal cat injected with clonidine i. v." *Brain Research* 50 (1973): 184–186.

Forssberg, H., Grillner, S., Rossignol, S. "Phase dependent reflex reversal during walking in chronic spinal cats." *Brain Research* 85 (1975): 103–107.

Fouad, K., Pearson, K. "Restoring walking after spinal cord injury." *Progress in Neurobiology* 73 (2004): 107–126.

Fung, J., Stewart, J. E., Barbeau, H. "The combined effects of clonidine and cyproheptadine with interactive training on the modulation of locomotion in spinal cord injured subjects." *Journal of Neurological Science* 100 (1990): 85–93.

Giroux, N., Chau, C., Barbeau, H., Reader, T. A., Rossignol, S. "Effects of intrathecal glutamatergic drugs on locomotion. II. NMDA and AP-5 in intact and late spinal cats." *Journal of Neurophysiology* 90 (2003): 1027–1045.

Giroux, N., Reader, T. A., Rossignol, S. "Comparison of the effect of intrathecal administration of clonidine and yohimbine on the locomotion of intact and spinal cats." *Journal of Neurophysiology* 85 (2001): 2516–2536.

Górska, T., Bem, T., Majczyński, H. "Locomotion in cats with ventral spinal lesions: support patterns and duration of support phases during unrestrained walking." *Acta Neurobiologiae Experimentalis* (Warsaw) 50 (1990): 191–199.

Górska, T., Bem, T., Majczyński, H., Zmysłowski, W. "Unrestrained walking in intact cats. *Brain Research Bulletin* 32 (1993a): 235–240.

Górska, T., Bem, T., Majczyński, H., Zmysłowski, W. "Unrestrained walking in cats with partial spinal lesions." *Brain Research Bulletin* 32 (1993b): 241–249.

Górska, T., Bem, T., Majczyński, H., Zmysłowski, W. "Different forms of impairment of the fore–hind limb coordination after partial spinal lesions in cats." *Acta Neurobiologiae Experimentalis* (Warsaw) 56 (1996): 177–188.

Górska, T., Chojnicka-Gittins, B., Majczyński, H., Zmysłwoski, W. "Overground locomotion after incomplete spinal lesions in the rat: quantitative gait analysis." *Journal of Neurotrauma* 24 (2007): 1198–1218.

Górska, T., Majczyński, H., Bem, T., Zmysłowski, W. "Hind limb swing, stance and step relationships during unrestrained walking in cats with lateral funicular lesion." *Acta Neurobiologiae Experimentalis (Warsaw)* 53 (1993c): 133–142.

Graybiel, A. M. "The basal ganglia." *Trends in Neuroscience* 18 (1995): 60–62.

Grill, R., Murai, K., Blesch, A., Gage, F. H., Tuszynski, M. H. "Cellular delivery of neurotrophin-3 promotes corticospinal axonal growth and partial functional recovery after spinal cord injury." *Journal of Neuroscience* 17 (1997b): 5560–5572.

Grillner, S. "Neurobiological bases of rhythmic motor acts in vertebrates." *Science* 228 (1985): 143–149.

Grillner, S., Rossignol, S. "Contralateral reflex reversal controlled by limb position in the acute spinal cat injected with clonidine i. v." *Brain Research* 144 (1978): 411–414.

Grillner, S., Zangger, P. "How detailed is the central pattern generation for locomotion?" *Brain Research* 88 (1975): 367–371.

Grillner, S., Zangger, P. "On the central generation of locomotion in the low spinal cat." *Experimental Brain Research* 34 (1979): 241–261.

Gruner, J. A., Yee, A. K., Blight, A. R. "Histological and functional evaluation of experimental spinal cord injury: evidence of a stepwise response to graded compression." *Brain Research* 729 (1996): 90–101.

Guertin, P., Angel, M. J., Perreault, M. C., McCrea, D. A. "Ankle extensor Group I afferents excite extensors throughout the hind limb during fictive locomotion in the cat." *Journal of Physiology* 487 (1995): 197–209.

Guevremont, L., Renzi, C. G., Norton J. A., Kowalczewski J., Saigal R., Mushahwar V. K. "Locomotor-related networks in the lumbosacral enlargement of the adult spinal cat: activation through intraspinal microstimulation." *IEEE Transactions on Neural Systems and Rehabilitation Engineering* 14 (2006): 266–272.

Hamers, F. P., Lankhorst, A. J., van Laar, T. J., Veldhuis, W. B., Gispen, W. H. "Automated quantitative gait analysis during overground locomotion in the rat: its application to spinal cord contusion and transection injuries." *Journal of Neurotrauma* 18 (2001): 187–201.

Holstege, J. C., Kuypers, H. G. "Brain stem projections to lumbar motoneurons in rat—I. An ultrastructural study using autoradiography and the combination of autoradiography and horseradish peroxidase histochemistry." *Neuroscience* 21 (1987): 345–367.

Jankowska, E., Gladden, M. H., Czarkowska-Bauch, J. "Modulation of responses of feline gamma-motoneurones by noradrenaline, tizanidine and clonidine." *Journal of Physiology* 512 (1998): 521–531.

Jankowska, E., Hammar, I., Chojnicka, B., Heden, C. H. "Effects of monoamines on interneurons in four spinal reflex pathways from Group I and/or Group II muscle afferents." *European Journal of Neuroscience* 12 (2000): 701–714.

Jankowska, E., Hammar, I., Djouhri, L., Heden, C., Szabo, L. Z., Yin, X. K. "Modulation of responses of four types of feline ascending tract neurons by serotonin and noradrenaline." *European Journal of Neuroscience* 9 (1997): 1375–1387.

Jankowska, E., Jukes, M. G., Lund, S., Lundberg, A. "The effect of Dopa on the spinal cord. 5. Reciprocal organization of pathways transmitting excitatory action to alpha motoneurones of flexors and extensors." *Acta Physiologica Scandinavica* 70 (1967a): 369–388.

Jankowska, E., Jukes, M. G., Lund, S., Lundberg, A. "The effect of Dopa on the spinal cord. 6. Half-centre organization of interneurones transmitting effects from the flexor reflex afferents." *Acta Physiologica Scandinavica* 70 (1967b): 389–402.

Jiang, W., Drew, T. "Effects of bilateral lesions of the dorsolateral funiculi and dorsal columns at the level of the low thoracic spinal cord on the control of locomotion in the adult cat. I. Treadmill walking." *Journal of Neurophysiology* 76 (1996): 849–866.

Jilge, B., Minassian, K., Rattay, F., Pinter, M. M., Gerstenbrand, F., Binder, H., Dimitrijevic, M. R. "Initiating extension of the lower limbs in subjects with complete spinal cord injury by epidural lumbar cord stimulation." *Experimental Brain Reserach* 154(3) (2004): 308–326.

Jordan, L. M. "Brain stem and spinal cord mechanisms for the initiation of locomotion." *In Neurobiological basis of Human Locomotion,* edited by M. Shimamaura, S. Grillner, V. R. Edgerton, 3–20. Tokyo: Japan Scientific Societies Press, 1991.

Jordan, L. M. "Initiation of locomotion in mammals." *Annals of the New York Academy of Science* 860 (1998): 83–93.

Jordan, L. M., Liu, J., Hedlund, P. B., Akay, T., Pearson, K. G. "Descending command systems for the initiation of locomotion in mammals." *Brain Research Review* 57 (2008): 183–191.

Jordan, L. M., Schmidt, B. J. "Propriospinal neurons involved in the control of locomotion: potential targets for repair strategies?" *Progress in Brain Research* 137 (2002): 125–139.

Jordan, L. M., Sławińska U. "Modulation of rhythmic movement: Control of coordination" *Progress in Brain Research* 188 (2011): 181–195.

Kaegi, S., Schwab, M. E., Dietz, V., Fouad, K. "Electromyographic activity associated with spontaneous functional recovery after spinal cord injury in rats." *European Journal of Neuroscience* 16 (2002): 249–258.

Kay-Lyons, M. "Central pattern generation of locomotion: a review of the evidence." *Physical Therapy* 82 (2002): 69–83.

Kern, H., McKay, W.B., Dimitrijevic, M. M., Dimitrijevic, M. R. "Motor control in the human spinal cord and the repair of cord function." *Current Pharmaceutical Design* 11(11) (2005): 1429–1439.

Kiehn, O., Sillar, K. T., Kjaerulff, O., McDearmid, J. R. "Effects of noradrenaline on locomotor rhythm-generating networks in the isolated neonatal rat spinal cord." *Journal of Neurophysiology* 82 (1999): 741–746.

Kiehn, O. "Locomotor circuits in the mammalian spinal cord." *Annual Review of Neuroscience* 29 (2006): 279–306.

Kjaerulff, O., Kiehn, O. "Distribution of networks generating and coordinating locomotor activity in the neonatal rat spinal cord in vitro: a lesion study." *Journal of Neuroscience* 16 (1996): 5777–5794.

Kloos, A. D., Fisher, L. C., Detloff, M. R., Hassenzahl, D. L., Basso, D. M. "Stepwise motor and all-or-none sensory recovery is associated with nonlinear sparing after incremental spinal cord injury in rats." *Experimental Neurology* 191 (2005): 251–265.

Kriellaars, D. J., Brownstone, R. M., Noga, B. R., Jordan, L. M. "Mechanical entrainment of fictive locomotion in the decerebrate cat." *Journal of Neurophysiology* 71 (1994): 2074–2086.

Kudo, N., Yamada, T. "N-methyl-D, L-aspartate-induced locomotor activity in a spinal cord–hind limb muscles preparation of the newborn rat studied in vitro." *Neuroscience Letters* 75 (1987): 43–48.

Kuypers, H. G. "The organization of the 'motor system." *International Journal of Neurology* 4 (1963): 78–91.

LaBella, L. A., Niechaj, A., Rossignol, S. "Low-threshold, short-latency cutaneous reflexes during fictive locomotion in the 'semi-chronic' spinal cat." *Experimental Brain Research* 91 (1992): 236–248.

Lafreniere-Roula, M., McCrea, D. A. "Deletions of rhythmic motoneuron activity during fictive locomotion and scratch provide clues to the organization of the mammalian central pattern generator." *Journal of Neurophysiology* 94 (2005): 1120–1132.

Leblond, H., Rossignol, S. "Intraspinal injections of yohimbine in midlumbar segments block spontaneous decerebrate locomotion in cats." *Society for Neuroscience* (2003) (Abstract 276.1).

Lemay, M.A., Grill, W. M. "Modularity of motor output evoked by intraspinal microstimulation in cats." *Journal of Neurophysiology* 91 (2004): 502–514

Liu, J., Jordan, L. M. "Stimulation of the parapyramidal region of the neonatal rat brain stem produces locomotor-like activity involving spinal 5-HT7 and 5-HT2A receptors." *Journal of Neurophysiology* 94 (2005): 1392–1404.

Loeb, G. E. "Ventral root projections of myelinated dorsal root ganglion cells in the cat." *Brain Research* 106 (1976): 159–165.

Loy, D. N., Magnuson, D. S., Zhang, Y. P., et al. "Functional redundancy of ventral spinal locomotor pathways." *Journal of Neuroscience* 22 (2002): 315–323.

Loy, D. N., Talbott, J. F., Onifer, S. M., et al. “Both dorsal and ventral spinal cord pathways contribute to overground locomotion in the adult rat.” *Experimental Neurology* 177 (2002): 575–580.

Lundberg, A. “Multisensory control of spinal reflex pathways.” *Progress in Brain Research* 50 (1979): 11–28.

Maclean, J. N., Cowley, K. C., Schmidt, B. J. “NMDA receptor-mediated oscillatory activity in the neonatal rat spinal cord is serotonin dependent.” *Journal of Neurophysiology* 79 (1998): 2804–2808.

Majczyński, H., Cabaj, A., Górska, T. “Intrathecal application of cyproheptadine impairs locomotion in intact rats.” *Neuroscience Letters* 381 (2005a): 16–20.

Majczyński, H., Cabaj, A., Sławińska, U., Górska, T. “Intrathecal administration of yohimbine impairs locomotion in intact rats.” *Behavioural Brain Research* 175 (2006): 315–322.

Majczyński, H., Maleszak, K., Cabaj, A., Sławińska, U. “Serotonin-related enhancement of recovery of hind limb motor functions in spinal rats after grafting of embryonic raphe nuclei.” *Journal of Neurotrauma* 22 (2005b): 590–604.

Majczyński, H., Maleszak, K., Górska, T., Sławińska, U. “Comparison of two methods for quantitative assessment of unrestrained locomotion in the rat.” *Journal of Neuroscience Methods* 163 (2007): 197–207.

Majczyński, H., Sławińska, U. “Locomotor recovery after thoracic spinal cord lesions in cats, rats and humans.” *Acta Neurobiologiae Experimentalis* (Warsaw) 67 (2007): 235–257.

McCrea, D. A. “Spinal circuitry of sensorimotor control of locomotion.” *Journal of Physiology* 533 (2001): 41–50.

Metz, G. A., Curt, A., van de Meent, H., Klusman, I., Schwab, M. E., Dietz, V. “Validation of the weight-drop contusion model in rats: a comparative study of human spinal cord injury.” *Journal of Neurotrauma* 17 (2000a): 1–17.

Metz, G. A., Dietz, V., Schwab, M. E., van de Meent, H. “The effects of unilateral pyramidal tract section on hind limb motor performance in the rat.” *Behavioural Brain Research* 96 (1998): 37–46.

Metz, G. A., Merkler, D., Dietz, V., Schwab, M. E., Fouad, K. “Efficient testing of motor function in spinal cord injured rats.” *Brain Research* 883 (2000b): 165–177.

Minassian, K., Jilge, B., Rattay, F., Pinter, M.M., Binder, H., Gerstenbrand, F., Dimitrijevic, M.R. “Stepping-like movements in humans with complete spinal cord injury induced by epidural stimulation of the lumbar cord: electromyographic study of compound muscle action potentials.” *Spinal Cord* 42(7) (2004): 401–416.

Minassian, K., Persy, I., Rattay, F., Pinter, M. M., Kern, H., Dimitrijevic, M. R. “Human lumbar cord circuitries can be activated by extrinsic tonic input to generate locomotor-like activity.” *Human Movement Science* 26(2) (2007): 275–95.

Miller, J. F., Paul, K. D., Lee, R. H., Rymer, W. Z., Heckman, C. J. “Restoration of extensor excitability in the acute spinal cat by the 5-HT2 agonist DOI.” *Journal of Neurophysiology* 75 (1996): 620–628.

Mori, S. “Integration of posture and locomotion in acute decerebrate cats and in awake, freely moving cats.” *Progress in Neurobiology* 28 (1987): 161–195.

Mori, S., Matsui, T., Kuze, B., Asanome, M., Nakajima, K., Matsuyama, K. “Stimulation of a restricted region in the midline cerebellar white matter evokes coordinated quadrupedal locomotion in the decerebrate cat." *Journal of Neurophysiology* 82 (1999): 290–300.

Mori, S., Matsuyama, K., Kohyama, J., Kobayashi, Y., Takakusaki, K. "Neuronal constituents of postural and locomotor control systems and their interactions in cats." *Brain Development* 14 Suppl (1992): S109–S120.

Muir, G. D., Whishaw, I. Q. "Complete locomotor recovery following corticospinal tract lesions: measurement of ground reaction forces during overground locomotion in rats." *Behavioural Brain Research* 103 (1999): 45–53.

Muir, G. D., Whishaw, I. Q. "Red nucleus lesions impair overground locomotion in rats: a kinetic analysis." *European Journal of Neuroscience* 12 (2000): 1113–1122.

Mushahwar, V.K., Jacobs, P.L., Normann, R.A., Triolo, R.J., Kleitman, N. "New functional electrical stimulation approaches to standing and walking". *Journal of Neural Engineering* 4(3) (2007): S181–197.

Nagano, N., Ono, H., Fukuda, H. "Functional significance of subtypes of 5-HT receptors in the rat spinal reflex pathway." *General Pharmacology* 19 (1988): 789–793.

Navarrete, R., Sławińska, U., Vrbová, G. "EMG activity patterns of hindlimb muscles during L-Dopa induced locomotion in neonatal rats." *Experimental Neurology* 173 (2002): 256–265.

Orlovsky, G. N. "Spontaneous and induced locomotion of the thalamic cat." *Biophysics* 14 (1969): 1154–1162.

Orlovsky, G. N. "Cerebellum and locomotion." In *Neurobiological Basis of Human Locomotion*, edited by M. Shimamaura, S. Grillner, V. R. Edgerton, 187–199. Tokyo: Japan Scientific Societies Press, 1991.

Pearson, K. G. "Common principles of motor control in vertebrates and invertebrates." *Annual Review of Neuroscience* 16 (1993): 265–297.

Pearson, K. G. "Generating the walking gait: role of sensory feedback." *Progress in Brain Research* 143 (2004): 123–129.

Ribotta, M. G., Provencher, J., Feraboli-Lohnherr, D., Rossignol, S., Privat, A., Orsal, D. "Activation of locomotion in adult chronic spinal rats is achieved by transplantation of embryonic raphe cells reinervating a precise lumbar level." *Journal of Neuroscience* 20 (2000): 5144–5152.

Rossignol, S., Barrière, G., Alluin, O., Frigon, A. "Re-expression of locomotor function after partial spinal cord injury." *Physiology* (Bethesda, Md.) 24 (2009): 127–139.

Rossignol, S., Bouyer, L., Barthelemy, D., Langlet, C., Leblond, H. "Recovery of locomotion in the cat following spinal cord lesions." *Brain Research Reviews* 40 (2002a): 257–266.

Rossignol, S., Bouyer, L., Langlet, C., et al. "Determinants of locomotor recovery after spinal injury in the cat." *Progress in Brain Research* 143 (2004): 163–172.

Rossignol, S., Chau, C., Giroux, N., et al. "The cat model of spinal injury." *Progress in Brain Research* 137 (2002b): 151–168.

Rossignol, S., Drew, T., Brustein, E., Jiang, W. "Locomotor performance and adaptation after partial or complete spinal cord lesions in the cat." *Progress in Brain Research* 123 (1999): 349–365.

Rossignol, S., Giroux, N., Chau, C., Marcoux, J., Brustein, E., Reader, T. A. "Pharmacological aids to locomotor training after spinal injury in the cat." *Journal of Physiology* 533 (2001): 65–74.

Rossignol, S., Saltiel, P., Perreault, M. C., Drew, T., Pearson, K. G., Belanger, M. "Intralimb and interlimb coordination in the cat during real and fictive rhythmic motor programs." *Seminars in Neuroscience* 5 (1993): 67–75.

Rossignol, S., Provencher, J., Jordan, L. M. "Effects of intrathecal cholinergic drugs on hind limb locomotion in the first two weeks after a complete spinalisation in cats." *Society for Neuroscience* (2005) (Abstract 865.3).

Rybak, I. A., Shevtsova, N. A., Lafreniere-Roula, M., McCrea, D. A. "Modelling spinal circuitry involved in locomotor pattern generation: insights from deletions during fictive locomotion." *Journal of Physiology* 577 (2006a): 617–639.

Rybak, I. A., Stecina, K., Shevtsova, N. A., McCrea, D. A. "Modelling spinal circuitry involved in locomotor pattern generation: insights from the effects of afferent stimulation." *Journal of Physiology* 577 (2006b): 641–658.

Schmidt, B. J., Jordan, L. M. "The role of serotonin in reflex modulation and locomotor rhythm production in the mammalian spinal cord." *Brain Research Bulletin* 53 (2000): 689–710.

Schucht, P., Raineteau, O., Schwab, M. E., Fouad, K. "Anatomical correlates of locomotor recovery following dorsal and ventral lesions of the rat spinal cord." *Experimental Neurology* 176 (2002): 143–153.

Sherrington, C. S. "Flexion-reflex of the limb, crossed extension-reflex, and reflex stepping and standing." *Journal of Physiology* 40 (1910): 28–121.

Shik, M. L., Orlovsky, G. N. "Neurophysiology of locomotor automatism." *Physiological Reviews* 56 (1976): 465–501.

Shik, M. L., Severin, F. V., Orlovsky, G. N. "Control of walking and running by means of electrical stimulation of the mesencephalon." *Electroencephalography & Clinical Neurophysiology* 26 (1969): 549.

Stecina, K., Quevedo, J., McCrea, D. A. "Parallel reflex pathways from flexor muscle afferents evoking resetting and flexion enhancement during fictive locomotion and scratch in the cat." *Journal of Physiology* 569 (2005): 275–290.

Sławińska, U., Majczyński, H., Djavadian, R. "Recovery of hind limb motor functions after spinal cord transection is enhanced by grafts of the embryonic raphe nuclei." *Experimental Brain Research* 132 (2000): 27–38.

Ulfhake, B., Arvidsson, U., Cullheim, S., Hokfelt, T., Visser, T. J. "Thyrotropin-releasing hormone (TRH)-immunoreactive boutons and nerve cell bodies in the dorsal horn of the cat L7 spinal cord." *Neuroscience Letters* 73 (1987): 3–8.

Wetzel, M. C., Stuart, D. G. "Ensemble characteristics of cat locomotion and its neural control." *Progress in Neurobiology* 7 (1976): 1–98.

Whelan, P. J. "Control of locomotion in the decerebrate cat." *Progress in Neurobiology* 49 (1996): 481–515.

Whelan, P. J., Hiebert, G. W., Pearson, K. G. "Stimulation of the Group I extensor afferents prolongs the stance phase in walking cats." *Experimental Brain Research* 103 (1995): 20–30.

White, S. R., Neuman, R. S. "Facilitation of spinal motoneurone excitability by 5-hydroxytryptamine and noradrenaline." *Brain Research* 188 (1980): 119–127.

White, S. R., Neuman, R. S. "Pharmacological antagonism of facilitatory but not inhibitory effects of serotonin and norepinephrine on excitability of spinal motoneurons." *Neuropharmacology* 22 (1983): 489–494.

Yakovenko, S., McCrea, D. A., Stecina, K., Prochazka, A. "Control of locomotor cycle durations." *Journal of Neurophysiology* 94 (2005): 1057–1065.

You, S. W., Chen, B. Y., Liu, H. L., et al. "Spontaneous recovery of locomotion induced by remaining fibers after spinal cord transection in adult rats." *Restorative Neurology & Neuroscience* 21 (2003): 39–45.

Zaporozhets, E., Jordan, L. M., Schmidt, B. J. "Noradrenergic, dopaminergic and serotonergic receptor antagonists block brain stem-evoked locomotion in the in vitro neonatal rat spinal cord." *Society for Neuroscience* (2003) (Abstract 277.11).

5

Summary of Strategies Used to Repair the Injured Spinal Cord

GERTA VRBOVÁ AND URSZULA SŁAWIŃSKA

CONTENTS

1. Introduction
2. Encouraging Regeneration of CNS Axons
   2.1. Overcoming the Unfavorable Environment for Regeneration of CNS Axons
   2.2. Providing Grafts of Peripheral Nerves to Support Regeneration
   2.3. Implanting Isolated Cell Populations to Promote Regeneration
      — Schwann cells
      — Olfactory ensheathing cells
      — Macrophages—immunobased therapy for SCI
      — Stem cells
3. Bypassing the Lesion Site by Grafts from Peripheral Nerves
4. Replacement of Damaged Adult CNS Tissue by Embryonic Grafts
   4.1. Grafts of Embryonic Spinal Cord
   4.2. Replacement of Motoneurones by Embryonic Grafts
      — Survival of grafted motoneurones
      — Depletion of the host motoneurones has been achieved by two different methods
      — Connecting the axons of grafted motoneurones to skeletal muscles
5. Activation of Existing Spinal Cord Circuitry—Intraspinal Grafting of Monoaminergic Cells
   5.1. The Importance of Serotoninergic Innervation for Normal Functions
   5.2. Restoration of Function by Intraspinal Grafting of Serotoninergic Embryonic Cells
6. Conclusions
References

At the Summer School for Biological Treatment of Chronic Spinal Cord Injury, held in Vienna in October 2008, some approaches tested on patients, based on experimental work on animals to encourage regeneration of axons in the CNS, were discussed. These included problems of (1) overcoming the effect of the unfavorable environment of the injured spinal cord on axon regeneration, (2) helping regeneration by implantation of various cell populations, and (3) bypassing the unfavorable environment of the spinal cord by grafts of peripheral nerves. This chapter summarizes experimental results that led to these trials on patients.

1. INTRODUCTION

Spinal cord injury produces variable deficits in movement, sensation, and autonomic functions. Traumatic injury to the spinal cord disrupts the long descending and ascending pathways, and causes degeneration of neurones in the lesioned area as well as destruction of the intrinsic spinal connections. The natural history of spinal cord injury involves the formation of a dense gliotic scar surrounding the lesion site and diffuse astrocytic gliosis. The degree of neurological impairment depends on the extent and site of the lesion, the species, and age. A variety of neurological deficits may evolve. In mammals, after spinal cord transection, different degrees of paralysis and other symptoms such as spasticity, incontinence, and loss of sensation below the lesion level develop. The effects of the CNS injury extend from the site of lesion to other parts of the nervous tissue. Many neurones outside the lesion site (even those of supraspinal origin) atrophy or die. At the injury site itself, the primary and secondary effects lead to cell loss. The formations of a glial scar or a cyst filled with fluid constitute a mechanical barrier for regenerating axons. Above all, due to absence of conduction across the injury site, the spinal cord circuitry below the lesion is deprived of supraspinal inputs so that it is not able to function properly. It is known that very little spontaneous regeneration across the lesion site occurs following spinal cord injury. Among many factors that are believed to contribute to this lack of regeneration are: (1) a glial scar (for review, see Fawcett and Asher, 1999; Fitch and Silver, 2008), (2) myelin inhibitory molecules (for review, see Huber and Schwab, 2000; Schwab, 2002), (3) cell death (Beattie et al., 2000; Beattie et al., 2002; Keane et al., 2006), (4) insufficient growth factor support, and (5) lack of permissive substrates for axonal regeneration. Recently, many experimental procedures have been employed to investigate these factors. Moreover, the strategies for reducing their impact were eagerly sought. Among them various grafting techniques were also introduced.

Although the first successful intracerebral transplantation was reported more than 100 years ago (Thompson, 1890), only the results of the investigations described during the last three decades have revealed revolutionary ideas concerning the developmental and compensatory plasticity of the mammalian CNS and challenged the dogma that survival of grafted neurones and regeneration of axons in the CNS is impossible. It was in the late 1970s when a new technique for repairing of a damaged neural circuitry by transplantation of embryonic neural tissue was successfully introduced (Björklund et al., 1976; Björklund and Stenevi, 1979; Stenevi and Björklund, 1978). Since that time, grafting strategies have been intensively explored in numerous studies on regeneration and functional recovery after CNS injury. However, despite the fact that many different approaches enhance the ability of neuronal regeneration, limited success in terms of functional recovery was achieved.

In this chapter we will present a selection of strategies that have been recently developed to obtain at least partial recovery after spinal cord injury.

2. ENCOURAGING REGENERATION OF CNS AXONS

2.1. Overcoming the Unfavorable Environment for Regeneration of CNS Axons

It is known that hardly any spontaneous regeneration of axons occurs following spinal cord injury. One of the possible reasons for this lack of spontaneous regeneration may be the non-permissive environment of the CNS for axon regeneration. Several factors that constitute the non-permissive environment of the CNS to prevent regeneration have been identified, and attempts have been made to overcome them. Strategies to digest extracellular matrix molecules that form a barrier to growing axons with enzymes such as chondroitinase ABC have proved to be moderately successful.

The central myelin produced by oligodendrocytes inhibits regeneration, and the mechanism of this effect has been analyzed. Each oligodendrocyte in the CNS myelinates several axons, and the central myelin produced contains several myelin associated proteins, including Nogo-66, Nogo-A, myelin associated glycoproteins (MAB), and oligodendrocyte glycoprotein (OMgp). These, taken together, are believed to act as growth inhibitory molecules that via a common NgR (Nogo receptor) activate a small cyclic gmp molecule (Rho), which brings about collapse of growth cones, probably by its action on cytoskeletal proteins (Fitch & Silver, 2008; Schwab, 2004). It is hoped that by overcoming these inhibitory influences, axon regeneration will be allowed to proceed. This regeneration could be aided by populations of cells that form a favorable environment for growing axons. The most favored of these are Schwann cells that do not express NgR, and olfactory ensheathing cells known to promote regeneration. Moreover, neurotrophic factors, inhibitors of NgR, p75 receptors, methods of increasing cAMP known to enhance regeneration can be used either on their own or in combination with other interventions to overcome the non-permissive environment of the CNS and encourage regeneration of CNS axons.

2.2. Providing Grafts of Peripheral Nerves to Support Regeneration

It has been long established that axons of peripheral nerves regenerate, while no such growth has been observed in the CNS. This lack of regeneration is not due to the intrinsic inability of axons of CNS neurones to grow, for conduits of peripheral nerves support growth of axons from central neurones. This was firmly established by Aguayo and his colleagues, who demonstrated that peripheral nerves implanted into the gray matter of the brain or spinal cord attract axons from neighboring neurones and provide an excellent environment for their long-distance regeneration (Aguayo et al., 1990; Aguayo et al., 1991).This approach followed earlier attempts to connect the two parts of spinal cord separated by injury by "a bridge" using a peripheral nerve. As reported by Ramon y Cajal in 1928 (Ramon y Cajal, 1928), Tello showed in 1911 that adult CNS neurones could regrow provided that they had access to the permissive environment of a previously degenerated sciatic nerve. Since that time, grafting techniques have been explored but have provided inconsistent and even ambiguous results.

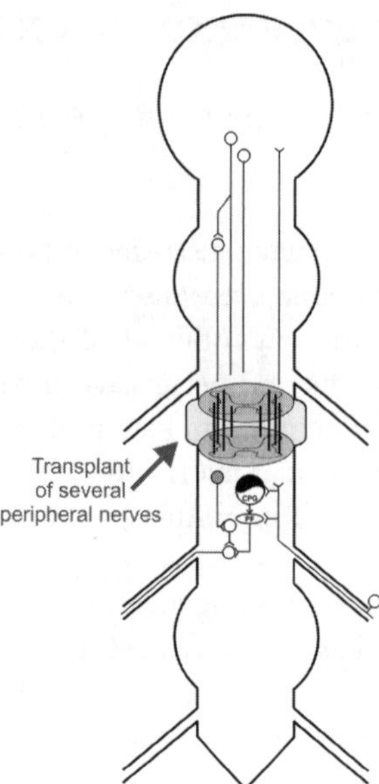

Figure 5–1 The bridge construction in the cavity of spinal cord lesion. This is a schematic drawing of the CNS. The lesion of the spinal cord is illustrated by brackets (*see arrow*). This strategy allows to encourage regeneration of axons throughout the bridge constructed of several peripheral nerves that connect the proximal white matter bundles to the gray matter of the distal stump, and vice versa. The regenerating axons can innervate the neural structures below the lesion and in this way enhance restoration the lost functions. In the figure there are schematically represented possible ways of connections to the motoneurones and to the structures that control locomotor movement. Abbreviations: CPG—the Central Pattern Generator; PF—the Pattern Formation.

In 1940, Sugar and Gerard (Sugar and Gerard, 1940) reported that functional recovery was achieved after using the degenerated sciatic nerve for constructing a "bridge" to reconnect the divided parts of the spinal cord (Figure 5–1). The bridge connected the white matter from above the lesion with the gray matter from below, and vice versa, by putting peripheral nerves into the cavity of the lesion. The grafted animals recovered voluntary hind limb toe movements during locomotion. Moreover, electrical stimulation of the brain stem elicited rhythmic stepping of hind limbs. However, at the time these, classical experiments could not be reproduced. Some negative results were observed by Bernard and Carpenter (1950), who have used both fresh or previously degenerated peripheral nerve auto- and homo-transplants to reconnect the sectioned rat spinal cord. Although no functional improvement in grafted animals was observed, morphological studies revealed that ten days after grafting, a few axons penetrated the implanted nerve, but none of these axons could be traced throughout the graft. Some other negative results were reported by Brown and McCouch (1947) as well as Feigin et al. (1951), who found no difference between the recovery of the grafted and control animals. Moreover, the anatomical analysis showed relatively poor fiber growth into the implant. Crude electrical stimulation of the brain stem and the cortex elicited either no or only a weak motor response in the hind limbs of both control and grafted animals. In conclusion, these authors claimed that no regeneration can occur through an intraspinal nerve bridge and suggested that Sugar and Gerard's positive results were due either to incomplete spinal cord transection or to misinterpretation (see also for earlier reviews: Nornes et al., 1983; Windle et al., 1956).

Augayo's experiments and a series of other papers that followed established that, although peripheral nerve grafts are good conduits for regenerating CNS axons, functional improvement was rarely seen. This was probably due to the fact that the growth of axons stopped when it left the graft and entered the host's CNS unfavorable environment. Nevertheless Cheng et al. (Cheng et al., 1996; Cheng et al., 1997; Cheng and Olson, 1995) reported that by using intercostal nerve grafts to connect the two parts of the severed spinal cord, some degree hind limb motor recovery could be achieved. In addition, the axonal regrowth through the "intraspinal bridge" was enhanced by the application of acidic fibroblast growth factor (aFGF). The restoration of hind limb movement was attributed to regenerated axons of long spinal tracts in adult rats following complete spinal cord transection (Cheng et al., 1996; Cheng et al., 1997). In more recent investigations (Lee et al., 2004; Lee et al., 2006), the presence of 5-HT-labeled axons below the lesion site at lumbar cord level was demonstrated and interpreted as successful regeneration of fibers from the raphe nuclei. At the same time, labeling of corticospinal tract axons at the graft site and below showed labeled neurones in the motor cortex, the red nucleus, the reticulospinal nuclei, the raphe nuclei, and the vestibular nuclei (Lee et al., 2004), confirming the possibility of axonal regeneration of these pathways. In the next study, the same authors described how the peripheral nerve graft and aFGF treatments improved hind limb locomotor ability, facilitated the regrowth of catecholaminergic fibers, and protected sympathetic preganglionic neurones. These effects ameliorated the autonomic dysfunction in a T8 spinal cord transected rat model (Lee et al., 2006). These results, taken together, show that the failure of CNS neurones to regenerate is not related to an intrinsic inability of the neurone to regenerate its processes, but is a feature of the environment that does not support regeneration.

A similar strategy tested in non-human primates after lateral hemisection did not show any functional improvement (Levi et al., 2002). Recently, the method of constructing a bridge using peripheral nerves was carried out in a group of patients in China. However, so far, this strategy has not provided any convincing benefits to people with SCI. Thus, to determine whether grafting peripheral nerve bridges can be safe and effective for enhancement of recovery in human spinal cord injury is uncertain.

2.3. Implanting Isolated Cell Populations to Promote Regeneration

Schwann cells

Another possible strategy to encourage regeneration of CNS axons is transplantation of a defined cell population into the site of the lesion (Figure 5–2). The transplanted cells can form a bridge for axonal regeneration, and some of them may additionally support axonal regeneration by secreting growth factors or other pro-regenerative molecules.

It has long been accepted that the injured axons in central nervous system of adult mammals do not regenerate. However results described in the previous section show

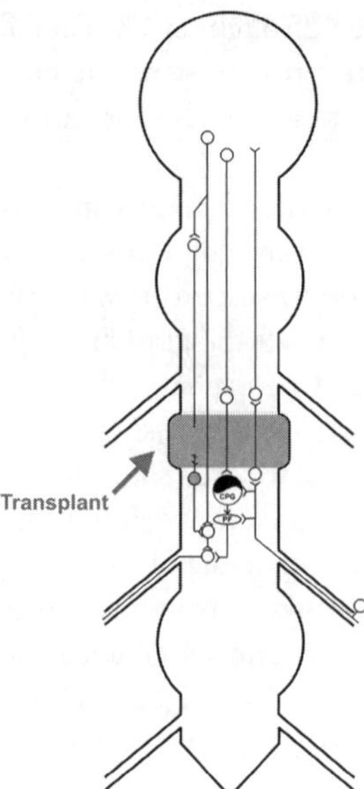

Figure 5–2 Transplantation into the cavity of lesion—Schwann cells or olfactory ensheathing cells. This is a schematic illustration of the CNS where the lesion of the spinal cord is represented by the shaded area, and illustrates another possible strategy to encourage regeneration of CNS axons. The transplantation of defined types of cells allows forming a kind of bridge for axonal regeneration, and some of them may additionally support the axonal regeneration by secretion of growth factors or other pro-regenerative molecules. The regenerating axons can innervate the neural structures below the lesion and in this way enhance restoration the lost functions. In the figure there are schematically represented possible ways of connections restored using this strategy to the motoneurones and to the structures that control locomotor movement. Abbreviations as in Fig. 5-1.

that they can regenerate if they are provided with a peripheral nerve graft. These findings indicate that given the appropriate environment such as Schwann cells, CNS neurones can regenerate their axons. Thus, the Schwann cells appeared to be ideal candidates for use in the damaged spinal cord to enhance axonal regeneration. Three decades ago, Richard P. Bunge proposed the possibility of isolating and culturing Schwann cells from a patient's peripheral nerve for autologous implantation into the injured spinal cord (Bunge, 1987; Bunge & Wood, 1987). Since that time, the methods for production of a large number of Schwann cells from both adult rat (Morrissey et al., 1991) and human (Casella et al., 1996; Levi et al., 1995) peripheral nerve for transplantation studies or therapy were developed.

The effectiveness of grafted Schwann cells in promoting axonal regeneration in the injured adult spinal cord has been studied in several experimental conditions (for review, see Bunge, 2001; Bunge, 1993; Thuret et al., 2006). Schwann cells were grafted into an injured spinal cord, where the lesion was produced either by compression (Martin et al., 1991; Martin et al., 1993), complete transection (Xu et al., 1995a; Xu et al., 1995b; Xu et al., 1997), or lateral hemisection (Bamber et al., 2001), as well as by creating a suction cavity in the corticospinal tract (Kuhlengel et al., 1990). In all these investigations, the effects of Schwann cell grafting were very similar and rather "beneficial" to the injured spinal cord. First, the grafted Schwann cells easily invaded the injured spinal cord. Depending on the number of grafted cells, they produced only a cluster of cells intermingled with scar tissue, or they filled completely a cavity of lesion by producing a very smooth interface between host and grafted tissue. Second, the tissue that connected the spinal cord stumps contained, in addition to the Schwann cells, also ensheathed unmyelinated and myelinated axons, blood vessels, fibroblasts, and meningeal cells (Oudega et al., 1997; Xu et al., 1997). Most important, nerve fibers originating from both stumps invaded the bridge. Thus, the grafted Schwann cells encouraged the growth and regeneration of lesioned fibers. However, retrograde tracing experiments revealed that, although axons of propriospinal origin grew into the graft tissue, they failed to enter the host spinal cord. Moreover, fibers of supraspinal brain stem structures (e.g., raphe nuclei, locus coeruleus) that are involved in motor control were rarely seen in the grafted tissue (Martin et al., 1991; Martin et al., 1993). Kuhlengel et al. (1990) found that the fibers of the corticospinal tract in injured neonatal rats grew their axons in fascicles along the border of the graft, but did not penetrate the graft.

The timing of the grafting procedure seems to be important. Grafting immediately after injury resulted in enhanced sprouting and ingrowth of host fibers but caused cyst formation in the spinal cord, and the reduction of gliosis was only moderate (Kuhlengel et al., 1990). Grafting performed two and four days after injury led to poor survival of the grafted tissue, probably because of release of cytotoxic factors in the lesioned cord (Martin et al., 1993). Delayed grafting (five or more days after injury) improved the survival and the integration of the graft into the host spinal cord and often resulted in a very good fusion between implant and host cord, with minimal glial scarring and no cyst formation (Kuhlengel et al., 1990). The functional investigations of grafted rats reported recovery of hind limb function in some (Takami et al., 2002) but not all lesioned animals. Thus, the message from experiments where the Schwann cells were transplanted into the cavity of the lesion is that although this strategy is able to induce some regeneration of supraspinal axons into the graft, the regenerated fibers are not able to grow from the graft in to the host spinal cord (Xu et al., 1997).

The transplantation of human Schwann cells into the transected spinal cord of rats with attenuated immune systems has also been reported to be successful. Although the brain stem axons regenerated into grafts and spinal axons regenerated distal to grafts, only a little functional improvement was reported (Guest et al., 1997b).

Thus the results of successful Schwann cell grafting show that transplanted Schwann cells have several beneficial effects, which influence the restorative process of the injured host spinal cord. They reduce glial scarring and are able to enhance to some extent the otherwise abortive axonal growth and regeneration. Unfortunately, grafts of Schwann cells cannot form functioning bridges between the injured parts of the spinal cord because long descending fibers do not usually enter the graft. Nevertheless, they are able to render the surrounding host spinal cord more permissive for axonal growth. Grafting Schwann cells to stimulate regeneration as opposed to remyelination in the spinal cord has not resulted in functional improvement, and their use for spinal cord injury patients is not yet applicable. Although purified and cultured Schwann cells can be maintained in tissue cell banks and are available from host peripheral nerves, they are still considered alien elements in the spinal cord under normal circumstances, and their long-term behavior is not known. Moreover, their almost unlimited capacity to proliferate within a CNS environment may be dangerous.

To improve the ability of Schwann cells to support axonal regeneration in the injured spinal cord, the Schwann cell bridge was enriched by neurotrophins. Infusion of BDNF (Brain-Derived Neurotrophic Factor) and NT-3 (Neurotrophic Factor-3) around the Schwann cell graft led to an increase in the number of myelinated axons in the graft. The number of axons that regenerated from propriospinal neurones into the graft was tripled in comparison to animals that did not receive Schwann cells enriched by neurotrophins (Xu et al., 1995a). In another study, Menei and colleagues (Menei et al., 1998) infected the Schwann cells with a retroviral vector carrying the human preproBDNF cDNA, and found more axons, including those from the brain stem, below the transection site. In another study, the delivery of BDNF and NT-3 via an adenoviral vector (Ad) distal to a Schwann cell graft in the completely transected adult rat thoracic spinal cord induced axonal growth beyond the level of transection (Blits et al., 2000). The rats from the neurotrophin group demonstrated significant improvement of hind limb functions compared with the control group. These experiments showed that the growth of injured axons could be further enhanced by combining the Schwann cells with neurotrophins.

Regeneration of axons into Schwann cell grafts can also be enhanced by increasing the levels of cAMP. In a study by Pearse and coworkers (Pearse et al., 2004), adult rats received Schwann cell grafts and intraspinal injection of dbcAMP one week after moderate spinal cord contusion. Some animals were also treated with rolipram, a compound that inhibits phosphodiesterase and allows cAMP to accumulate. There was greater sparing of myelinated axons and an overall increase in myelinated axons within the graft, and most important, a number of serotoninergic fibers that grew across the lesion site in animals that received treatment with either dbcAMP or rolipram. Thus elevation of cAMP could increase the regenerative capacity of injured axons.

Olfactory ensheathing cells

The next strategy introduced to achieve regeneration of fibers in the injured spinal cord combined grafting of Schwann cells with olfactory ensheathing glia (for reviews, see Boyd et al., 2005; Franklin & Barnett, 2000; Ramon-Cueto et al., 2000). Olfactory ensheathing cells (OECs) are unique, for they are responsible for the continual regeneration and remyelination of olfactory axons throughout the life of adult mammals (for review, see Boyd et al., 2003; Doucette, 1995; Ramon-Cueto & Avila, 1998; Ramon-Cueto & Valverde, 1995).

Olfactory ensheathing cells from the olfactory bulb have some common phenotypic properties with Schwann cells and astrocytes. They express glial fibrillary acidic protein (GFAP, an astrocyte marker) and form end-feet around blood vessels. They also express the low-affinity NGF receptor and produce laminin, characteristic of Schwann cells. However, they should be considered a distinct glial cell type in the CNS. In the adult mammalian olfactory bulb, where OECs are present, normal and injured olfactory axons are able to elongate and establish synaptic contacts with other neurones throughout the subject's lifetime. These features indicated that grafted olfactory cells might be good candidates for supporting regeneration in other parts of the CNS as well.

The first evidence of their possible usefulness came from experiments *in vitro*. They showed that the morphological and immunological characteristics of cultured cells from the olfactory nerve and glomerular layers were similar to those of Schwann cells, and the similarities could account for the permissiveness to axonal growth of the olfactory bulb (Ramon-Cueto & Nieto-Sampedro, 1992). The finding that the rat embryonic OECs co-cultured with dorsal root ganglion neurones can assemble a myelin sheath followed (Devon & Doucette, 1995).

In vivo studies showed that olfactory-ensheathing glia cells can promote the growth of axotomized dorsal root axons into the adult rat spinal cord (Ramon-Cueto & Nieto-Sampedro, 1994). Ensheathing glial cells were used here to bridge the gap between the spinal cord and the cut dorsal root. The grafted cells readily migrated into the spinal cord and were followed by regenerating dorsal root axons. Only in the presence of OECs did regenerating axons reach the spinal cord, suggesting that the presence of these cells in the spinal cord was important for successful regeneration. Subsequently it was shown that remyelination of axons by OECs in the posterior columns could enhance axonal conduction across the previously demyelinated area (Imaizumi et al., 1998). Thus OECs encouraged axonal growth as well as their remyelination.

In another series of experiments, Ramon-Cueto and colleagues (Ramon-Cueto et al., 2000; Ramon-Cueto & Avila, 1998) injected olfactory glia suspensions into the proximal and distal spinal cord stumps. Grafted olfactory glial cells migrated from the injection sites toward more rostral and caudal regions and induced significant functional recovery in paralyzed animals. Animals supported their body weight, displayed voluntary hind limb movements, and their hind limbs responded to sensory stimuli. The conclusion from these and many other investigations is that OECs can promote long-distance regeneration of several descending and ascending tracts after spinal cord injury (Lu et al., 2001; Lu et al., 2002; Ramon-Cueto et al., 2000; Ramon-Cueto, 2000; Ramon-Cueto & Avila, 1998; Santos-Benito & Ramon-Cueto, 2003). This functional improvement suggested that OECs could be the choice of cells to be grafted into injured human spinal cords.

Unexpectedly, other research from several laboratories has failed to replicate the promising effects of OEC transplantation after dorsal rhizotomy (Gomez et al., 2003; Ramer et al., 2004b; Riddell et al., 2004) and have questioned the possibility that OECs are directly responsible for either myelinating axons or inducing their regeneration. In view of this inconsistency, the role of OECs in promoting axon regeneration might require redefinition.

It was suggested that OECs have to collaborate with additional cell types in order to promote beneficial effects on remyelinating denuded axons within the spinal cord (Barnett & Chang, 2004; Boyd et al., 2005; Lakatos et al., 2003). It was proposed that OECs in collaboration with host Schwann cells contribute to a three-dimensional matrix within the damaged spinal cord. This matrix may contain growth factors and extracellural matrix molecules that create a substrate conducive to axonal regrowth and remyelination. This alternative interpretation of earlier experiments should not detract from our appreciation of earlier studies that suggested a beneficial effect of OEC implantation on axon regeneration (Boyd et al., 2004; Garcia-Alias et al., 2004; Keyvan-Fouladi et al., 2003; Li et al., 1997; Li et al., 1998; Li et al., 2003; Li & Raisman, 1997; Lu et al., 2001; Lu et al., 2002; Navarro et al., 1999; Plant et al., 2003; Ramer et al., 2004a; Ramon-Cueto & Avila, 1998; Ramon-Cueto & Nieto-Sampedro, 1994;

Verdu et al., 2003) and on remyelination (Akiyama et al., 2004; Barnett et al., 2000; Franklin & Gilson, 1996; Imaizumi et al., 1998; Imaizumi et al., 2000; Kato et al., 2000; Lakatos et al., 2003; Li et al., 1998; Li & Raisman, 1997; Sasaki et al., 2004). The exact mechanisms underlying the beneficial effects of OEC grafts after spinal cord injury need to be reevaluated in the context of the unique cooperation between invading host Schwann cells and OECs (Boyd et al., 2005).

Together with olfactory ensheathing glial cells there are also other candidates for cell transplantation into the area of the injured site of the spinal cord: pituicytes and tanycytes. These cell types are either precursors or members of a family of Schwann-like macroglia that are referred to as *aldynoglia;* that is, the kind of cells that are able to make the CNS microenvironment more hospitable to growing axons (Gudino-Cabrera & Nieto-Sampedro, 2000). Grafted tanycytes (undifferentiated neuronal precursor cells in the CNS) and OECs promote the growth of axons after being grafted into the CNS of adult rats (Li et al., 1997; Li et al., 1998; Ramon-Cueto et al., 2000; Ramon-Cueto & Avila, 1998; Ramon-Cueto & Nieto-Sampedro, 1994; Ramon-Cueto & Valverde, 1995). All three types of Schwann cell–like macroglia are able to myelinate DRG neurites *in vitro* (Gudino-Cabrera & Nieto-Sampedro, 2000). There is also a relatively unexplored area concerning the cellular interaction between OECs and astrocytes, or even the possibility that OECs could differentiate into astrocyte-like cells (Boyd et al., 2003).

Based on the results of research described above, several clinical trials worldwide have been initiated and have used autologous transplantation of olfactory tissue containing OECs into the damaged spinal cords of humans. However, it has to be emphasized that the translation of results from animal experiments to the human situation is not straightforward and requires caution.

Macrophages—immunobased therapy for SCI

The lack of axonal regeneration and the poor recovery of function in the mammalian CNS differs from the peripheral nervous system (PNS), where regeneration is possible. Some understanding of the mechanisms responsible for PNS axon regeneration may help us find ways to facilitate regeneration in the CNS, as discussed above. In the PNS, during the early phase after nervous system injury, macrophages seem to be important for axonal regeneration and recovery of function.

It has been well established that macrophages play a major role in the early inflammatory response in all soft-tissue wounds (Perry & Gordon, 1991). In the PNS, an early and robust accumulation of macrophages is believed to be crucial for the regeneration of injured axons (for review, see Perry et al., 1993). In the injured CNS, however, an early and robust accumulation of macrophages causes damage that exceeds the beneficial effects of the inflammatory reaction (Blight, 1985; Blight, 1992; Blight, 1994; Giulian et al., 1989; Giulian & Robertson, 1990). In the PNS, circulating monocytes infiltrate the distal degenerated part of the nerve approximately 24 hours after injury (Lazar et al., 1999), while in the CNS, a significant macrophage/microglia response is obtained only 14 to 18 days (or even three weeks) after injury (George & Griffin, 1994; Lazar et al., 1999). In the PNS, a reduction in the responses of macrophages after peripheral nerve injury impaired axonal regeneration (Bedi et al., 1992; Brown et al., 1991; Dailey et al., 1998; Lazar et al., 1999). Thus, the response of monocytes (microglia/macrophages) to axon damage is different in the adult mammalian central nervous system from that in the peripheral nervous system.

Moreover, it is now known that, in contrast to the PNS, in the CNS the inflammatory reactions can cause or increase tissue injury (Popovich et al., 2002) and inhibit axonal growth (Lacroix et al., 2002). However, new evidence indicates that after CNS injury, the inflammatory cells, among them macrophages, can provide neuroprotection and control of the regenerative response. Although the nature of their role is still a matter of discussion, it seems to be clear that immune cells can release both neuroprotective and neurodestructive molecules at the site of the injury (Kerschensteiner et al., 2009).

Recent data show that the same mode of activation of macrophages promotes axon regeneration as well as cell death (Gensel et al., 2009; Stoll et al., 2002). Thus the net effect on neuronal regeneration seems to be determined by a balance between the destructive and protective factors released during the neuroimmune response. In order to develop more specific therapeutic interventions in the future, the identification of the regulatory switches that govern the balance between protective and destructive responses in different immune cell populations is needed. It is therefore important to understand the consequences of macrophage invasion in the nervous system.

Macrophages are needed to remove myelin debris known to inhibit axonal regrowth (Cadelli et al., 1992; Schnell & Schwab, 1990), to recycle lipid degradation products (Harel et al., 1989; Muller et al., 1985; Stoll & Muller, 1986), and as a source of cytokines and growth factors (Heumann et al., 1987b). In the CNS, activated macrophages/microglia are responsible for creating a favorable environment for regeneration by degrading specific inhibitory molecules on adult mammalian central myelin and astrocytes, which prevent axonal growth and reactive neurite sprouting (Avellino et al., 1995; Caroni & Schwab, 1988; David et al., 1990; Davies et al., 1997; George & Griffin, 1994; Siegal et al., 1990; Stoll et al., 1989; Z'Graggen et al., 1998). Macrophages/microglia also upregulate molecules that promote axonal growth, such as nerve growth factor (Brown et al., 1991; Heumann et al., 1987a; Hikawa & Takenaka, 1996). Thus active macrophages are needed for regrowth of injured axons. It seems that, in general, active macrophages have multiple actions in healing processes. First, macrophages are responsible for phagocytosis, needed for removal of inhibitory elements including myelin debris, which would otherwise block the process of regrowth (Cadelli et al., 1992; Schnell & Schwab, 1990). Second, activated macrophages are able to provide apolipoproteins, the lipid-associated proteins involved in lipid metabolism and membrane reconstruction (Harel et al., 1989; Muller et al., 1985; Stoll & Muller, 1986), as well as the growth factors and cytokines needed to make the neuronal environment permissive to and supportive of regeneration (Benveniste, 1992; David et al., 1990; Eitan et al., 1992; Heumann et al., 1987b; Schwartz et al., 1989). Macrophages not only produce and release many hydrolytic enzymes useful for debridement of dead and dying cells, they are also a particularly rich source of growth factors and cytokines useful for promoting intracellular signaling, mitosis, and extracellular matrix production (Gordon, 1995; Lotan & Schwartz, 1994; Perry & Gordon, 1991). The responses of the CNS and the PNS to injury are also mediated by specific molecular products secreted by macrophages following their activation (David et al., 1990; Franzen et al., 1998; Lazarov-Spiegler et al., 1996; Prewitt et al., 1997). It is believed that macrophages, activated at different regions of the nervous system, produce and secrete variable types and amounts of molecular products, thereby stimulating or preventing the regenerative ability of the nervous tissue (Lazarov-Spiegler et al., 1996).

Thus, it might be that suitably activated macrophages can contribute positively to the homeostasis of the CNS by the recruitment of adaptive immunity from the periphery. The successful activation of microglia and macrophages is the key to efficient phagocytic removal of myelin debris from the injured CNS (Rotshenker, 2003; Vallieres et al., 2006). However, it has to be pointed out that this part of the physiological repair mechanism needs to be rigorously controlled in terms of the timing and intensity of the cellular response (for review, see: Popovich & Longbrake, 2008; Schwartz & Yoles, 2006).

As a potential treatment, transplantation of macrophages has further important advantages in that the cells can be derived autologously and noninvasively. An effective multipotent therapy for CNS injuries might therefore involve optimizing this procedure in order to achieve the growth of many axons (Lazarov-Spiegler et al., 1996). It is therefore not surprising that attempts were made to implant activated macrophages into the spinal cord after injury.

Some studies have shown that activated macrophages implanted into the transected adult spinal cords promote axonal regeneration and behavioral recovery (Bomstein et al., 2003; Rapalino et al., 1998). At least two different methods were used to activate macrophages. Autologous macrophages can be activated to a wound-healing phenotype through co-incubation with peripheral nerve segments (Lazarov-Spiegler et al., 1998) or with the skin (Bomstein et al., 2003). Transplantation of macrophages activated by either method led to a significant motor recovery in rats with transected spinal cords (Bomstein et al., 2003; Rapalino et al., 1998). Moreover, it was shown that the injection of skin-coincubated macrophages into contused spinal cord of rats not only resulted in improved motor recovery, but also in the reduction of the spinal cyst formation (Bomstein et al., 2003).

Based on these results, an experimental therapy, ProCord™, has been introduced, which was designed to enhance the repair capacity of macrophages grafted into the traumatically injured human spinal cord. The scientific rationale for this approach stemmed from data in animal models described above. Despite the technical success of ProCord™ that was quickly evolved with the Phase I clinical trials completed (Knoller et al., 2005), there are still questions about the rationale behind this approach. Some argue that there is no apparent need to augment the macrophages' response after SCI, because there is no clear evidence of the beneficial effects of the activated macrophages injected into the lesioned spinal cord (Popovich & Longbrake, 2008). It is possible that, like their endogenous counterparts, transplanted macrophages will undergo progressive changes in function in response to the various micro-environmental signals produced in the injured spinal cord (Pan et al., 2002; Pineau & Lacroix, 2007; Popovich & Longbrake, 2008; Schnell et al., 1999a; Schnell et al., 1999b; Stout et al., 2005; Streit et al., 1998). Additional studies are required to determine whether this is the case.

Stem cells

It is widely believed that stem cells could be a source for new neurones or glial cells in the injured or damaged CNS. Stem cells have several advantages for prospective therapy because they may support regeneration as well as differentiate into neurones, glia, or other cell types due to their multipotent potential. Gaiano and Fishel (1998) raised hopes for the possible role of stem cells in CNS repair by suggesting that once the stem cells were transplanted into the brain, they are able to differentiate into appropriate neural and glial cell populations. Subsequently, some studies reported a functional impact for this approach. McDonald and colleagues (McDonald et al., 1999) described an improvement of locomotor hind limb movements after grafting embryonic stem cells into the injured spinal cord of rats. This study reported a replacement of oligodendrocytes by grafted embryonic stem cells. However, it is not clear whether the grafted stem cells themselves, or their beneficial influence on the host cells, contributed to the structural reorganization and repair.

Apart from embryonic stem cells, a source of multipotential stem cells was identified in adult bone marrow stromal cells (MSCs). These cells can differentiate into astrocytes, oligodendrocytes, and cells expressing markers of immature neurones such as nestin, when transplanted into rodents CNS (Akiyama et al., 2002; Kopen et al., 1999; Woodbury et al., 2000). Moreover, bone marrow transplants were reported to provide tissue protection and directional guidance for axons after contusive spinal cord injury in rats (Ankeny et al., 2004). MSCs grafted into the cavity of spinal cord lesion enhanced hind limb air stepping associated with activation of the stepping control circuitry; however, they did not influence the overground locomotor recovery (Ankeny et al., 2004).

Adult bone marrow stromal cells provide a very small number of multipotential stromal cells, and therefore the presence of stem cells in the human umbilical cord offered hope for another rich source of stem cells. Due to their primitive nature and ability to develop into non-hematopoietic cells of various tissue lineages, it was hoped that these cells might be useful as an alternative cell source for cell-based therapies requiring the replacement of individual cell types or substitution of missing substances (Garbuzova-Davis et al., 2006). Dasari and coworkers (2008) reported recently that the human umbilical-cord-blood stem cells after delivery into the contusion site of the rat spinal cord migrate up to 2 mm rostrocaudally in the white and gray matter and survive up to five weeks after transplantation in the injured neural tissue. According to this report, differentiated neurones and oligodendrocytes were mostly observed in the dorsal region of the epicentrum, up to 2 mm rostrocaudally. The highest density of human umbilical-cord-derived stem cells was found at the area of primary injury, and was gradually reduced as the border with intact spinal cord tissue was approached. No such cells were found in areas of the intact spinal cord (Dasari et al., 2008). These results suggest that such a strategy promotes preferential survival and/or differentiation of human umbilical cord stem cells toward oligodendrocyte and neural lineage. In paraplegic rats that received grafts of umbilical cord, a gradual restoration of hind limb motor functions slowly appeared. Scores that tested the animals' motor hind limb abilities (Basso et al., 1995) were significantly higher at five and six weeks after injury in rats with an umbilical graft. Moreover, the ability of the animals to maintain their balance while walking on beams was better and consistently improving compared with the injured control rats during the whole time of testing. This functional improvement was related to the enhanced neuronal and oligodendrocyte preservation in grafted rats. These results were interpreted to show that the presence of the human umbilical cord stem cells induces an increase in the numbers of neurones and oligodendrocytes, which might be involved in enhancing functional recovery after SCI in rats (Dasari et al., 2008).

There are several mechanisms that may account for the positive effect of the grafted human umbilical cord stem cells, including remyelination and regeneration of axons as well as formation of neurones and oligodendrocytes. The positive outcome correlates with the ability of human umbilical cord stem cells to reduce apoptotic cell death. Long-term studies on positive effects of human umbilical-cord-blood stem cells are needed to provide further evidence regarding their therapeutic potentials after SCI (Dasari et al., 2008), particularly in view of careful recent studies of human umbilical cord cells and their ability to differentiate into neurones. The umbilical cord stem cells form a mixed population of various cell types, of which the mesenchymal cells displayed the most encouraging features for giving rise to a neuronal lineage (Zwart et al., 2009). However, even in these cells, it was impossible to induce neurone-like characteristics using various established methods (Hill et al., 2009). Nevertheless, implantation of human umbilical-cord-derived stem cells into the damaged optic tract had some beneficial effect on retinal cells destined to die. This was due to release of growth factors by the grafted cells. It is therefore likely that the beneficial effects produced by grafted human umbilical cords in paraplegic rats may be due to the release of neurotrophic factors.

Another reason why the use of stem cells for repair of CNS injury has to be regarded with some reservation are findings of previous studies on grafting of embryonic tissue into an adult host. When assessing the most suitable age of the embryonic graft for transplantation into the adult CNS, it was established that successful grafting can only be achieved when the differentiation of the grafted cell types is completed before surgery. If the grafted tissue used had not completed differentiation, the grafts of embryonic tissue did not survive (Björklund et al., 1983c; Sieradzan & Vrbová, 1989; and others—see also the following chapter about the age of the graft). It is regrettable that this very promising approach will still need much work before it will be useful for treatment of the damaged CNS.

3. BYPASSING THE LESION SITE BY GRAFTS FROM PERIPHERAL NERVES

Spinal cord injury leads to alterations of motor and somatosensory functions that are mediated by CNS structures located in the spinal cord below the lesion. Results from experiments on animals show that implantation of a peripheral nerve graft or reimplantation of avulsed ventral roots into the spinal cord allow axonal regrowth of injured spinal neurones into a peripheral nerve conduit (Bray et al., 1987; Cullheim et al., 1989; Horvat et al., 1989; Nógrádi & Vrbová, 1994; Nógrádi & Vrbová, 1996a; Sieradzan & Vrbová, 1989). The possibility that a peripheral nerve conduit can lead axons from neurones above the lesion of the spinal cord towards the paralyzed parts of body, and in this way reestablish the supraspinal control of lost function, has been explored.

Attempts were made to achieve the recovery of lost motor function after spinal cord injury by connecting the ventral roots of the spinal cord rostral to the lesion site directly to the muscles with the interposition of a nerve graft. One cut end of an isolated peripheral nerve was connected to the ventral root or inserted into the spinal cord rostral to the lesion, while the other end of the nerve graft was then sutured either to a nerve, through which axons will eventually reach one or more paralyzed muscles, or directly to muscles (Figure 5–3). This approach was used by Brunelli et al., (1983). They provided a regeneration pathway toward the periphery, not for motor axons but for descending supraspinal axons that were interrupted at the

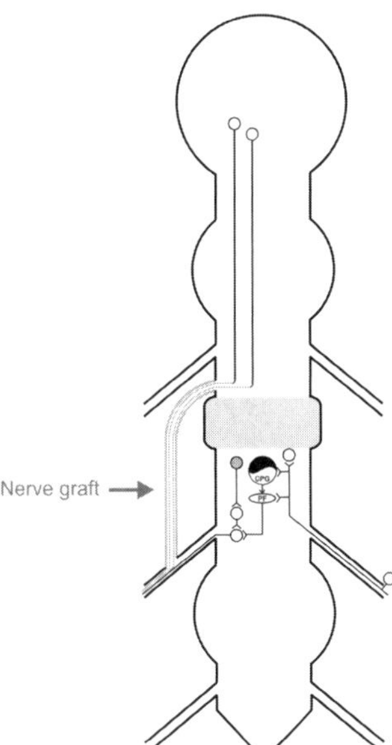

Figure 5–3 The bridge construction through spinal root. Using this strategy, attempts were made to achieve the recovery of lost motor function after spinal cord injury by connecting the spinal cord rostral to the lesion site directly to the muscles with the interposition of a nerve graft. The distal stump of the nerve graft can then be sutured either to a nerve, through which axons will eventually reach one or bigger number of paralyzed muscles, or directly to muscles, and in this way to enhance the restoration of lost functions. This strategy allows the cortico-muscle connection to be reestablished. Abbreviations as in Fig. 5-1.

lesion site. In their study on rats, they reported that axons from supraspinal neurones could grow along a peripheral nerve graft, bypass the motoneurone, reach skeletal muscles, and reinnervate them. The same authors reported that this procedure provided a partial recovery of function. Earlier experiments carried out by the same group in nonhuman primates bypassed the site of the spinal cord lesion by guiding axons from supraspinal neurones to skeletal muscles via muscular nerve branches inserted into the severed lateral bundle of the spinal cord (Brunelli, 2001; Brunelli & Brunelli, 1996). The authors reported that this procedure led to muscle reinnervation and restoration of motor function. They concluded that the regrowth of axons descending from central noncholinergic neurones was responsible for functional muscle reinnervation. In view of previous experimental evidence, first described by Langley & Anderson (1904), that only cholinergic neurones can effectively innervate skeletal muscles, the possibility that glutamatergic supraspinal neurones can provide effective reinnervation of striated muscles and form neuromuscular junctions expressing AMPA glutamate receptors has to be reviewed with caution.

Thus unless further, more compelling and thorough physiological and pharmacological evidence is presented, these findings cannot be taken to form a basis for the use of these grafting procedures in human patients.

Another possibility for constructing a bridge through which axon regeneration could proceed was the use of a thoracic nerve above the injured spinal cord that was

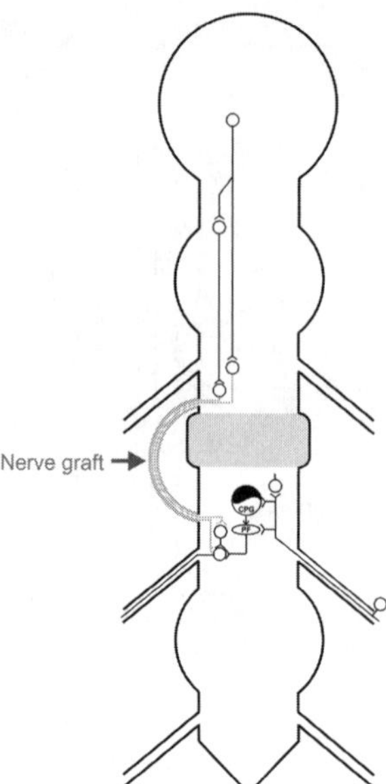

Figure 5–4 The bridge construction. This strategy uses one of the thoracic nerves and implants it into the lumbar gray matter below the level of spinal cord injury. This kind of strategy allows motoneurones above the lesion to reach the cells that are the pre-motor to the motoneurones below the lesion. Shaded area illustrates the site of the lesion. Abbreviations as in Fig. 5-1.

detached from the muscle it innervates and then the cut distal end implanted into the lumbar gray matter below the level of the spinal cord injury (Campos et al., 2004; Campos et al., 2008). This approach enables the regeneration of axons from supraspinal neurones to reach the neural circuitry and in this way reestablish the descending supraspinal influence that was interrupted at the lesion site (Figure 5–4). One month after the cut end of the distal stump of the ventral root was inserted into the spinal cord below the site of the lesion, projections from supraspinal regions were present in the ventral motor laminae of the cord, including identified synapses established directly on motoneurones. Moreover, the bridge circuit could be activated by electrical stimulation of neural pathways rostral to its origin, which evoked motor responses. (Campos et al., 2004; Campos et al., 2008).

Encouraged by these results from animal experiments, attempts were made to apply this approach to paraplegic patients. The first operation was performed in a young lady four months after complete SC lesion at T9. First voluntary movements of the connected muscles were obtained after 17 months, and 27 months after the operation, she was able to walk up to 60 steps with the help of a walker and to climb steps in the water.

The other method that used a peripheral nerve graft to bridge the rostral spinal cord above with the caudal part below the lesion has been used by Carlson and Sundin (Carlsson & Sundin, 1980). In two paraplegic patients who had traumatic lesions of the conus medullaris spinal root, a functioning ventral root above the lesion was cut and its distal end connected to the S2 and S3 ventral and dorsal roots to restore lost bladder control. In both patients the micturition reflex and bladder function were restored. Moreover, both patients could feel the urge to void, and could initiate micturition voluntarily to empty their bladders. However, the relatively good bladder functions might be a result of either regeneration of the newly constructed nervous pathways or spontaneously developed reflex bladders in partial upper neurone lesions. In 2002, Tadie with his colleagues (Tadie et al., 2002) reported that through the nerve autografts implanted between the rostral spinal ventral horn and the caudal ventral roots, rostral spinal motoneurone can reach peripheral targets, leading to some return of muscle function of the patient three years after spinal cord traumatic injury at the T9 level. During surgery, three segments from an autologous sural nerve were implanted into the right and left antero-lateral quadrant of the cord at T7–T8 levels, then connected to homolateral L2–L4 lumbar ventral roots, respectively. Eight months after surgery, voluntary contractions of bilateral adductors and of the left quadriceps, together with related motor unit activity potentials were observed (Tadie et al., 2002). It seems that methods of spinal cord–nerve roots bypasses might provide a strategy for repairing both motor and sensory pathways after spinal cord injury.

4. REPLACEMENT OF DAMAGED ADULT CNS TISSUE BY EMBRYONIC GRAFTS

The success of neural transplantation of embryonic or immature tissue into the adult CNS depends on several factors, among which both the donor and the host have to be taken into account. Concerning the host, any initial damage or depletion of existing structures at the site where the graft is to be transplanted seems to be the most important factor. Concerning the donor tissue, although adult peripheral nerves survive transplantation into the mature host brain, transplantation of structures or cells from the central nervous system is viable only if taken from suitably aged embryonic, or in certain circumstances, neonatal donors (Björklund et al., 1983c). Relevant populations of neurones that have not yet differentiated are not suitable for grafting, while older neurones that have developed extensive connections so that dissection involves axotomy and unavoidable trauma are also unsuitable for grafting. The optimum donor age of embryo seems to vary according to species as well as the different parts of the nervous system. Results from many experiments agree that the neural tissue most suitable for grafting should be taken during the time when neurogenesis of the specific populations of cells to be used for grafting is completed. For example, in the rat, transplants of the substantia nigra, which contains dopaminergic cells, produce the best reinnervation of the caudate nucleus when taken from donors on the fourteenth and fifteenth gestational days. When donors only 12 to 36 hours older were tested, graft survival was markedly reduced (Björklund et al., 1980). Similarly, grafts of tissue from the cerebellum survive best if taken from young embryos (Sotelo 1986; Sotelo & Alvarado-Mallart, 1986; 1987a). These results indicate that optimum neuronal survival after grafting coincides with the period of proliferation, migration, and early differentiation for each neuronal type. Nevertheless, it seems possible that, after transplantation, embryonic tissue still possesses some capacity for continued neurogenesis.

The success of transplantation of embryonic neural tissue into adult donors in the midbrain (Björklund et al., 1983a; 1983b; 1983d; 1985; Björklund & Stenevi, 1984) and cerebellum (Sotelo et al., 1990; Sotelo & Alvarado-Mallart, 1986; 1987b) encouraged others to use this technique to repair the damaged spinal cord.

4.1. Grafts of Embryonic Spinal Cord

Grafts of embryonic spinal cord were used to provide permissive conditions for axonal growth. In newborn rats, these grafts placed into the lesion site were able to restore some segmental and intersegmental connections as well as some recovery of supraspinal projections that led to improved locomotor functions. After neonatal cervical spinal cord injury, transplantation of embryonic tissue into the injury site restored rhythmic alternating movements involved in locomotion, as well as the development and recovery of skilled forelimb movements involved in target-directed reaching and grooming behaviors (for review, see Bregman, 1998).

Following these successful results in neonatal animals, grafts of embryonic spinal cord were used to provide permissive conditions for axonal growth in adults after spinal cord injury. It was hoped that solid grafts of embryonic spinal cord, or relevant populations of neurones taken from embryonic spinal cord, might develop connections with the host neural circuitry, form a bridge between the two separated parts of the spinal cord, and in this way enhance restoration of CNS function (Figure 5–5).

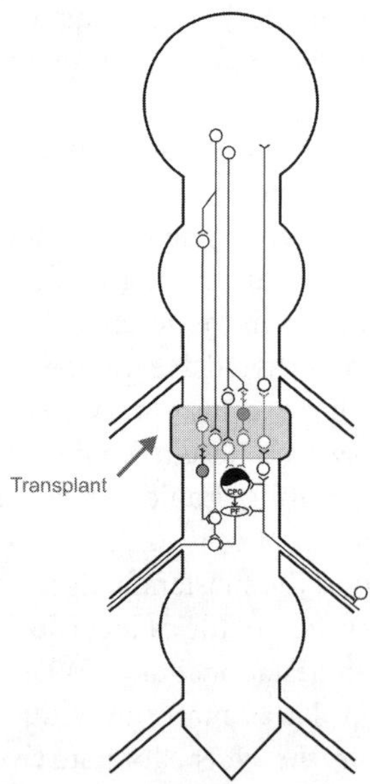

Figure 5–5 Schematic representation of the damaged spinal cord from adult rats where either solid grafts of embryonic spinal cord or cell suspension from embryonic spinal cord (illustrated in the dark-gray color) were inserted into the lesion (a shaded light gray area) to test the ability of CNS to establish a new network of neural connections (open circles—neurones; lines—the axons and dendrites; in dark-gray—grafted neurones establishing the new connections; in black—the host network). Abbreviations as in Fig. 5-1.

In contrast to results obtained in neonatal rats, in the injured spinal cord of adults, only a few short-distance connections between the graft and the host were established at the segmental level. Nevertheless, application of various trophic factors in combination with the graft increased both the density and extent of serotonergic and corticospinal axonal growth into the transplanted tissue (for review, see Bregman et al., 2002). Moreover, application of these trophic factors not only increased the growth within the transplant but also modified the cell body response to injury by upregulating growth-associated cellular programs and preventing the atrophy of the injured neurones. Thus, after partial spinal cord injury, both regenerating and sprouting axons contribute to functional recovery. In the case of total transection, the neural tissue transplants in the presence of neurotrophic factors are also able to dramatically enhance axonal regrowth into the spinal cord below the lesion. These restorations of anatomical connections across the injury site were correlated with recovery of hind limb locomotor functions. The animals demonstrated hind limb body-weight support and plantar stepping. This treatment was successful even when it was applied two to four weeks after spinal cord transection (Bregman et al., 2002; Coumans et al., 2001). Surprisingly, the amount of axonal regrowth and the extent of the recovery of motor functions were even better in the chronic animals than in the acute ones.

Not only application of trophic factors, but increasing the levels of cAMP using the phosphodiesterase inhibitor rolipram also significantly enhanced axon regrowth into the grafted spinal cord and functional recovery (Nikulina et al., 2004). The growth of injured supraspinal pathways across the transplant and into the host spinal cord caudal to the transection was confirmed by retrograde tracing, which revealed Fluoro-Gold-labeled neurones within the transplant itself and in the spinal cord rostral to the transplant as well. In addition, the labeled neurones were clearly identified within the cortex and in the brain stem nuclei, indicating the presence of axons from supraspinal and brain stem neurones that regenerated through the embryonic grafted tissue into the caudal part of the host cord. In control spinal animals (without a graft, or with a graft but without neurotrophins), there were no retrogradely labeled neurones in any of the brain stem nuclei or in the host spinal cord rostral to the lesion Bregman et al., 2002). Thus the main conclusion from these experiments is that the transplant of embryonic spinal cord tissue and the neurotrophic factors can both provide a bridge and act as a relay to restore supraspinal input to the spinal cord circuitry below the lesion across the transection site. While it is clear from these data (Bregman et al., 2002) that the anatomical connections established across the transplant in the presence of neurotrophic support contribute to the recovery of motor functions after complete spinal cord transection, whether this is related to the induced regeneration and sprouting of axons of host origin is not certain. The authors suggest that plasticity within the spinal cord caudal to the lesion and plasticity at supraspinal levels also may contribute to the recovery (Bregman et al., 2002).

4.2. Replacement of Motoneurones by Embryonic Grafts

Motoneurones are unusual cells in that that their cell body, dendrites, and the very proximal part of their axons are in the CNS (spinal cord and brain stem), while the main part of the lengthy axon that connects the neurone to its target muscle is outside the CNS. When the proximal part of the axon is injured, as is often the case in spinal cord injury, the affected motoneurones die (Lieberman, 1971). Due to this, the connection between the spinal cord and muscles can be irretrievably lost after certain types of spinal cord injury. Findings that lost motoneurones can be replaced by embryonic grafts may therefore be important for encouraging recovery after spinal cord injury.

Sieradzan and Vrbová (1989) demonstrated that motoneurone-enriched grafts of embryonic spinal cord are able to survive in the spinal cord of adult rats. However, the success of grafts of embryonic motoneurones in restoring function depends on the following factors: (1) survival of the grafted cells in the adult spinal cord, (2) the ability of the axons of the grafted motoneurones to reach and reinnervate paralyzed muscles, and (3) the integration of the grafted cells into the neuronal circuitry of the host.

Survival of grafted motoneurones

The successful survival of grafted motoneurones in the spinal cord depends both on the host environment and on the donor cells. Grafted motoneurones are usually expected to replace lost motoneurones of the host, and it has been found that a motoneurone-depleted host spinal cord provides a more favorable environment for the survival of grafted motoneurones than an undamaged spinal cord (Sieradzan & Vrbová, 1991). Regarding the donor cells, the developmental age of the donor cells used for grafting is important. The ideal time-window during development when motoneurones can be obtained with the least possible damage is between the formation of motoneurone columns and the progressive growth of their processes. In rats, this period is between days E11 and E13 in the lumbosacral cord (Altman & Bayer, 1984; Nornes & Das, 1974). Another important factor that determines the survival of the grafted motoneurones is the provision of a target muscle that they can innervate and interact with. It is well established that embryonic and neonatal motoneurones cannot survive without interacting with their target (Greensmith & Vrbová,1991; 1992). It was therefore important to provide a conduit for the axons of grafted embryonic motoneurones to allow them to establish connections with skeletal muscle fibers. Some of these conditions were fulfilled in a series of experiments on rats carried out by Sieradzan and Vrbová (for review, see Nógrádi & Szabo, 2008).

Depletion of the host motoneurones has been achieved by two different methods

First, cutting the sciatic nerve in neonatal animals permanently depletes the lumbosacral cord at the level of L4–L5 of 90% of its motoneurones. Using this method provided a host spinal cord depleted of its own motoneurones during early stages of development and ready to accept grafted cells at any developmental stage (Sieradzan & Vrbová, 1989). In these animals, however, the ventral roots of L4–L5 segments degenerated, and muscles supplied by these nerves were permanently denervated. Therefore, in these animals it was impossible to guide the axons of any neurones from the CNS towards the muscles originally supplied by the lost motoneurones of the host.

Second, another method that would allow the reconnection of grafted cells to the denervated muscles of the host was used to deplete the host spinal cord of its own motoneurones. In adult animals, ventral root avulsion results in up to 90% loss of the injured motoneurones (Lieberman, 1971) and provides a favorable environment for grafted motoneurones (Nógrádi & Vrbová, 1996b).

Connecting the axons of grafted motoneurones to skeletal muscles

Two basic strategies have been used to connect the grafted motoneurones to skeletal muscles. These experiments were designed (a) to provide the grafted motoneurones with a target muscles, and (b) to test their ability to reinnervate denervated muscles of the host. In the model where depletion of the cord was achieved during the neonatal period by injuring the sciatic nerve, a hind limb muscle from the contralateral leg was removed together with its nerve and placed paravertebraly, alongside the vertebral column, close to the site of the graft. The central end of the peripheral nerve was inserted into the cord close to the graft, with the expectation that the axons of the grafted motoneurones would enter the peripheral nerve conduit and reinnervate the muscle provided. This model was successful in that the axons of the grafted motoneurones reinnervated the muscle, induced the development of neuromuscular junctions, maintained the structural integrity of the muscle, and led to the differentiation of fiber types in the muscle innervated by the grafted motoneurones. In addition, many more grafted motoneurones survived in animals where the axons reinnervated the muscle than in animals where no muscle was provided for the graft (Clowry & Vrbová, 1992; Sieradzan & Vrbová, 1993b). In these experiments, a considerable number of grafted motoneurones expressed acetylcholinesterase, and a few of them, ChAT (cholinacetyltransferase). Interestingly, while axons of grafted cells exited the spinal cord via a peripheral nerve conduit, no axons were seen to enter the ventral root of the host (Clowry & Vrbová, 1992), and reinnervate the denervated skeletal muscles. This may have been caused by the non-permissive environment of the CNS for axon regeneration (see above).

In a different set of experiments, the spinal cord was depleted of its motoneurones in adult animals by avulsion of the ventral roots. Embryonic motoneurones were placed into the motoneurone depleted cord and the proximal part of the damaged ventral root, which is known to provide a permissive environment for axon growth (Carlstedt et al., 1989; Carlstedt & Cullheim, 2000; Cullheim et al., 1989), was reinserted into the cord close to the graft (Nógrádi & Vrbová, 1996b). The recovery of motor function and reinnervation of previously denervated muscle was followed. Retrograde labeling revealed that a large number of axons from grafted motoneurones pre-labeled with BrdU (bromodeoxyuridine) at the time of grafting, entered the reimplanted ventral root. The regenerating axons reinnervated the denervated muscles, reversed the atrophy that occurred during denervation, and reversed the paralysis suffered by the animals following ventral root avulsion.

An important issue was to examine the phenotype of the grafted cells. The grafted cells were therefore examined for markers characteristic of mature motoneurones such as the peptide CGRP, expressed in only a subgroup of motoneurones but absent in any other cell type, and ChAT, which labels all intact motoneurones. The results revealed that some but not all motoneurones of graft origin displayed these markers. This indicates that some but not all grafted motoneurones displayed these neurochemical features of mature motoneurones (Nógrádi & Vrbová, unpublished results).

These results taken together show that grafted embryonic motoneurones: (a) survive and develop in a motoneurone-depleted adult spinal cord; (b) are able to extend their axons into a suitable conduit that will guide them to the muscle; (c) reinnervate denervated skeletal muscles of the host. Potentially therefore, they are suitable candidates for replacement of motoneurones after spinal cord injury in those cases where the loss of motoneurones occurs. For meaningful recovery, however, it is essential that such grafted cells should become integrated into the spinal cord circuitry of the host. So far, this aspect of the problem is waiting to be solved.

5. ACTIVATION OF EXISTING SPINAL CORD CIRCUITRY—INTRASPINAL GRAFTING OF MONOAMINERGIC CELLS

5.1. The Importance of Serotoninergic Innervation for Normal Functions

The locomotor functions in mammals are controlled by networks of neurones located in the spinal cord and constituting the circuitry called a central pattern generator (CPG). The activity of this circuitry is controlled by descending inputs from supraspinal structures and the afferent information from the periphery. Although the locomotor movement of hind limbs can be elicited even if the CPG circuitry is separated from supraspinal and afferent inputs, the descending monoaminergic supraspinal projections are very important for the modulation of the spinal locomotor pattern-generating mechanisms and for the regulation of spinal reflex activities (see Grillner, 1985; 1996; 2002; Hultborn & Nielsen, 2007; Jordan et al., 1979; Jordan, 1998; Jordan et al., 2008). It has been shown that acute spinal cats could generate fictive locomotion after intravenous injection of L-dopa (Grillner & Zangger, 1975; Jankowska et al., 1967a; Jankowska et al., 1967b) and stepping movement on a treadmill after administration of the α_2-noradrenergic agonist clonidine (Forssberg & Grillner, 1973). It became clear that the monoaminergic projections regulate the lumbosacral neuronal circuitry that control hind limb movements (Jankowska et al., 1993; Jankowska et al., 1994; Jankowska et al., 1995; Jankowska et al., 1997; Jankowska et al., 1998). At least two descending projections of the monoaminergic system; that is, serotoninergic and noradrenergic, play a crucial role in the control of the excitability of the spinal circuitry. The supraspinal serotonergic descending projections are involved in the initiation and control of locomotor hind limb movements (Jordan et al., 2008).There is ample evidence to show that descending serotonergic pathways make synaptic contact with motoneurones (Holstege & Kuypers, 1987; Jordan & Schmidt, 2002; Ulfhake et al., 1987) and increase their excitability (Jordan & Schmidt, 2002; White & Neuman, 1980; White & Neuman, 1983). Moreover, local application of these monoamines modulates the transmission between primary afferents and premotor interneurones. This has a particularly strong impact on reflex actions because these interneurones directly excite or inhibit motoneurones (Jankowska et al., 2000).

In addition to hind limb locomotor movements, the urogenital and bladder functions as well as penile erection are controlled by the neural circuitry of the spinal cord, and the normal bladder function requires spinal and supraspinal control. Micturition requires coordinated activation of the smooth muscle of the bladder (detrusor) and striated muscle of the external urethral sphincter. This is achieved by the integration of excitatory, inhibitory, and sensory nerve activity in control centers in the spinal cord, pons, and forebrain. The spinal cord at the L6–S1 level of rats contains the autonomic preganglionic neurones that control urogenital function. Moreover, the ventral horn of the L5–L6 segment of the spinal cord contains motoneurones that supply pelvic striated muscles; for example, the ischiocavernosus and bulbospongiosus muscles (Faden et al., 1988; Schroder, 1980; Schroder & Skagerberg, 1985), and these particular neurones receive strong serotoninergic projections.

The reduced release of noradrenaline and serotonin after spinal cord injury markedly alters the locomotor functions as well as the bladder, bowl control, and sexual reflexes. Total spinal cord transection induces almost complete disappearance of monoaminergic neurotransmitters below the lesion (Faden et al., 1988). After spinal cord transection, extensor excitability is sharply reduced, and the stretch reflex is almost abolished, and subsequent administration of serotonin precursors or agonists can restore their functions considerably (Ahlman et al., 1971; Ellaway & Trott, 1975). Trials with systemic administration (intravenous or intraperitoneal) of monoamine agonists demonstrated some modifications of spinal reflexes and improvement of locomotor performance of animals that had their spinal cord transected (Barbeau & Rossignol, 1987; 1990; 1991; 1994). It has to be pointed that, although the systemic administration of monoaminergic drugs positively modulates many neurological functions, it also affects the peripheral autonomic nervous system and has serious side effects (Fung et al., 1990). Therefore, various methods for local intraspinal application of monoaminergic drugs are being explored.

5.2. Restoration of Function by Intraspinal Grafting of Serotoninergic Embryonic Cells

A promising approach is the grafting of embryonic cells destined to release monoamines taken from the brain stem into the spinal cord below the site of the lesion (see Figure 5–6). These embryonic cells can survive and release monoamines in their new environment. One can then assume that neurotransmitters, such as serotonin or noradrenaline, released from intraspinally grafted monoaminergic neurones, would be able to locally stimulate neural structures and in this way regulate lost neural functions. It might be that the complex sequences of the locomotor-like hind limb movement as well as the penile reflexes that are dramatically altered after spinal cord injury in mammals could be significantly restored using this therapy.

The results of first homologous fetal brain grafts were published almost 30 years ago (Nygren et al., 1977). It was shown that immature cells containing noradrenaline (NA) from locus coeruleus and 5-hydroxytryptamine (5-HT) from raphe nuclei could survive transplantation into an adult spinal cord previously deprived of their noradrenergic and serotonergic inputs by a total transection of the spinal cord. Since then, two different methods of transplantation have been developed. In one, a solid piece of embryonic tissue was grafted into the lumbar spinal cord (Commissiong, 1983; Nygren et al., 1977; Sławińska et al., 2000); in another, cell suspension was used for intraspinal grafting (i.e., Björklund et al., 1983c; Buchanan & Nornes, 1986; Foster et al., 1989; Privat et al., 1986; Rajaofetra et al., 1992a). In both cases, the defined region of the brain stem containing the raphe and/or locus coeruleus nuclei was dissected from rat embryos (E14–E15) of the same inbred strain as the host (for methods, see Cooper et al., 1996; Rajaofetra et al., 1992b; Sławińska et al., 2000).

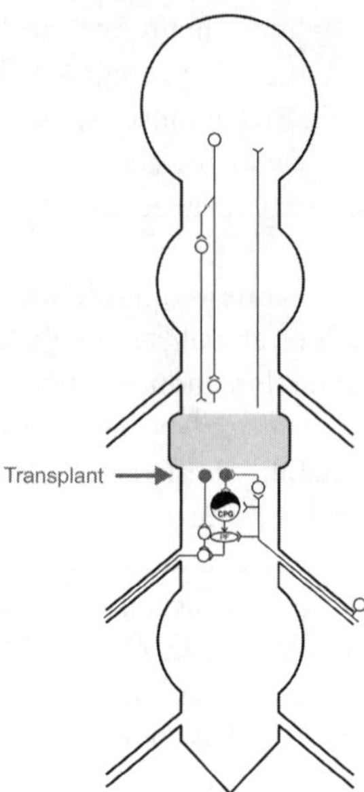

Figure 5–6 Transplantation of embryonic serotonergic cells into the spinal cord below the site of the lesion. This strategy is able to enhance the restoration of motor function by the reestablished monoaminergic innervations of the host spinal cord circuitry by the axons of the grafted cells. The grafted cells provide a relatively precise targeting of serotoninergic influences over the host spinal cord and can not only act as a source of a diffusely released neurotransmitter, but can also selectively activate or inhibit the appropriate cell populations of the host spinal cord that control hind limb locomotor movement. In the figures, there are schematically represented possible ways of connections restored using this strategy to the motoneurones and to the structures that control locomotor movement. Abbreviations as in Fig. 5–1.

This age of fetuses corresponds to the time when most of the neurogenesis in the embryonic brain stem nuclei is completed.

It is important to note that in the spinal cord of adult mammals the only source of monoaminergic fibers is from axons and terminals of neurones from supraspinal structures. Thus, the spinal cord of rats below the site of total transection is completely devoid of monoaminergic innervation. Following intraspinal transplantation of the raphe nuclei, the 5-HT-immunoreactive neurones usually are distributed in the host cord in two locations: (a) within the solid tissue implants, and (b) in the host gray matter near the injection site (Buchanan & Nornes, 1986; Sławińska et al., 2000). The question of whether the transplantation of cell suspension or that of a solid piece of tissue is more effective is still open. The former seems to hold greatest promise for extensive reinnervation of the larger areas of the cord due to a better chance for migration of single cells from the injection site. However, it has been reported that many serotoninergic cells grafted in a solid piece of tissue migrated from the graft over a distance of up to 1.2 mm from the site of injection (Sławińska et al., 2000). Moreover, it seems that there are certain advantages of grafting a solid piece of tissue over cell suspension grafts into a spinal cord. First, the grafted solid tissue has an intact structure with the supporting glial and other cells, which protects the serotoninergic neurones from damage. Second, the solid graft is naturally less likely to be flushed away by cerebrospinal fluid at the time of surgery. Third, the solid transplant can be monitored post-grafting by *in vivo* magnetic resonance imaging (Akesson et al., 2001). It was also reported that human solid grafts of embryonic spinal cord have a more restricted growth pattern than the grafted cell suspension (Akesson et al., 2001). Nevertheless, in case of both techniques discussed, the serotoninergic or noradrenergic cells extended their axons into the distal part of the transected spinal cord, spreading rostrally up to the level of transection, and caudally for a considerable distance. In both cases the longest of the serotoninergic axons reached a distance of 15 mm–20 mm from the level at which serotoninergic perikarya were still visible (Foster et al., 1989; Privat et al., 1989; Sławińska et al., 2000). Thus, these results demonstrate that the effectiveness of reinnervation by serotoninergic cells grafted into the spinal cord as suspension or as solid pieces of tissue was very similar.

The first attempt to investigate the functional improvement in hind limb movement recovery related to grafted noradrenergic cells was undertaken by Buchanan and Nornes (Buchanan & Nornes, 1986), who tested the force of the hind limb flexion reflex after acute spinal transection. This reflex is strongly enhanced by catecholamines (Grossmann et al., 1975; Nygren & Olson, 1976), and consistent with this in rats with grafted noradrenergic cells, the flexion reflexes were significantly stronger than in the controls. Further evidence that the increase in the strength of the flexion reflex was mediated via noradrenergic inputs was provided by results that showed that these effects were blocked by α-adrenergic receptors. These results demonstrated that grafts of embryonic locus coeruleus cells survive, grow, and expand catecholamine containing processes, and affect the functional activity of the spinal cord.

The first investigators of functional improvement after grafting serotoninergic cells into the spinal cord of paraplegic rats (Privat et al., 1988) focused their attention on the control of sexual reflexes. In contrast to animals without a graft, in paraplegic rats that have received the graft of raphe cells, penis stimulation was followed by ejaculation (Privat et al., 1988). Thus, in addition to good survival of grafted cells, in paraplegic rats, sexual reflexes were also restored.

Studies of the effects of raphe grafts on hind limb locomotor abilities tested rats suspended over a moving treadmill or examined fictive motor activities (Yakovleff et al., 1989; Yakovleff et al., 1995). In contrast to control paraplegic rats, in paraplegic rats that received a graft of embryonic locus coeruleus neurones, a bilateral, alternating, rhythmic locomotor-like activity was recorded in muscle nerves. This effect was mediated by 5-HT-containing neurones, since removal of noradrenergic cells by 6-hydroxydopamine had no effect on the restored locomotor-like activity. These results led to the conclusion that the reestablished serotoninergic innervation was the most important factor for the restoration of locomotor function of hind limb muscles in adult paraplegic rats. The recovery of motor function in adult rats with their spinal cord transected at the thoracic level was investigated using several behavioral tests, including kinematic and electromyographic analysis of hind limb movement during bipedal locomotion (Majczyński et al., 2005; Ribotta et al., 2000; Sławińska et al., 2000), as well as some simple spinal reflexes (Sławińska et al., 2000). Results from these studies revealed an improved recovery of hind limb motor function in the adult paraplegic rats independently of whether the grafting was performed one week or one month after spinal cord transection. Moreover, it was demonstrated that the improved hind limb locomotor function restoration brought about by grafted serotonin-releasing cells was mediated by 5-HT2 receptors, since cyproheptadine (5-HT2 antagonist) i.p. application significantly affected the hind limb movement restored by the graft (Majczyński et al., 2005).

The enhanced recovery of hind limb motor functions is probably due to the increased excitability of the neuronal circuitry in the injured spinal cord. The greater excitability of the spinal neural circuitry in paraplegic rats that have received the graft of the embryonic brain stem containing raphe nuclei was indicated by the appearance of (a) the coordinated locomotor pattern, (b) the spontaneous air stepping, and (c) the low threshold for evoking simple hind limb reflexes. Thus the new monoaminergic connections between the grafted cells and host spinal cord provide a relatively precise targeting of serotoninergic influences over the host spinal cord. The grafted cells therefore not only act as a source of a diffusely released neurotransmitter, but can also selectively activate or inhibit the appropriate cell populations of the host spinal cord.

6. CONCLUSIONS

Although some of the interventions described above enhance functional recovery in various animal models the improvement may not be the same in humans, or may not be of sufficient magnitude to improve the everyday quality of life of individuals with spinal cord injury. Therefore a combination of effective and safe therapeutic interventions will be required. These interventions should combine biological interventions with methods used to induce recovery of function by externally driven devices that activate the neuronal circuitry of the spinal cord as described in other Chapters of this book. Moreover, due to the unpredictability of the consequences of the injury of different parts of the spinal cord, to obtain the best functional recovery, different strategies for neural tissue repair need to be coordinated in space and in time. Moreover, the outcome of the effects of any new interventions has to be assessed with caution to avoid the risk of inducing unjustified hopes in patients suffering from spinal cord trauma or any other CNS injury.

References

Aguayo, A. J., Bray, G. M., Carter, D. A., Villegas-Perez, M. P., Vidal-Sanz, M., Rasminsky, M. "Regrowth and connectivity of injured central nervous system axons in adult rodents." *Acta Neurobiologiae Experimentalis* (Warsaw) 50 (1990): 381–389.

Aguayo, A. J., Rasminsky, M., Bray, G. M., et al. "Degenerative and regenerative responses of injured neurons in the central nervous system of adult mammals." *Philosophical Transactions of the Royal Society: B. Biological Sciences* 331 (1991): 337–343.

Ahlman, H., Grillner, S., Udo, M. "The effect of 5-HTP on the static fusimotor activity and the tonic stretch reflex of an extensor muscle." *Brain Research* 27 (1971): 393–396.

Akesson, E., Holmberg, L., Jonhagen, M. E., et al. "Solid human embryonic spinal cord xenografts in acute and chronic spinal cord cavities: A morphological and functional study." *Experimental Neurology* 170 (2001): 305–316.

Akiyama, Y., Lankford, K., Radtke, C., Greer, C. A., Kocsis, J. D. "Remyelination of spinal cord axons by olfactory ensheathing cells and Schwann cells derived from a transgenic rat expressing alkaline phosphatase marker gene." *Neuron Glia Biology* 1 (2004): 47–55.

Akiyama, Y., Radtke, C., Kocsis J. D. "Remyelination of the rat spinal cord by transplantation of identified bone marrow stromal cells." *Journal of Neuroscience* 22 (2002): 6623–6630.

Altman, J., Bayer, S. A. "The development of the rat spinal cord." *Advances in Anatomy, Embryology, and Cell Biology* 85 (1984): 1–164.

Ankeny, D. P., McTigue, D. M., Jakeman, L. B. "Bone marrow transplants provide tissue protection and directional guidance for axons after contusive spinal cord injury in rats." *Experimental Neurology* 190 (2004): 17–31.

Avellino, A. M., Hart, D., Dailey, A. T., Mackinnon, M., Ellegala, D., Kliot, M. "Differential macrophage responses in the peripheral and central nervous system during Wallerian degeneration of axons." *Experimental Neurology* 136 (1995): 183–198.

Bamber, N. I., Li, H., Lu, X., Oudega, M., Aebischer, P., Xu, X. M. "Neurotrophins BDNF and NT-3 promote axonal re-entry into the distal host spinal cord through Schwann cell–seeded mini-channels." *European Journal of Neuroscience* 13 (2001): 257–268.

Barbeau, H., Rossignol, S. "Recovery of locomotion after chronic spinalization in the adult cat." *Brain Research* 412 (1987): 84–95.

Barbeau, H., Rossignol, S. "The effects of serotonergic drugs on the locomotor pattern and on cutaneous reflexes of the adult chronic spinal cat." *Brain Research* 514 (1990): 55–67.

Barbeau, H., Rossignol, S. "Initiation and modulation of the locomotor pattern in the adult chronic spinal cat by noradrenergic, serotonergic and dopaminergic drugs." *Brain Research* 546 (1991): 250–260.

Barbeau, H., Rossignol, S. "Enhancement of locomotor recovery following spinal cord injury." *Current Opinion in Neurology* 7 (1994): 517–524.

Barnard, J. W., Carpenter, W. "Lack of regeneration in spinal cord of rat." *Journal of Neurophysiology* 13 (1950): 223–228.

Barnett, S. C., Alexander, C. L., Iwashita, Y., et al. "Identification of a human olfactory ensheathing cell that can effect transplant-mediated remyelination of demyelinated CNS axons." *Brain* 123 (2000): 1581–1588.

Barnett, S. C., Chang, L. "Olfactory ensheathing cells and CNS repair: Going solo or in need of a friend?" *Trends in Neuroscience* 27 (2004): 54–60.

Basso, D. M., Beattie, M. S., Bresnahan, J. C. "A sensitive and reliable locomotor rating scale for open field testing in rats." *Journal of Neurotrauma* 12 (1995): 1–21.

Beattie, M. S., Hermann, G. E., Rogers, R. C., Bresnahan, J. C. "Cell death in models of spinal cord injury." *Progress in Brain Research* 137 (2002): 37–47.

Beattie, M. S., Li, Q., Bresnahan, J. C. "Cell death and plasticity after experimental spinal cord injury." *Progress in Brain Research* 128 (2000): 9–21.

Bedi, K. S., Winter, J., Berry, M., Cohen, J. "Adult rat dorsal root ganglion neurons extend neurites on predegenerated but not on normal peripheral nerves in vitro." *European Journal of Neuroscience* 4 (1992): 193–200.

Benveniste, E. N. "Inflammatory cytokines within the central nervous system: Sources, function, and mechanism of action." *American Journal of Physiology* 263 (1992): C1–C16.

Björklund, A., Gage, F. H., Schmidt, R. H., Stenevi, U., Dunnett, S. B. "Intracerebral grafting of neuronal cell suspensions. VII. Recovery of choline acetyltransferase activity and acetylcholine synthesis in the denervated hippocampus reinnervated by septal suspension implants." *Acta Physiologica Scandinavica* Suppl 522 (1983a): 59–66.

Björklund, A., Gage, F. H., Stenevi, U., Dunnett, S. B. "Intracerebral grafting of neuronal cell suspensions. VI. Survival and growth of intrahippocampal implants of septal cell suspensions." *Acta Physiologica Scandinavica* Suppl 522 (1983b): 49–58.

Björklund, A., Gage, F. H., Stenevi, U., Dunnett, S. B., Kelly, P. A. "Intracerebral neural grafting in animal models of aging brain: Strategies, rationale and preliminary results." *Danish Medical Bulletin* 32 Suppl 1 (1985): 35–39.

Björklund, A., Schmidt, R. H., Stenevi, U. "Functional reinnervation of the neostriatum in the adult rat by use of intraparenchymal grafting of dissociated cell suspensions from the substantia nigra." *Cell Tissue Research* 212 (1980): 39–45.

Björklund, A., Stenevi, U. "Reconstruction of the nigrostriatal dopamine pathway by intracerebral nigral transplants." *Brain Research* 177 (1979): 555–560.

Björklund, A., Stenevi, U. "Intracerebral neural implants: Neuronal replacement and reconstruction of damaged circuitries." *Annual Review of Neuroscience* 7 (1984): 279–308.

Björklund, A., Stenevi, U., Schmidt, R. H., Dunnett, S. B., Gage, F. H. "Intracerebral grafting of neuronal cell suspensions. I. Introduction and general methods of preparation." *Acta Physiologica Scandinavica* Suppl 522 (1983c): 1–7.

Björklund, A., Stenevi, U., Schmidt, R. H., Dunnett, S. B., Gage, F. H. "Intracerebral grafting of neuronal cell suspensions. II. Survival and growth of nigral cell suspensions implanted in different brain sites." *Acta Physiologica Scandinavica* Suppl 522 (1983d): 9–18.

Björklund, A., Stenevi, U., Svendgaard, N. "Growth of transplanted monoaminergic neurones into the adult hippocampus along the perforant path." *Nature* 262 (1976): 787–790.

Blakemore, W. F., Crang, A. J. "The use of cultured autologous Schwann cells to remyelinate areas of persistent demyelination in the central nervous system." *Journal of the Neurological Sciences* 70 (1985): 207–223.

Blight, A. R. "Delayed demyelination and macrophage invasion: A candidate for secondary cell damage in spinal cord injury." *Central Nervous System Trauma* 2 (1985): 299–315.

Blight, A. R. "Macrophages and inflammatory damage in spinal cord injury." *Journal of Neurotrauma* 9 Suppl 1 (1992): S83–S91.

Blight, A. R. "Effects of silica on the outcome from experimental spinal cord injury: Implication of macrophages in secondary tissue damage." *Neuroscience* 60 (1994): 263–273.

Blits, B., Dijkhuizen, P. A., Boer, G. J., Verhaagen, J. "Intercostal nerve implants transduced with an adenoviral vector encoding neurotrophin-3 promote regrowth of injured rat corticospinal tract fibers and improve hind limb function." *Experimental Neurology* 164 (2000): 25–37.

Bomstein, Y., Marder, J. B., Vitner, K., et al. "Features of skin-coincubated macrophages that promote recovery from spinal cord injury." *Journal of Neuroimmunology* 142 (2003): 10–16.

Boyd, J. G., Doucette, R., Kawaja, M. D. "Defining the role of olfactory ensheathing cells in facilitating axon remyelination following damage to the spinal cord." *Journal of the Federation of American Societies for Experimental Biology* 19 (2005): 694–703.

Boyd, J. G., Lee, J., Skihar, V., Doucette, R., Kawaja, M. D. "LacZ-expressing olfactory ensheathing cells do not associate with myelinated axons after implantation into the compressed spinal cord." *Proceedings of the National Academy of Sciences* (U.S.) 101 (2004): 2162–2166.

Boyd, J. G., Skihar, V., Kawaja, M., Doucette, R. "Olfactory ensheathing cells: Historical perspective and therapeutic potential." *Anatomical Record (Part B: New Anatomy)* 271 (2003): 49–60.

Bray, G. M., Villegas-Perez, M. P., Vidal-Sanz, M., Aguayo, A. J. "The use of peripheral nerve grafts to enhance neuronal survival, promote growth and permit terminal reconnections in the central nervous system of adult rats." *Journal of Experimental Biology* 132 (1987): 5–19.

Bregman, B. S. "Regeneration in the spinal cord." *Current Opinion in Neurobiology* 8 (1998): 800–807.

Bregman, B. S., Coumans, J. V., Dai, H. N., et al. "Transplants and neurotrophic factors increase regeneration and recovery of function after spinal cord injury." *Progress in Brain Research* 137 (2002): 257–273.

Brown, J. O., McCouch, G. P. "Abortive regeneration of the transected spinal cord." *Journal of Comparative Neurology* 87 (1947): 131–137.

Brown, M. C., Perry, V. H., Lunn, E. R., Gordon, S., Heumann, R. "Macrophage dependence of peripheral sensory nerve regeneration: Possible involvement of nerve growth factor." *Neuron* 6 (1991): 359–370.

Brunelli, G., Milanesi, S., Bartolaminelli, P., De, F. G., Brunelli, F., Bottonelli, P. V. "Experimental grafts in spinal cord lesions (preliminary report)." *Italian Journal of Orthopaedics and Traumatology* 9 Suppl. (1983): 53–56.

Brunelli, G. A. "Direct neurotization of muscles by presynaptic motoneurons." *Journal of Reconstructive Microsurgery* 17 (2001): 631–636.

Brunelli, G. A., Brunelli, G. R. "Experimental surgery in spinal cord lesions by connecting upper motoneurons directly to peripheral targets." *Journal of Peripheral Nervous System* 1 (1996): 111–118.

Buchanan, J. T., Nornes, H. O. "Transplants of embryonic brain stem containing the locus coeruleus into spinal cord enhance the hindlimb flexion reflex in adult rats." *Brain Research* 381 (1986): 225–236.

Bunge, M. B. "Bridging areas of injury in the spinal cord." *Neuroscientist* 7 (2001): 325–339.

Bunge, R. P. "Tissue culture observations relevant to the study of axon–Schwann cell interactions during peripheral nerve development and repair." *Journal of Experimental Biology* 132 (1987): 21–34.

Bunge, R. P. "Expanding roles for the Schwann cell: Ensheathment, myelination, trophism and regeneration." *Current Opinion in Neurobiology* 3 (1993): 805–809.

Bunge, R. P., Wood, P. M. "Tissue culture studies of interactions between axons and myelinating cells of the central and peripheral nervous system." *Progress in Brain Research* 71 (1987): 143–152.

Cadelli, D. S., Bandtlow, C. E., Schwab, M. E. "Oligodendrocyte- and myelin-associated inhibitors of neurite outgrowth: Their involvement in the lack of CNS regeneration." *Experimental Neurology* 115 (1992): 189–192.

Campos, L., Meng, Z., Hu, G., Chiu, D. T., Ambron, R. T., Martin, J. H. "Engineering novel spinal circuits to promote recovery after spinal injury." *Journal of Neuroscience* 24 (2004): 2090–2101.

Campos, L. W., Chakrabarty, S., Haque, R., Martin, J. H. "Regenerating motor bridge axons refine connections and synapse on lumbar motoneurons to bypass chronic spinal cord injury." *Journal of Comparative Neurology* 506 (2008): 838–850.

Carlsson, C. A., Sundin, T. "Reconstruction of afferent and efferent nervous pathways to the urinary bladder in two paraplegic patients." *Spine* 5 (1980): 37–41.

Carlstedt, T., Cullheim, S. "Spinal cord motoneuron maintenance, injury and repair." *Progress in Brain Research* 127 (2000): 501–514.

Carlstedt, T., Cullheim, S., Risling, M., Ulfhake, B. "Nerve fibre regeneration across the PNS-CNS interface at the root-spinal cord junction." *Brain Research Bulletin* 22 (1989): 93–102.

Caroni, P., Schwab, M. E. "Two membrane protein fractions from rat central myelin with inhibitory properties for neurite growth and fibroblast spreading." *Journal of Cell Biology* 106 (1988): 1281–1288.

Casella, G. T., Bunge, R. P., Wood, P. M. "Improved method for harvesting human Schwann cells from mature peripheral nerve and expansion in vitro." *Glia* 17 (1996): 327–338.

Cheng, H., Almstrom, S., Gimenez-Llort, L., et al. "Gait analysis of adult paraplegic rats after spinal cord repair." *Experimental Neurology* 148 (1997): 544–557.

Cheng, H., Cao, Y., Olson, L. "Spinal cord repair in adult paraplegic rats: Partial restoration of hind limb function." *Science* 273 (1996): 510–513.

Cheng, H., Olson, L. "A new surgical technique that allows proximodistal regeneration of 5-HT fibers after complete transection of the rat spinal cord." *Experimental Neurology* 136 (1995): 149–161.

Clowry, G. J., Vrbová, G. "Observations on the development of transplanted embryonic ventral horn neurones grafted into adult rat spinal cord and connected to skeletal muscle implants via a peripheral nerve." *Experimental Brain Research* 91 (1992): 249–258.

Commissiong, J. W. "Fetal locus coeruleus transplanted into the transected spinal cord of the adult rat." *Brain Research* 271 (1983): 174–179.

Cooper, R. N., Feraboli-Lohnherr, D., Butler-Browne, G., Orsal, D., Ribotta, M., Privat, A. "Intraspinal injection of embryonic neurons maintains muscle phenotype in adult chronic spinal rats." *Journal of Neuroscience Research* 46 (1996): 324–329.

Coumans, J. V., Lin, T. T., Dai, H. N., et al. "Axonal regeneration and functional recovery after complete spinal cord transection in rats by delayed treatment with transplants and neurotrophins." *Journal of Neuroscience* 21 (2001): 9334–9344.

Cullheim, S., Carlstedt, T., Linda, H., Risling, M., Ulfhake, B. "Motoneurons reinnervate skeletal muscle after ventral root implantation into the spinal cord of the cat." *Neuroscience* 29 (1989): 725–733.

Dailey, A. T., Avellino, A. M., Benthem, L., Silver, J., Kliot, M. "Complement depletion reduces macrophage infiltration and activation during Wallerian degeneration and axonal regeneration." *Journal of Neuroscience* 18 (1998): 6713–6722.

Dasari, V. R., Spomar, D. G., Li, L., Gujrati, M., Rao, J. S., Dinh, D. H. "Umbilical cord blood stem cell mediated downregulation of fas improves functional recovery of rats after spinal cord injury." *Neurochemical Research* 33 (2008): 134–149.

David, S., Bouchard, C., Tsatas, O., Giftochristos, N. "Macrophages can modify the nonpermissive nature of the adult mammalian central nervous system." *Neuron* 5 (1990): 463–469.

Davies, S. J., Fitch, M. T., Memberg, S. P., Hall, A. K., Raisman, G., Silver, J. "Regeneration of adult axons in white matter tracts of the central nervous system." *Nature* 390 (1997): 680–683.

Devon, R., Doucette, R. "Olfactory ensheathing cells do not require L-ascorbic acid in vitro to assemble a basal lamina or to myelinate dorsal root ganglion neurites." *Brain Research* 688 (1995): 223–229.

Doucette, R. "Olfactory ensheathing cells: Potential for glial cell transplantation into areas of CNS injury." *Histology and Histopathology* 10 (1995): 503–507.

Eitan, S., Zisling, R., Cohen, A., et al. "Identification of an interleukin 2-like substance as a factor cytotoxic to oligodendrocytes and associated with central nervous system regeneration." *Proceedings of the National Academy of Sciences* (U.S.) 89 (1992): 5442–5446.

Ellaway, P. H., Trott, J. R. The mode of action of 5-hydroxytryptophan in facilitating a stretch reflex in the spinal cat. *Experimental Brain Research* 22 (1975): 145–162.

Faden, A. I., Gannon, A., Basbaum, A. I. "Use of serotonin immunocytochemistry as a marker of injury severity after experimental spinal trauma in rats." *Brain Research* 450 (1988): 94–100.

Fawcett, J. W., Asher, R. A. "The glial scar and central nervous system repair." *Brain Research Bulletin* 49 (1999): 377–391.

Feigin, I., Geller, E. H., Wolf, A. "Absence of regeneration in the spinal cord of the young rat." *Journal of Neuropathology and Experimental Neurology* 10 (1951): 420–425.

Fitch, M. T., Silver, J. "CNS injury, glial scars, and inflammation: Inhibitory extracellular matrices and regeneration failure." *Experimental Neurology* 209 (2008): 294–301.

Forssberg, H., Grillner, S. "The locomotion of the acute spinal cat injected with clonidine i.v." *Brain Research* 50 (1973): 184–186.

Foster, G. A., Roberts, M. H., Wilkinson, L. S., et al. "Structural and functional analysis of raphe neurone implants into denervated rat spinal cord." *Brain Research Bulletin* 22 (1989): 131–137.

Franklin, R. J., Barnett, S. C. "Olfactory ensheathing cells and CNS regeneration: The sweet smell of success?" *Neuron* 28 (2000): 15–18.

Franklin, R. J., Gilson, J. M. "Remyelination in the CNS of the hypothyroid rat." *Neuroreport* 7 (1996): 1526–1530.

Franzen, R., Schoenen, J., Leprince, P., Joosten, E., Moonen, G., Martin, D. "Effects of macrophage transplantation in the injured adult rat spinal cord: A combined immunocytochemical and biochemical study." *Journal of Neuroscience Research* 51(1998): 316–327.

Fung, J., Stewart, J. E., Barbeau, H. "The combined effects of clonidine and cyproheptadine with interactive training on the modulation of locomotion in spinal cord injured subjects." *Journal of Neurological Sciences* 100 (1990): 85–93.

Gaiano, N., Fishell, G. "Transplantation as a tool to study progenitors within the vertebrate nervous system." *Journal of Neurobiology* 36 (1998): 152–161.

Garbuzova-Davis, S., Willing, A. E., Saporta, S., et al. "Novel cell therapy approaches for brain repair." *Progress in Brain Research* 157 (2006): 207–222.

Garcia-Alias, G., Lopez-Vales, R., Fores, J., Navarro, X., Verdu, E. "Acute transplantation of olfactory ensheathing cells or Schwann cells promotes recovery after spinal cord injury in the rat." *Journal of Neuroscience Research* 75 (2004): 632–641.

Gensel, J. C., Nakamura, S., Guan, Z., van Rooijen, N., Ankeny, D. P., Popovich, P. G. "Macrophages promote axon regeneration with concurrent neurotoxicity." *Journal of Neuroscience* 29 (2009): 3956–3968.

George, R., Griffin, J. W. "Delayed macrophage responses and myelin clearance during Wallerian degeneration in the central nervous system: The dorsal radiculotomy model." *Experimental Neurology* 129 (1994): 225–236.

Giulian, D., Chen, J., Ingeman, J. E., George, J. K., Noponen, M. "The role of mononuclear phagocytes in wound healing after traumatic injury to adult mammalian brain." *Journal of Neuroscience* 9 (1989): 4416–4429.

Giulian, D., Robertson, C. "Inhibition of mononuclear phagocytes reduces ischemic injury in the spinal cord." *Annals of Neurology* 27 (1990): 33–42.

Gomez, V. M., Averill, S., King, V., et al. "Transplantation of olfactory ensheathing cells fails to promote significant axonal regeneration from dorsal roots into the rat cervical cord." *Journal of Neurocytology* 32 (2003): 53–70.

Gordon, S. "The macrophage." *Bioessays* 17 (1995): 977–986.

Greensmith, L., Vrbová, G. "Neuromuscular contacts in the developing rat soleus depend on muscle activity." *Brain Research: Developmental Brain Research* 62 (1991): 121–129.

Greensmith, L., Vrbová, G. "Alterations of nerve-muscle interaction during postnatal development influence motoneurone survival in rats." *Brain Research: Developmental Brain Research* 69 (1992): 125–131.

Grillner, S. "Neurobiological bases of rhythmic motor acts in vertebrates." *Science* 228 (1985): 143–149.

Grillner, S. "Neural networks for vertebrate locomotion." *Scientific American* 274 (1996): 64–69.

Grillner, S. "The spinal locomotor CPG: A target after spinal cord injury." *Progress in Brain Research* 137 (2002): 97–108.

Grillner, S., Zangger, P. "How detailed is the central pattern generation for locomotion?" *Brain Research* 88 (1975): 367–371.

Grossmann, W., Jurna, I., Nell, T. "The effect of reserpine and DOPA on reflex activity in the rat spinal cord." *Experimental Brain Research* 22 (1975): 351–361.

Gudino-Cabrera, G., Nieto-Sampedro, M. "Schwann-like macroglia in adult rat brain." *Glia* 30 (2000): 49–63.

Guest, J. D., Rao, A., Olson, L., Bunge, M. B., Bunge, R. P. "The ability of human Schwann cell grafts to promote regeneration in the transected nude rat spinal cord." *Experimental Neurology* 148 (1997b): 502–522.

Harel, A., Fainaru, M., Shafer, Z., Hernandez, M., Cohen, A., Schwartz, M. "Optic nerve regeneration in adult fish and apolipoprotein A-I." *Journal of Neurochemistry* 52 (1989): 1218–1228.

Heumann, R., Korsching, S., Bandtlow, C., Thoenen, H. "Changes of nerve growth factor synthesis in nonneuronal cells in response to sciatic nerve transection." *Journal of Cell Biology* 104 (1987a): 1623–1631.

Heumann, R., Lindholm, D., Bandtlow, C., et al. "Differential regulation of mRNA encoding nerve growth factor and its receptor in rat sciatic nerve during development, degeneration, and regeneration: Role of macrophages." *Proceedings of the National Academy Science* (U.S.) 84 (1987b): 8735–8739.

Hikawa, N., Takenaka, T. "Sensory neurons regulate immunoglobulin secretion of spleen cells: Cellular analysis of bidirectional communications between neurons and immune cells." *Journal of Neuroimmunology* 70 (1996): 191–198.

Hill, A. J., Zwart, I., Tam, H. H., et al. "Human umbilical cord blood-derived mesenchymal stem cells do not differentiate into neural cell types or integrate into the retina after intravitreal grafting in neonatal rats." *Stem Cells Development* 18 (2009): 399–409.

Holstege, J. C., Kuypers, H. G. "Brain stem projections to lumbar motoneurons in rat. I. An ultrastructural study using autoradiography and the combination of autoradiography and horseradish peroxidase histochemistry." *Neuroscience* 21 (1987): 345–367.

Horvat, J. C., Pecot-Dechavassine, M., Mira, J. C., Davarpanah, Y. "Formation of functional endplates by spinal axons regenerating through a peripheral nerve graft. A study in the adult rat." *Brain Research Bulletin* 22 (1989): 103–114.

Huber, A. B., Schwab, M. E. "Nogo-A, a potent inhibitor of neurite outgrowth and regeneration." *Biological Chemistry* 381 (2000): 407–419.

Hultborn, H., Nielsen, J. B. "Spinal control of locomotion—from cat to man." *Acta Physiologica* (Oxford, UK) 189 (2007): 111–121.

Imaizumi, T., Lankford, K. L., Kocsis, J. D. "Transplantation of olfactory ensheathing cells or Schwann cells restores rapid and secure conduction across the transected spinal cord." *Brain Research* 854 (2000): 70–78.

Imaizumi, T., Lankford, K. L., Waxman, S. G., Greer, C. A., Kocsis, J. D. "Transplanted olfactory ensheathing cells remyelinate and enhance axonal conduction in the demyelinated dorsal columns of the rat spinal cord." *Journal of Neuroscience* 18 (1998): 6176–6185.

Jankowska, E., Gladden, M. H., Czarkowska-Bauch, J. "Modulation of responses of feline gamma-motoneurones by noradrenaline, tizanidine and clonidine." *Journal of Physiology* 512 (1998): 521–531.

Jankowska, E., Hammar, I., Chojnicka, B., Heden, C. H. "Effects of monoamines on interneurons in four spinal reflex pathways from group I and/or group II muscle afferents." *European Journal of Neuroscience* 12 (2000): 701–714.

Jankowska, E., Hammar, I., Djouhri, L., Heden, C., Szabo, L. Z., Yin, X. K. "Modulation of responses of four types of feline ascending tract neurons by serotonin and noradrenaline." *European Journal of Neuroscience* 9 (1997): 1375–1387.

Jankowska, E., Jukes, M. G., Lund, S., Lundberg, A. "The effect of DOPA on the spinal cord. 5. Reciprocal organization of pathways transmitting excitatory action to alpha motoneurones of flexors and extensors." *Acta Physiologica Scandinavica* 70 (1967a): 369–388.

Jankowska, E., Jukes, M. G., Lund, S., Lundberg, A. "The effect of DOPA on the spinal cord. 6. Half-centre organization of interneurones transmitting effects from the flexor reflex afferents." *Acta Physiologica Scandinavica* 70 (1967b): 389–402.

Jankowska, E., Krutki, P., Lackberg, Z. S., Hammar, I. "Effects of serotonin on dorsal horn dorsal spinocerebellar tract neurons." *Neuroscience* 67 (1995): 489–495.

Jankowska, E., Lackberg, Z. S., Dyrehag, L. E. "Effects of monoamines on transmission from group II muscle afferents in sacral segments in the cat." *European Journal of Neuroscience* 6 (1994): 1058–1061.

Jankowska, E., Riddell, J. S., Skoog, B., Noga, B. R. "Gating of transmission to motoneurones by stimuli applied in the locus coeruleus and raphe nuclei of the cat." *Journal of Physiology* 461 (1993): 705–722.

Jordan, L. M. "Initiation of locomotion in mammals." *Annals of the New York Academy of Science* 860 (1998): 83–93.

Jordan, L. M., Liu, J., Hedlund, P. B., Akay, T., Pearson, K. G. "Descending command systems for the initiation of locomotion in mammals." *Brain Research Review* 57 (2008): 183–191.

Jordan, L. M., Pratt, C. A., Menzies, J. E. "Locomotion evoked by brain stem stimulation: Occurrence without phasic segmental afferent input." *Brain Research* 177 (1979): 204–207.

Jordan, L. M., Schmidt, B. J. "Propriospinal neurons involved in the control of locomotion: Potential targets for repair strategies?" *Progress in Brain Research* 137 (2002): 125–139.

Kato, T., Honmou, O., Uede, T., Hashi, K., Kocsis, J. D. "Transplantation of human olfactory ensheathing cells elicits remyelination of demyelinated rat spinal cord." *Glia* 30 (2000): 209–218.

Keane, R. W., Davis, A. R., Dietrich, W. D. "Inflammatory and apoptotic signaling after spinal cord injury." *Journal of Neurotrauma* 23 (2006): 335–344.

Kerschensteiner, M., Meinl, E., Hohlfeld, R. "Neuro-immune crosstalk in CNS diseases." *Neuroscience* 158 (2009): 1122–1132.

Keyvan-Fouladi, N., Raisman, G., Li, Y. "Functional repair of the corticospinal tract by delayed transplantation of olfactory ensheathing cells in adult rats." *Journal of Neuroscience* 23 (2003): 9428–9434.

Knoller, N., Auerbach, G., Fulga, V., et al. "Clinical experience using incubated autologous macrophages as a treatment for complete spinal cord injury: Phase I study results." *Journal of Neurosurgery of Spine* 3 (2005): 173–181.

Kopen, G. C., Prockop, D. J., Phinney, D. G. "Marrow stromal cells migrate throughout forebrain and cerebellum, and they differentiate into astrocytes after injection into neonatal mouse brains." *Proceedings of the National Academy of Sciences* (U.S.) 96 (1999): 10711–10716.

Kuhlengel, K. R., Bunge, M. B., Bunge, R. P., Burton, H. "Implantation of cultured sensory neurons and Schwann cells into lesioned neonatal rat spinal cord. II. Implant characteristics and examination of corticospinal tract growth." *Journal of Comparative Neurology* 293 (1990): 74–91.

Lacroix, S., Chang, L., Rose-John, S., Tuszynski, M. H. "Delivery of hyper-interleukin-6 to the injured spinal cord increases neutrophil and macrophage infiltration and inhibits axonal growth." *Journal of Comparative Neurology* 454 (2002): 213–228.

Lakatos, A., Smith, P. M., Barnett, S. C., Franklin, R. J. "Meningeal cells enhance limited CNS remyelination by transplanted olfactory ensheathing cells." *Brain* 126 (2003): 598–609.

Langley, J. N., Anderson, H. K. "On autogenetic regeneration in the nerves of the limbs." *Journal of Physiology* 30 (1904): 418–428.

Lazar, D. A., Ellegala, D. B., Avellino, A. M., Dailey, A. T., Andrus, K., Kliot, M. "Modulation of macrophage and microglial responses to axonal injury in the peripheral and central nervous systems." *Neurosurgery* 45 (1999): 593–600.

Lazarov-Spiegler, O., Solomon, A. S., Schwartz, M. "Peripheral nerve-stimulated macrophages simulate a peripheral nerve-like regenerative response in rat transected optic nerve." *Glia* 24 (1998): 329–337.

Lazarov-Spiegler, O., Solomon, A. S., Zeev-Brann, A. B., Hirschberg, D. L., Lavie, V., Schwartz, M. "Transplantation of activated macrophages overcomes central nervous system regrowth failure." *Journal of the Federation of American Societies for Experimental Biology* 10 (1996): 1296–1302.

Lee, Y. S., Li, C. Y., Robertson, R. T., Hsiao, I., Lin, V. W. "Motor recovery and anatomical evidence of axonal regrowth in spinal cord-repaired adult rats." *Journal of Neuropathology and Experimental Neurology* 63 (2004): 233–245.

Lee, Y. S., Lin, C. Y., Robertson, R. T., et al. "Re-growth of catecholaminergic fibers and protection of cholinergic spinal cord neurons in spinal repaired rats." *European Journal of Neuroscience* 23 (2006): 693–702.

Levi, A. D., Bunge, R. P., Lofgren, J. A., et al. "The influence of heregulins on human Schwann cell proliferation." *Journal of Neuroscience* 15 (1995): 1329–1340.

Levi, A. D., Dancausse, H., Li, X., Duncan, S., Horkey, L., Oliviera, M. "Peripheral nerve grafts promoting central nervous system regeneration after spinal cord injury in the primate." *Journal of Neurosurgery* 96 (2002): 197–205.

Li, Y., Decherchi, P., Raisman, G. "Transplantation of olfactory ensheathing cells into spinal cord lesions restores breathing and climbing." *Journal of Neuroscience* 23 (2003): 727–731.

Li, Y., Field, P. M., Raisman, G. "Repair of adult rat corticospinal tract by transplants of olfactory ensheathing cells." *Science* 277 (1997): 2000–2002.

Li, Y., Field, P. M., Raisman, G. "Regeneration of adult rat corticospinal axons induced by transplanted olfactory ensheathing cells." *Journal of Neuroscience* 18 (1998): 10514–10524.

Li, Y., Raisman, G. "Integration of transplanted cultured Schwann cells into the long myelinated fiber tracts of the adult spinal cord." *Experimental Neurology* 145 (1997): 397–411.

Lieberman, A. R. "The axon reaction: A review of the principal features of perikaryal responses to axon injury." *International Review of Neurobiology* 14 (1971): 49–124.

Lotan, M., Schwartz, M. "Cross talk between the immune system and the nervous system in response to injury: Implications for regeneration." *Journal of the Federation of American Societies for Experimental Biology* 8 (1994): 1026–1033.

Lu, J., Feron, F., Ho, S. M., Kay-Sim, A., Waite, P. M. "Transplantation of nasal olfactory tissue promotes partial recovery in paraplegic adult rats." *Brain Research* 889 (2001): 344–357.

Lu, J., Feron, F., Kay-Sim, A., Waite, P. M. "Olfactory ensheathing cells promote locomotor recovery after delayed transplantation into transected spinal cord." *Brain* 125 (2002): 14–21.

Majczyński, H., Maleszak, K., Cabaj, A., Sławińska, U. "Serotonin-related enhancement of recovery of hind limb motor functions in spinal rats after grafting of embryonic raphe nuclei." *Journal of Neurotrauma* 22 (2005): 590–604.

Martin, D., Schoenen, J., Delree, P., Leprince, P., Rogister, B., Moonen, G. "Grafts of syngenic cultured, adult dorsal root ganglion-derived Schwann cells to the injured spinal cord of adult rats: Preliminary morphological studies." *Neuroscience Letters* 124 (1991): 44–48.

Martin, D., Schoenen, J., Delree, P., et al. "Syngenic grafting of adult rat DRG-derived Schwann cells to the injured spinal cord." *Brain Research Bulletin* 30 (1993): 507–514.

McDonald, J. W., Liu, X. Z., Qu, Y., et al. "Transplanted embryonic stem cells survive, differentiate and promote recovery in injured rat spinal cord." *Nature Medicine* 5 (1999): 1410–1412.

Menei, P., Montero-Menei, C., Whittemore, S. R., Bunge, R. P., Bunge, M. B. "Schwann cells genetically modified to secrete human BDNF promote enhanced axonal regrowth across transected adult rat spinal cord." *European Journal of Neuroscience* 10 (1998): 607–621.

Morrissey, T. K., Kleitman, N., Bunge, R. P. "Isolation and functional characterization of Schwann cells derived from adult peripheral nerve." *Journal of Neuroscience* 11 (1991): 2433–2442.

Muller, H. W., Gebicke-Harter, P. J., Hangen, D. H., Shooter, E. M. "A specific 37,000-dalton protein that accumulates in regenerating but not in nonregenerating mammalian nerves." *Science* 228 (1985): 499–501.

Navarro, X., Valero, A., Gudino, G., et al. "Ensheathing glia transplants promote dorsal root regeneration and spinal reflex restitution after multiple lumbar rhizotomy." *Annals of Neurology* 45 (1999): 207–215.

Nikulina, E., Tidwell, J. L., Dai, H. N., Bregman, B. S., Filbin, M. T. "The phosphodiesterase inhibitor rolipram delivered after a spinal cord lesion promotes axonal regeneration and functional recovery." *Proceedings of the National Academy of Sciences* (U.S.) 101 (2004): 8786–8790.

Nógradi, A., Szabo, A. "Transplantation of embryonic neurones to replace missing spinal motoneurones." *Restorative Neurology and Neuroscience* 26 (2008): 215–223.

Nógrádi, A., Vrbová, G. "The use of embryonic spinal cord grafts to replace identified motoneuron pools depleted by a neurotoxic lectin, volkensin." *Experimental Neurology* 129 (1994): 130–141.

Nógrádi, A., Vrbová, G. "Improved motor function of denervated rat hindlimb muscles induced by embryonic spinal cord grafts." *European Journal of Neuroscience* 8 (1996a): 2198–2203.

Nógrádi, A., Vrbová, G. "Reinnervation of denervated hindlimb muscles by axons of grafted motoneurons via the reimplanted L4 ventral root." *Neurobiology* 4 (1996b): 231–232.

Nornes, H., Björklund, A., Stenevi, U. "Reinnervation of the denervated adult spinal cord of rats by intraspinal transplants of embryonic brain stem neurons." *Cell Tissue Research* 230 (1983): 15–35.

Nornes, H. O., Das, G. D. "Temporal pattern of neurogenesis in spinal cord of rat. I. An autoradiographic study—time and sites of origin and migration and settling patterns of neuroblasts." *Brain Research* 73 (1974): 121–138.

Nygren, L. G., Olson, L. "On spinal noradrenaline receptor supersensitivity: Correlation between nerve terminal densities and flexor reflexes various times after intracisternal 6-hydroxydopamine." *Brain Research* 116 (1976): 455–470.

Nygren, L. G., Olson, L., Seiger, A. "Monoaminergic reinnervation of the transected spinal cord by homologous fetal brain grafts." *Brain Research* 129 (1977): 227–235.

Oudega, M., Xu, X. M., Guenard, V., Kleitman, N., Bunge, M. B. "A combination of insulin-like growth factor-I and platelet-derived growth factor enhances myelination but diminishes axonal regeneration into Schwann cell grafts in the adult rat spinal cord." *Glia* 19 (1997): 247–258.

Pan, J. Z., Ni, L., Sodhi, A., Aguanno, A., Young, W., Hart, R. P. "Cytokine activity contributes to induction of inflammatory cytokine mRNAs in spinal cord following contusion." *Journal of Neuroscience Research* 68 (2002): 315–322.

Pearse, D. D., Pereira, F. C., Marcillo, A. E., et al. "cAMP and Schwann cells promote axonal growth and functional recovery after spinal cord injury." *Nature Medicine* 10 (2004): 610–616.

Perry, V. H., Andersson, P. B., Gordon, S. "Macrophages and inflammation in the central nervous system." *Trends in Neuroscience* 16 (1993): 268–273.

Perry, V. H., Gordon, S. "Macrophages and the nervous system." *International Review of Cytology* 125 (1991): 203–244.

Pineau, I., Lacroix, S. "Proinflammatory cytokine synthesis in the injured mouse spinal cord: Multiphasic expression pattern and identification of the cell types involved." *Journal of Comparative Neurology* 500 (2007): 267–285.

Plant, G. W., Christensen, C. L., Oudega, M., Bunge, M. B. "Delayed transplantation of olfactory ensheathing glia promotes sparing/regeneration of supraspinal axons in the contused adult rat spinal cord." *Journal of Neurotrauma* 20 (2003): 1–16.

Popovich, P. G., Guan, Z., McGaughy, V., Fisher, L., Hickey, W. F., Basso, D. M. "The neuropathological and behavioral consequences of intraspinal microglial/macrophage activation." *Journal of Neuropathology and Experimental Neurology* 61 (2002): 623–633.

Popovich, P. G., Longbrake, E. E. "Can the immune system be harnessed to repair the CNS?" *Nature Reviews Neuroscience* 9 (2008): 481–493.

Prewitt, C. M., Niesman, I. R., Kane, C. J., Houle, J. D. "Activated macrophage/microglial cells can promote the regeneration of sensory axons into the injured spinal cord." *Experimental Neurology* 148 (1997): 433–443.

Privat, A., Mansour, H., Geffard, M. "Transplantation of fetal serotonin neurons into the transected spinal cord of adult rats: Morphological development and functional influence." *Progress in Brain Research* 78 (1988): 155–166.

Privat, A., Mansour, H., Pavy, A., Geffard, M., Sandillon, F. "Transplantation of dissociated foetal serotonin neurons into the transected spinal cord of adult rats." *Neuroscience Letters* 66 (1986): 61–66.

Privat, A., Mansour, H., Rajaofetra, N., Geffard, M. "Intraspinal transplants of serotonergic neurons in the adult rat." *Brain Research Bulletin* 22 (1989): 123–129.

Prockop, D. J. "Marrow stromal cells as stem cells for nonhematopoietic tissues." *Science* 276 (1997): 71–74.

Rajaofetra, N., Konig, N., Poulat, P., et al. "Fate of B1-B2 and B3 rhombencephalic cells transplanted into the transected spinal cord of adult rats: Light and electron microscopic studies." *Experimental Neurology* 117 (1992a): 59–70.

Rajaofetra, N., Poulat, P., Marlier, L., et al. "Transplantation of embryonic serotonin immunoreactive neurons into the transected spinal cord of adult monkey (*Macaca fascicularis*)." *Brain Research* 572 (1992b): 329–334.

Ramer, L. M., Au, E., Richter, M. W., Liu, J., Tetzlaff, W., Roskams, A. J. "Peripheral olfactory ensheathing cells reduce scar and cavity formation and promote regeneration after spinal cord injury." *Journal of Comparative Neurology* 473 (2004a): 1–15.

Ramer, L. M., Richter, M. W., Roskams, A. J., Tetzlaff, W., Ramer, M. S. "Peripherally-derived olfactory ensheathing cells do not promote primary afferent regeneration following dorsal root injury." *Glia* 47 (2004b): 189–206.

Ramon y Cajal, S. *Degeneration and Regeneration of the Nervous System*. Oxford, U.K.: Oxford University Press, 1928.

Ramon-Cueto, A. "Olfactory ensheathing glia transplantation into the injured spinal cord." *Progress in Brain Research* 128 (2000): 265–272.

Ramon-Cueto, A., Avila, J. "Olfactory ensheathing glia: Properties and function." *Brain Research Bulletin* 46 (1998): 175–187.

Ramon-Cueto, A., Cordero, M. I., Santos-Benito, F. F., Avila, J. "Functional recovery of paraplegic rats and motor axon regeneration in their spinal cords by olfactory ensheathing glia." *Neuron* 25 (2000): 425–435.

Ramon-Cueto, A., Nieto-Sampedro, M. "Glial cells from adult rat olfactory bulb: Immunocytochemical properties of pure cultures of ensheathing cells." *Neuroscience* 47 (1992): 213–220.

Ramon-Cueto, A., Nieto-Sampedro, M. "Regeneration into the spinal cord of transected dorsal root axons is promoted by ensheathing glia transplants." *Experimental Neurology* 127 (1994): 232–244.

Ramon-Cueto, A., Valverde, F. "Olfactory bulb ensheathing glia: A unique cell type with axonal growth-promoting properties." *Glia* 14 (1995): 163–173.

Rapalino, O., Lazarov-Spiegler, O., Agranov, E., et al. "Implantation of stimulated homologous macrophages results in partial recovery of paraplegic rats." *Nature Medicine* 4 (1998): 814–821.

Ribotta, M. G., Provencher, J., Feraboli-Lohnherr, D., Rossignol, S., Privat, A., Orsal, D. "Activation of locomotion in adult chronic spinal rats is achieved by transplantation of embryonic raphe cells reinnervating a precise lumbar level." *Journal of Neuroscience* 20 (2000): 5144–5152.

Riddell, J. S., Enriquez-Denton, M., Toft, A., Fairless, R., Barnett, S. C. "Olfactory ensheathing cell grafts have minimal influence on regeneration at the dorsal root entry zone following rhizotomy." *Glia* 47 (2004): 150–167.

Rotshenker, S. "Microglia and macrophage activation and the regulation of complement-receptor-3 (CR3/MAC-1)-mediated myelin phagocytosis in injury and disease." *Journal of Molecular Neuroscience* 21 (2003): 65–72.

Santos-Benito, F. F., Ramon-Cueto, A. "Olfactory ensheathing glia transplantation: A therapy to promote repair in the mammalian central nervous system." *Anatomical Record (Part B: New Anatomy)* 271 (2003): 77–85.

Sasaki, M., Lankford, K. L., Zemedkun, M., Kocsis, J. D. "Identified olfactory ensheathing cells transplanted into the transected dorsal funiculus bridge the lesion and form myelin." *Journal of Neuroscience* 24 (2004): 8485–8493.

Schnell, L., Fearn, S., Klassen, H., Schwab, M. E., Perry, V. H. "Acute inflammatory responses to mechanical lesions in the CNS: Differences between brain and spinal cord." *European Journal of Neuroscience* 11 (1999a): 3648–3658.

Schnell, L., Fearn, S., Schwab, M. E., Perry, V. H., Anthony, D. C. "Cytokine-induced acute inflammation in the brain and spinal cord." *Journal of Neuropathology and Experimental Neurology* 58 (1999b): 245–254.

Schnell, L., Schwab, M. E. "Axonal regeneration in the rat spinal cord produced by an antibody against myelin-associated neurite growth inhibitors." *Nature* 343 (1990): 269–272.

Schroder, H. D. "Organization of the motoneurons innervating the pelvic muscles of the male rat." *Journal of Comparative Neurology* 192 (1980): 567–587.

Schroder, H. D., Skagerberg, G. "Catecholamine innervation of the caudal spinal cord in the rat." *Journal of Comparative Neurology* 242 (1985): 358–368.

Schwab, M. E. "Increasing plasticity and functional recovery of the lesioned spinal cord." *Progress in Brain Research* 137 (2002): 351–359.

Schwab, M. E. "Nogo and axon regeneration." *Current Opinion in Neurobiology* 14 (2004): 118–124.

Schwartz, M., Cohen, A., Stein-Izsak, C., Belkin, M. "Dichotomy of the glial cell response to axonal injury and regeneration." *The Journal of the Federation of American Societies for Experimental Biology* 3 (1989): 2371–2378.

Schwartz, M., Yoles, E. "Immune-based therapy for spinal cord repair: Autologous macrophages and beyond." *Journal of Neurotrauma* 23 (2006): 360–370.

Siegal, J. D., Kliot, M., Smith, G. M., Silver, J. "A comparison of the regeneration potential of dorsal root fibers into gray or white matter of the adult rat spinal cord." *Experimental Neurology* 109 (1990): 90–97.

Sieradzan, K., Vrbová, G. "Replacement of missing motoneurons by embryonic grafts in the rat spinal cord." *Neuroscience* 31 (1989): 115–130.

Sieradzan, K., Vrbová, G. "Factors influencing survival of transplanted embryonic motoneurones in the spinal cord of adult rats." *Experimental Neurology* 114 (1991): 286–299.

Sieradzan, K., Vrbová, G. "The ability of developing spinal neurons to reinnervate a muscle through a peripheral nerve conduit is enhanced by cografted embryonic spinal cord." *Experimental Neurology* 122 (1993b): 232–243.

Sotelo, C. "Neuronal transplantation: Purkinje cell replacement and reconstruction of a defective cerebellar circuitry in mice with heredo-degenerative ataxia." *Bollettino-Societa Italiana Biologia Sperimentale* 62 (1986): 1479–1485.

Sotelo, C., Varado-Mallart, R. M. "Growth and differentiation of cerebellar suspensions transplanted into the adult cerebellum of mice with heredodegenerative ataxia." *Proceedings of the National Academy of Sciences* (U.S.) 83 (1986): 1135–1139.

Sotelo, C., Varado-Mallart, R. M. "Cerebellar transplantations in adult mice with heredo-degenerative ataxia." *Annals of the New York Academy of Science* 495 (1987a): 242–267.

Sotelo, C., Varado-Mallart, R. M. "Embryonic and adult neurons interact to allow Purkinje cell replacement in mutant cerebellum." *Nature* 327 (1987b): 421–423.

Sotelo, C., Varado-Mallart, R. M., Gardette, R., Crepel, F. "Fate of grafted embryonic Purkinje cells in the cerebellum of the adult 'Purkinje cell degeneration' mutant mouse. I. Development of reciprocal graft–host interactions." *Journal of Comparative Neurology* 295 (1990): 165–187.

Stenevi, U., Björklund, A. "Transplantation techniques for the study of regeneration in the central nervous system." *Progress in Brain Research* 48 (1978): 101–112.

Stoll, G., Jander, S., Schroeter, M. "Detrimental and beneficial effects of injury-induced inflammation and cytokine expression in the nervous system." *Advances in Experimental Medicine and Biology* 513 (2002): 87–113.

Stoll, G., Muller, H. W. "Macrophages in the peripheral nervous system and astroglia in the central nervous system of rat commonly express apolipoprotein E during development but differ in their response to injury." *Neuroscience Letters* 72 (1986): 233–238.

Stoll, G., Trapp, B. D., Griffin, J. W. "Macrophage function during Wallerian degeneration of rat optic nerve: Clearance of degenerating myelin and Ia expression." *Journal of Neuroscience* 9 (1989): 2327–2335.

Stout, R. D., Jiang, C., Matta, B., Tietzel, I., Watkins, S. K., Suttles, J. "Macrophages sequentially change their functional phenotype in response to changes in microenvironmental influences." *Journal of Immunology* 175 (2005): 342–349.

Streit, W. J., Semple-Rowland, S. L., Hurley, S. D., Miller, R. C., Popovich, P. G., Stokes, B. T. "Cytokine mRNA profiles in contused spinal cord and axotomized facial nucleus suggest a beneficial role for inflammation and gliosis." *Experimental Neurology* 152 (1998): 74–87.

Sugar, O., Gerard, R. W. "Spinal cord regeneration in the rat." *Journal of Neurophysiology* 3 (1940): 1–19.

Sławińska, U., Majczyński, H., Djavadian, R. "Recovery of hindlimb motor functions after spinal cord transection is enhanced by grafts of the embryonic raphe nuclei." *Experimental Brain Research* 132 (2000): 27–38.

Tadie, M., Liu, S., Robert, R., et al. "Partial return of motor function in paralyzed legs after surgical bypass of the lesion site by nerve autografts three years after spinal cord injury." *Journal of Neurotrauma* 19 (2002): 909–916.

Takami, T., Oudega, M., Bates, M. L., Wood, P. M., Kleitman, N., Bunge, M. B. "Schwann cell but not olfactory ensheathing glia transplants improve hindlimb locomotor performance in the moderately contused adult rat thoracic spinal cord." *Journal of Neuroscience* 22 (2002): 6670–6681.

Thompson, G. "Successful brain grafting." *New York Medical Journal* 51 (1890): 701–702.

Thuret, S., Moon, L. D., Gage, F. H. "Therapeutic interventions after spinal cord injury." *Nature Reviews Neuroscience* 7 (2006): 628–643.

Ulfhake, B., Arvidsson, U., Cullheim, S., et al. "An ultrastructural study of 5-hydroxytryptamine-, thyrotropin-releasing hormone- and substance P–immunoreactive axonal boutons in the motor nucleus of spinal cord segments L7–S1 in the adult cat." *Neuroscience* 23 (1987): 917–929.

Vallieres, N., Berard, J. L., David, S., Lacroix, S. "Systemic injections of lipopolysaccharide accelerates myelin phagocytosis during Wallerian degeneration in the injured mouse spinal cord." *Glia* 53 (2006): 103–113.

Verdú, E., Garcia-Alias, G., Forés J., López-Vales, R., Navarro, X. "Olfactory ensheathing cells transplanted in lesioned spinal cord prevent loss of spinal cord parenchyma and promote functional recovery." *Glia* 42 (2003): 275–286.

White, S. R., Neuman, R. S. "Facilitation of spinal motoneurone excitability by 5-hydroxytryptamine and noradrenaline." *Brain Research* 188 (1980): 119–127.

White, S. R., Neuman, R. S. "Pharmacological antagonism of facilitatory but not inhibitory effects of serotonin and norepinephrine on excitability of spinal motoneurons." *Neuropharmacology* 22 (1983): 489–494.

Windle, W. F., Littrell, J. L., Smart, J. O., Joralemon J. "Regeneration in the cord of spinal monkeys." *Neurology* 6 (1956): 420–428.

Woodbury, D., Schwarz, E. J., Prockop, D. J., Black, I. B. "Adult rat and human bone marrow stromal cells differentiate into neurons." *Journal of Neuroscience Research* 61 (2000): 364–370.

Xu, X. M., Chen, A., Guenard, V., Kleitman, N., Bunge, M. B. "Bridging Schwann cell transplants promote axonal regeneration from both the rostral and caudal stumps of transected adult rat spinal cord." *Journal of Neurocytology* 26 (1997): 1–16.

Xu, X. M., Guenard, V., Kleitman, N., Aebischer, P., Bunge, M. B. "A combination of BDNF and NT-3 promotes supraspinal axonal regeneration into Schwann cell grafts in adult rat thoracic spinal cord." *Experimental Neurology* 134 (1995a): 261–272.

Xu, X. M., Guenard, V., Kleitman, N., Bunge, M. B. "Axonal regeneration into Schwann cell–seeded guidance channels grafted into transected adult rat spinal cord." *Journal of Comparative Neurology* 351 (1995b): 145–160.

Yakovleff, A., Cabelguen, J. M., Orsal, D., et al. "Fictive motor activities in adult chronic spinal rats transplanted with embryonic brain stem neurons." *Experimental Brain Research* 106 (1995): 69–78.

Yakovleff, A., Roby-Brami, A., Guezard, B., Mansour, H., Bussel, B., Privat, A. "Locomotion in rats transplanted with noradrenergic neurons." *Brain Research Bulletin* 22 (1989): 115–121.

Z'Graggen, W. J., Metz, G. A., Kartje, G. L., Thallmair, M., Schwab, M. E. "Functional recovery and enhanced corticofugal plasticity after unilateral pyramidal tract lesion and blockade of myelin-associated neurite growth inhibitors in adult rats." *Journal of Neuroscience* 18 (1998): 4744–4757.

Zwart, I., Hill, A. J., Al-Allaf, F., et al. "Umbilical cord blood mesenchymal stromal cells are neuroprotective and promote regeneration in a rat optic tract model." *Experimental Neurology* 216 (2009): 439–448.

6

The Reconstructive Neurosurgery of Spinal Cord Injury

JUSTIN M. BROWN

CONTENTS

1. Introduction
2. Reconstructive Neurosurgery
3. The Current State of Functional Neurosurgery
4. The Traumatized Spinal Cord
5. Pathology of the Injured Metamere
   5.1. Consequences of the Pathological Changes
   5.2. Intervention at the Injured Metamere
6. Pathology of the Sublesional Segment
   6.1. Spasticity Reduction and Functional Neurosurgery
      — Therapy
      — Stimulation
      — Pharmacological interventions
      — Ablative procedures
   6.2. Functional Augmentation: The Restorative Approach
      — Reduction of pathological inputs
      — Optimization of physiological inputs
      — The restorative approach: additional thoughts
7. Focal Interventions for Function Recovery and the Expanding Role of Nerve Transfers
   7.1. Tendon Transfer Surgery
   7.2. Nerve Transfer Surgery
   7.3. Managing Focal Spasticity
8. Conclusion
References

1. INTRODUCTION

It has been suggested that there are two primary categories of neurosurgical procedures: anatomical and functional (Iskandar & Nashold, 1995). *Anatomical procedures* address abnormalities based upon their deviation from normal and "healthy" anatomy. Examples of this include shunting hydrocephalus, clipping aneurysms, and stabilizing spinal fractures. These procedures generally aim to interrupt a destructive process in order to save life or *preserve* function. *Functional procedures* attempt to *improve* function by altering the underlying physiology. For the most part, these procedures have been ablative in nature. Whether resecting or disconnecting an epileptogenic focus to eliminate seizures, interrupting pain transmission in spinothalamic tractotomy, or inhibiting globus pallidus function in a patient with Parkinsonian tremors, functional interventions target structures that are either the source of or contribute to the propagation of a "dysfunction." When addressing involuntary movements and spasms, functional neurosurgery has traditionally addressed these motor outputs as a dysfunction that must be eliminated instead of as a consequence of disordered motor control, which might be reordered to provide improved function.

2. RECONSTRUCTIVE NEUROSURGERY

"Reconstructive surgery" has traditionally referred to techniques of reapproximation, redistribution, or augmentation of a patient's tissues to render a more functional outcome. Unlike bone or soft tissues, neural components are less amenable to rearrangement to compensate for a lacking function. Because of the sophistication of the substrate, surgeons have typically been satisfied to successfully remove a destructive lesion without producing further dysfunction. Thus a reconstructive subdiscipline within neurosurgery has emerged only slowly. However, surgical interventions to improve neurological function have been developed, beginning with the ablative and inhibitory procedures of traditional functional neurosurgery and progressing to what is now known as *reconstructive neurosurgery.*

One of the earliest uses of the term "reconstructive neurosurgery" is in a manuscript addressing the management of war-related peripheral nerve injuries by two military neurosurgeons, Captain Stanley Potter & Major Edmund Croce, in 1947 (Potter & Croce, 1947). The next appearance of this phrase occurs in the 1980s, also in reference to restorative procedures of the peripheral nervous system (Narakas, 1981; Shibib et al., 1985). Since that time, the term has been applied to a variety of central and peripheral nervous system manipulations aimed at improving functional neurological status (see Table 6–1). These procedures include ablative procedures and the implantation of neuromodulation devices, as well as nervous tissue reconstruction, reorganization, and transplantation (Doczi & Teasdale, 2003; Chiu et al., 2008).

The term has been increasingly applied to cellular therapies, primarily those directed at replacing dopaminergic cells in order to reverse the movement disorder associated with Parkinson's disease (Polgar et al., 2003; Polgar & Morris, 2005). Interventions aimed at bridging disruptions between the central and peripheral nervous systems, such as nerve root reimplantation following traumatic cervical nerve root avulsion injuries, have also utilized this term (Kliot et al., 1992; Carlstedt et al., 2000). Recently it has been suggested that any reconstructive procedure performed by a neurosurgeon, including spinal column and vascular procedures, falls within this category of reconstructive neurosurgery (Katayama, 2009). We will limit our

Table 6–1 Prior References to Reconstructive Neurosurgery

Reconstructive Neurosurgery Intervention	Publication
Peripheral nerve reconstruction	Potter and Croce, 1947
	Narakas, 1981
	Shibib, 1985
Cell transplantation	Doczi and Teasdale, 2003
	Chiu et al., 2008
	Polgar et al., 2003 and 2005
Implant-based stimulation of neural structures	Doczi and Teasdale, 2003
	Chiu et al., 2008
Spinal nerve root reimplantation	Carlstedt et al., 2000 Kliot et al., 1992

discussions to procedures applied to the central or peripheral nervous system that correct deficits by augmenting neural control, restoring neural connectivity, and redistributing intact residual functions. Essentially, reconstructive neurosurgery is the functional neurosurgical counterpart to restorative neurology.

3. THE CURRENT STATE OF FUNCTIONAL NEUROSURGERY

As an understanding of the physiology and corresponding anatomy underlying a number of neurological dysfunctions has emerged, interventions have expanded accordingly. The number of anatomical targets available for manipulation has increased to include the cortex, basal ganglia, cerebellum, spinal cord, nerve roots, peripheral nerves, and autonomic ganglia. Localization techniques provide three-dimensional targeting of deep structures, both invasively and noninvasively. Interventions now include numerous permutations of what can be broadly classified as ablative interventions, neurostimulation, and targeted pharmacological administration. These advances have provided functional interventions for the six basic categories of dysfunction: abnormal *involuntary* movements, spasticity, pain, psychiatric disorders, epilepsy, and neuroendocrine disorders (Iskandar & Nashold, 1995).

A seventh category of dysfunction has emerged—one that pertains to abnormal voluntary movements, or *impaired motor control.* In the second half of the last century, the discipline of restorative neurology arose in response to this category of dysfunction (Dimitrijevic, 1985; Dimitrijevic et al., 1997), and more recently, reconstructive neurosurgery has emerged as its surgical subdiscipline. Restorative neurology and reconstructive neurosurgery emphasize the use of neurophysiological methods to characterize residual and even subclinical functions. These findings are then used to direct a clinical plan to maximize a given patient's motor control. Stroke, multiple sclerosis, cerebral palsy, traumatic brain injury, and spinal cord injury, among other entities, were addressed based not on what was missing, as was the case with conventional medicine, but on what was present—the residual functional capacities—in order to capitalize on these latent capabilities. In keeping with the goal of this book, we are going to focus upon the reconstructive neurosurgery of spinal cord injury.

4. THE TRAUMATIZED SPINAL CORD

Traumatic spinal cord injury, above the level of the cauda equina, results in three distinct regions of the spinal cord: the *supralesional segment* (SLS), the *injured metamere* (IM), and the *infralesional segment* (ILS) (Figure 6–1). Following the initial trauma, a period of healing ensues, and a new, stable, structural and functional organization of the central nervous system eventually emerges and persists (Dimitrijevic et al., 1997). The functions of this new system are expressed as alternative but characteristic motor control (Kern et al., 2005). By better defining the three components of the "new" central nervous system, a practical approach to maximizing its functional output can be achieved.

The SLS resulting from a spinal cord injury includes the brain, brain stem, and all components of the central nervous system rostral to the site of injury

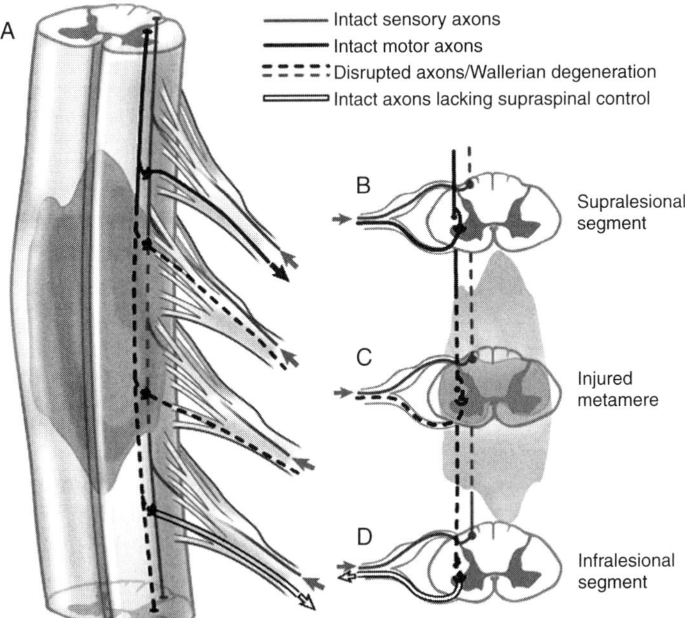

Figure 6–1 When a spinal cord is injured above the level of the cauda equina, white matter tracts are interrupted and gray matter commonly is lost secondary to both the initial insult and the consequent central hemorrhagic necrosis (*A*). As a result, three regions of the spinal cord emerge: (*B*) the *supralesional segment* proximal to the trauma, which maintains essentially normal motor control; (*C*) the *injured metamere*, which is directly impacted by the trauma and suffers a mixed injury with decreased input from above as well as reduced output due to its disrupted gray matter; and (*D*) the *infralesional segment* whose function is primarily determined by the degree of white matter disruption at the site of trauma.

(see Figure 6–1B). This region maintains volitional control of its directly associated myotomes and generally receives uncorrupted direct afferent input. This region, though, is deprived of some degree of ascending information from both the IM and the caudal segments, the ILS. Effects of this can be seen in alterations of motor unit firing rates of the strong, intact supralesional muscle groups (Shefner et al., 1995). Plasticity within the neural circuitry of the SLS ensues to maximize the functionality of the residual tracts, both ascending and descending, that span the lesion. Cortical reorganization assigns significantly more area of motor cortex to control of the supralesional musculature. Additionally, residual information ascending from the IM and ILS may be amplified and, in some cases, lead to pain syndromes (though a complete discussion of this is beyond the scope of this chapter) (Beric, 1993; Siddall, 2009). The SLS represents the residual "healthy" component of the altered nervous system.

The IM is the region directly affected by the trauma and is characterized by tissue destruction, which may extend several levels above and below the actual site of impact (Coulet et al., 2002) (see Figure 6–1C). Other regions are commonly indirectly affected (this is further discussed later in the chapter). This region generally suffers a mixed injury, including a preponderance of central gray matter destruction (Kakulas, 2004). The myotomes corresponding to this segment may be affected by upper motor neuron (UMN) dysfunction, lower motor neuron (LMN) dysfunction, or some mixture of the two, secondary to the spinal cord contusion alone. Additional damage to nerve roots at the IM is common (Benzel & Larson, 1986). Residual spinal cord compression may persist, or scarring and tethering of the spinal cord may develop at this site. These pathologies can also lead to secondary cystic or myelomalacic myelopathy (Falcone et al., 1994; Holly et al., 2000; Falci et al., 2009). The LMN injuries at this segment are commonly overlooked because of the more salient UMN injuries. The injuries affecting this segment can result in pathological spontaneous activity, which is conducted to the SLS as neuropathic pain and/or to the ILS as spontaneous spasms (Sjolund, 2002).

The last region, the ILS, consists of the spinal cord and associated peripheral nervous system below the lesion (see Figure 6–1D). This region, like the SLS, may be functionally intact, but receives reduced input from the SLS and IM. The ILS generally retains its properties as a processor to respond to both peripheral and descending input in order to generate a corresponding motor output. This segment, though, suffers from a deprivation of descending inputs and, similarly to the SLS, undergoes plasticity of its own. The gray matter, the propriospinal fibers within the fasciculus proprius, and the primary sensory input are usually present and healthy (Kern et al., 2005). Although healthy, intact peripheral connections may for the most part persist, a "functional deafferentation" (activity-dependant input deprivation) may be a consequence of a reduced motor output, which results from the diminished UMN drive. This reduction in movement limits afferent input to the spinal cord from several sources, including reduced load-bearing, reduced proprioceptive inputs, and reduced cutaneous stimuli (Dietz, 2010).

5. PATHOLOGY OF THE INJURED METAMERE

In most traumatic spinal injuries, at least a bridge of white matter remains to connect the ILS to the SLS, with complete transections being relatively rare (Kostyk &

Popovich, 2010). Within this white matter, the proportion of these axons that retains function is variable. Evidence of demyelination and remyelination is generally present here. A portion of this remyelination is often provided by Schwann cells that have migrated into the damaged tissue. These may be accompanied by a disorganized array of peripheral axons as well. Within this bridge of white matter, the number of retained traversing axons often does not correlate well with the degree of retained function (Kakulas, 2004). *Which axons are preserved* (anterior white matter being preferable) and *whether those residual axons are effectively conducting* are important (Kostyk & Popovich, 2010).

5.1. Consequences of the Pathological Changes

An oversimplification of the resulting motor control can be represented by three basic conditions: supralesional normal volitional control (see Figure 6–1B); lesional flaccid paralysis from loss of the LMN and muscular denervation (see Figure 6–1C); infralesional spastic paralysis with an intact LMN but loss of central control resulting from white matter damage (UMN) (see Figure 6–1D). In reality, though, there is a gradation with overlap of these three conditions and variations in the severity of each. Some studies of this phenomenon report that very few muscle groups sustain a complete LMN injury (Peckham et al., 1976). Others document large regions of complete denervation spanning multiple levels of the spinal cord (Mulcahey et al., 1999). Corresponding postmortem studies of the associated ventral roots have demonstrated the persistence of only small-diameter myelinated or unmyelinated axons, consistent with complete muscle denervation (Thomas & Grumbles, 2005). Our clinical observations have reflected the findings of each of these studies. Although some patients may have several muscle groups with no detectable innervation, others have signs of partial LMN injury scattered across many muscle groups. In addition to LMN damage from central gray matter destruction, associated brachial plexus injuries and nerve root compression may also contribute to the LMN injury and flaccid paralysis within and adjacent to the IM (Benzel & Larson, 1986; McGowin et al., 1989; Midha, 1997).

5.2. Intervention at the Injured Metamere

Whether or not surgical decompression of a traumatically compromised spinal canal in the acute setting is appropriate—and, if so, when—remains hotly debated (El Masry & Meerkotter, 1992; Cadotte et al., 2010). Arguments for early intervention cite animal studies demonstrating improved functional outcomes with earlier relief of spinal cord compression and clinical data regarding benefits of early mobilization and rehabilitation (Gupta et al., 2010; Hall, 2010; Carreon & Dimar, 2011). Arguments against surgery document that imaging parameters of the degree of spinal canal compression do not correlate with ultimate functional recovery (El Masry & Meerkotter, 1992). They explain that the physiological instability of the injured spinal cord leads to "silent deterioration" when the expected degree of neurological recovery is not achieved in a subset of patients who have undergone early decompression. Today we have methods to answer these concerns. For example, transcutaneously placed epidural electrodes in combination with transcranial stimulation at the bedside in an ICU setting can be used to assess the degree of translesional connectivity and monitor changes that occur with and without surgical intervention: documenting, for example, the event corresponding with the loss of the D-wave. These concepts are further developed in Chapter 9.

Once the physiological instability and vascular changes have resolved, untoward effects of a surgical intervention are less of a concern. Unfortunately, interest in surgical intervention is generally lacking. The "damage is done" concept is widely accepted. Interestingly, the benefits of nerve root decompression have been cited by multiple authors (Benzel & Larson, 1986; Yablon et al. 1991; Stauffer 1975). In fact, both nerve root and spinal cord functional improvement have been documented after late decompression, even in patients with chronic incomplete injury, while chronic complete injury generally demonstrated only nerve root recovery (McAfee et al., 1985; Transfeldt et al., 1990; Anderson & Bohlman, 1992; Bohlman & Anderson 1992; Bohlman et al. 1994). In these cases, though, there was a trend toward better recovery when decompression was performed within a year.

The functional recovery noted in these cases can be accounted for in part by reversal of conduction block, which occurs in both the spinal cord and nerve roots as a result of compression (Wright & Palmer, 1969; Tani et al., 1999; Ishida et al., 2003). Conduction block can result from focal ischemia, demyelination, and temporal dispersion (Taylor & Willison, 2005). When compression is relieved, ischemia is reversed immediately, and these associated conduction blocks often resolve rapidly. At times such recovery is recognized immediately upon the patient's awakening from surgery and may progress over the following days. Conduction blocks due to demyelination may resolve in the following weeks to months as remyelination progresses and matures. When pressure is not relieved, though, a conduction block often progresses to an axotomy, which corresponds with the decreasing efficacy of these decompression operations after significant time has elapsed. In some cases, the patient with an incomplete spinal cord injury, with continued spinal cord compression, may therefore be considered to have two concomitant injuries: the injury resulting from the initial trauma and a second injury equivalent to spondylotic myelopathy. In addition to some functional improvement, patients who underwent such decompression operations frequently noted an associated reduction in pain and spasticity as this "pathological input" to the IM was eliminated (Anderson & Bohlman, 1992). In keeping with this strategy, an important study showed dramatic results in ASIA-A (American Spinal Injury Association—complete SCI) patients after spinal canal optimization (Zhu et al, 2008).

In addition to residual compression, simple tethering of the IM so that it is unable to pulsate within the cerebrospinal fluid as a result of collagenous scar formation or arachnoiditis can also have detrimental effects (Klekamp et al., 1997; Lee et al., 1997; Falci et al., 2009). These can impede neurological recovery, but are most notorious as a source of late deterioration from the development of an expanding syrinx or myelomalacic myelopathy (Brodbelt & Stoodley, 2003; Morikawa et al., 2006). An expanding syrinx in the setting of late neurological deterioration remains one of the few widely accepted criteria for late surgical intervention following traumatic spinal cord injury. Of note, the procedures discussed above, if indicated, should obviate these complications.

The potential for recovery of affected *nerve roots* may be assessed by direct stimulation of the associated paralyzed muscle groups or compound motor action potentials (CMAPs). The nerve roots whose associated muscles respond to stimulation or whose associated nerves provide robust CMAPs, and particularly those with a corresponding region of partial sensory preservation, are likely to include traversing axons affected by neurapraxia. This can at times be difficult to discriminate from intact peripheral nerves paralyzed as a result of the UMN injury, but the lack of spasticity helps favor the peripheral conduction block as the source. If these axons are indeed present but affected by a conduction block, they should recover as perfusion is restored and remyelination proceeds.

The degree of *spinal cord* recovery following a decompression operation is not as easily predicted. While we know that an incomplete injury is more likely to respond than a complete one, further prognostication is difficult. Studies have indicated that somatosensory evoked potentials may be capable of demonstrating a conduction block within the spinal cord (Tani et al., 1999; Ishida et al., 2003). Regardless, the surgical goal for the spinal cord, as in spondylotic myelopathy, is to prevent progression of functional decline, with the hope of some degree of improvement.

6. PATHOLOGY OF THE SUBLESIONAL SEGMENT

Following spinal cord injury, the ILS is affected by Wallerian degeneration as the disconnected fibers that previously provided input to the gray matter die back. In this process the axons distal to the injury disintegrate and their myelin sheaths lyse, forming globules. Macrophages take up the debris, and astrocytes lay down fibers parallel to the lost axons, resulting in "isomorphic gliosis" (Kakulas, 2004). Names have been given to identify patterns of residual motor and sensory functions after specific lesions of the spinal cord. Such syndromes include central cord, anterior cord, posterior cord, and Brown-Sequard, among others. Generally, though, with closed spinal trauma, these specific syndromes are less pronounced, and a very heterogenous set of injury patterns and severities results.

In an attempt to provide a useful classification for such injuries, Dimitrijevic proposed two basic categories of injury: "reduced anatomy" and "new anatomy" (Dimitrijevic et al., 1997) (Figure 6–2). The *reduced anatomy* condition represents a spinal cord that has retained its ability to activate discrete motor groups below the level of injury. The motor control remains organized but specificity is reduced, co-contractions occur, and efficiency is affected. In the *new anatomy* condition, alternatively, the few remaining descending axons act on spinal networks to produce primarily diffuse activation or inhibition. The propriospinal system, which is capable of augmenting input by recruiting additional motor cells within the spinal cord, becomes an important network for integrating sensorimotor activities in the spinal cord deprived of supraspinal control (Dimitrijevic et al., 1983).

Much like the computer adage "garbage in equals garbage out," the output of the SLS is based on its residual inputs. The rarer the input, the more the "gain" is increased to "discern" any residual, weak descending input. As a result, the response to any input is more pronounced. With less input, there is less discrete activation and more co-activation. This results from a number of underlying mechanisms, including

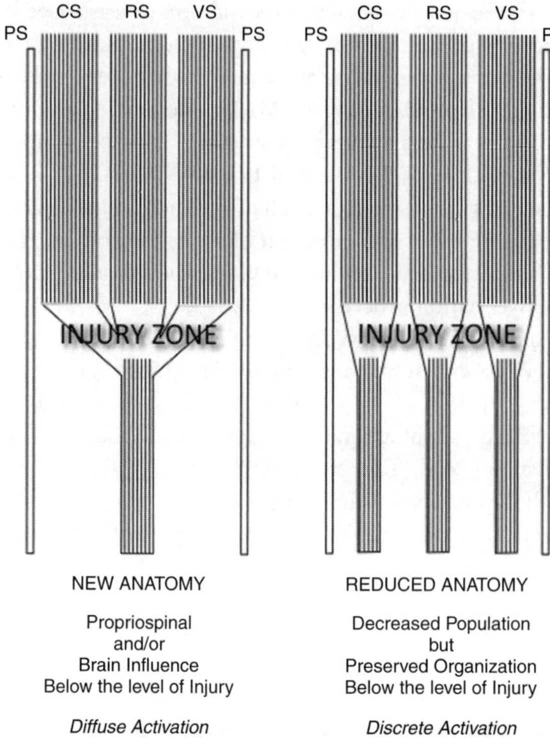

Figure 6–2 Simplified classification of the descending control exerted upon the infralesional segment following a spinal cord injury, discriminating whether a degree of *discrete control* persists (*left*) or simply *influence,* such as diffuse activation (*right*). Tracts represented include: CS = corticospinal, PS = propriospinal, RS = rubrospinal, VS = ventral spinocerebellar. (Adapted from Dimitrijevic, M. R., McKay, W. B., Sherwood, A. M, "Motor control physiology below spinal cord injury: residual volitional control of motor units in paretic and paralyzed muscles." In *Advances in Neurology, vol. 72. Neuronal Regeneration, Reorganization, and Repair*, edited by F. J. Seil, 1997, p. 337.)

sprouting of the residual local afferents to occupy vacated terminals of the prior descending axons; reduction in presynaptic inhibition; and enhancement in the excitability of motoneurons due in part to the activation of persistent inward currents (PICs) (McCouch et al., 1958; Elbasiouny et al., 2010). Additionally, the propriospinal system recruits additional motor neurons within the spinal cord, responding to both peripheral and central inputs and resulting in a more diffuse activation (Dimitrijevic et al., 1983).

With the increasing severity of a lesion, instead of receiving a robust descending drive, the cord receives a weaker descending input, which may be lost in the random peripheral "noise." Given that both central and peripheral inputs converge on the premotor center to produce the final motor command, even when appropriate descending efferents exist they can be masked by or must compete with the peripheral input (Kern et al., 2005; Dietz, 2010). As a result, the movements expressed often do not reflect the subject's intention and may not be easily attenuated. Therefore, traumatic spinal cord injury tends to result in two basic outputs from the infralesional segment: functional/volitional outputs representing the response to residual appropriate descending input and "recognizable" peripheral input, and dysfunctional/spastic outputs representing the response to erratic peripheral input and potentially additional spontaneous discharges from regions of disrupted tissue within the IM (Figure 6–3). Given that the same processor produces both outputs, reducing one without reducing the other becomes a challenge.

Peripheral inputs are received from a number of sources, including skin, joint, and muscle receptors; load receptors; and nociception. Central inputs consist of the residual white matter tracts that successfully traverse the IM to synapse within the SLS. Additionally, some authors argue that spontaneous activity from the injured spinal cord tissue at the IM would constitute an additional input (Loeser et al., 1968). To influence the motor output of the system, neurological interventions should primarily modify these inputs, reducing the pathological inputs and augmenting or supplementing the healthy inputs (Figure 6–3).

6.1. Spasticity Reduction and Functional Neurosurgery

The following is a review of the fundamental interventions available today for the management of spasticity, with a focus on functional neurosurgical procedures and their development.

Therapy

Without adequate preservation of passive range of motion and muscular intrinsic properties, even the restoration of a perfect nervous system would not be expressed. As such, stretching, casting, bracing, and other methods are primary interventions.

The presence and appropriateness of sensory input plays a crucial role in motor control following spinal cord injury (Barbeau et al., 2006). In fact, the input from simply positioning a patient in the standing position (activation of load receptors, stretching of flexor musculature, and alteration of sensory input) provides some degree of spasticity reduction and spontaneous activity of antigravity muscles (Stevenson, 2010). When active movement is not possible, phasic and sustained passive movement has also proven beneficial as can be accomplished through modalities such as passive cycling (Harkema et al., 1997; Krause et al., 2008; Mazzocchio et al., 2008). Finally, reproducing the entirety of the gait cycle with body-weight-support treadmill training with manually assisted foot placement can produce much more robust effects (Figure 6–4).

Stimulation

Artificially increasing input through electrical stimulation is known to be of benefit as well. When used improperly, however, some paradigms have actually demonstrated an increase in spasticity, as one would expect with increasing "noise" (Robinson et al., 1988). Both the stimulation parameters and their timing are critical (Szecsi & Schiller, 2009).

By creating a more physiological signal, afferent excitation via stimulation of peripheral nerves can restore reflex modulation during walking (Muir & Steeves, 1997) (Figure 6–5). Passive cycling in motor complete spinal cord injury patients, when driven by functional electrical stimulation (FES) of leg muscles, has a significantly greater effect on spasticity (Krause et al., 2008). Similarly, coupling

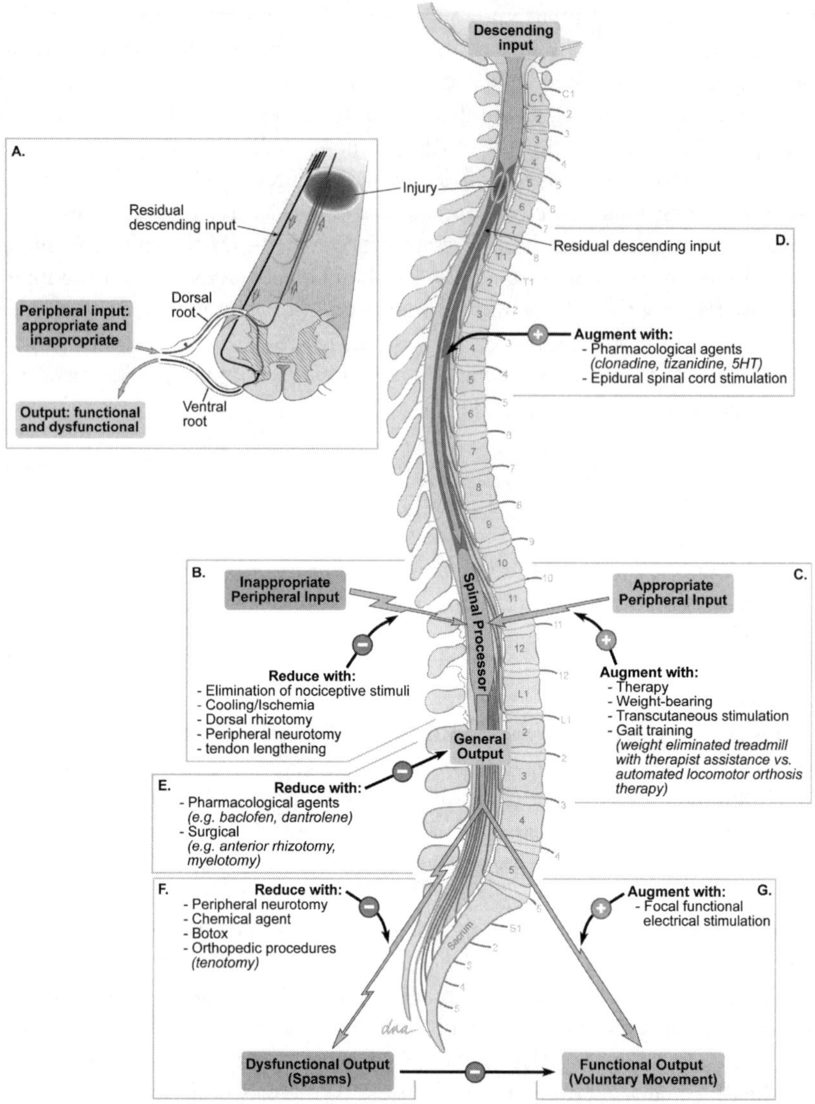

Figure 6–3 The infralesional segment of the spinal cord is typically a healthy processor whose outputs are often dysfunctional as a result of the altered inputs. While inputs are limited to those arriving from residual tracts that traverse the IM and those arriving via the dorsal roots, the latter provides a much greater influence than before injury; output through intact ventral roots remains essentially unaffected (*A*). A primary method of altering the output of the processor, therefore, is either reducing inappropriate inputs (*B*) or augmenting appropriate peripheral inputs (*C*). Advances are being made in providing input to the processor that either replaces lost descending neurotransmitters or mimics familiar descending electrical activity (*D*). Many of the spasticity treatments that are utilized today cause a general suppression of functional and dysfunctional output, reducing spasms and hindering potential ambulation (*E*). Alternatively, treatments are available that can specifically reduce dysfunctional output (*F*) or augment functional output (*G*). (*See* color insert.)

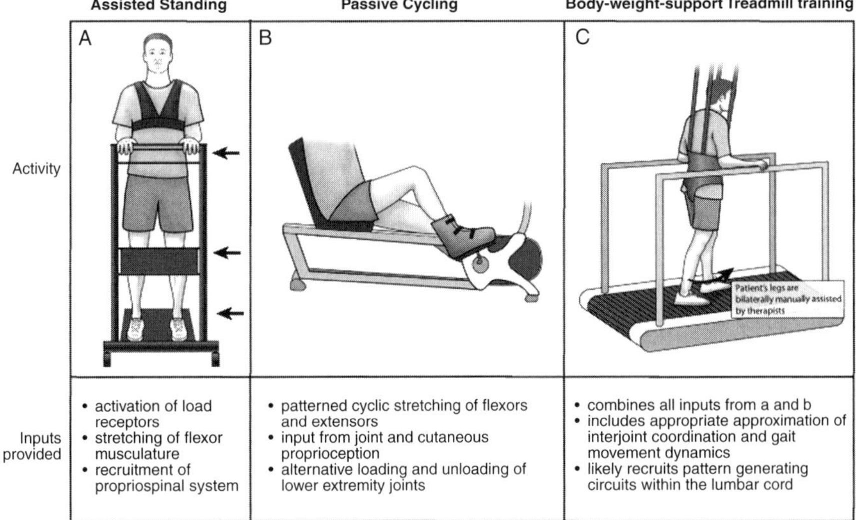

Figure 6–4 Optimizing appropriate peripheral input: incremental therapies. Therapy alone can provide significant useful inputs to the spinal cord, which can reduce spasticity, augment function, and help drive plasticity. Each modality provides a subset of the normal complement of peripheral inputs to the ILS. Standing alone activates load receptors at the hips, knees, and ankles (*A*). Implementation of passive physiological movements provides a number of additional inputs, including joint, muscular, and cutaneous proprioceptive feedback in a physiological pattern (*B*). Assisted treadmill training may provide the most physiological set of inputs, combining each of those provided by the first two modalities (*C*).

stimulation paradigms with gait training has been demonstrated to improve intralimb coordination (Field-Fote & Tepavac, 2002; Hesse et al., 2004).

Pharmacological interventions

The mainstay of contemporary spasticity management in spinal cord injury has been the use of pharmacological agents. The most commonly employed medications include dantrolene, diazepam, tizanidine, and baclofen (Fiedler & Jeffrey, 2002; Elbasiouny et al., 2010; Adams & Hicks, 2005). Dantrolene works on the muscle itself to reduce contractility; the others act centrally. With increasing severity of spasticity, increasingly large doses of these medications are required to have a useful effect. Unfortunately, side effects can be quite disabling with such doses, and methods of targeted application have therefore been devised.

Surgical placement of a programmable pump for intrathecal administration of baclofen has been the most widely accepted functional neurosurgical intervention for spasticity management and has now been incorporated into the spasticity algorithm of most rehabilitation centers. Clinical studies have demonstrated its efficacy and reliability, and clinicians and patients alike are more comfortable with it than with other surgical interventions because it is reversible (Azouvi et al., 1996; Dario & Tomei, 2004; Jagatsinh, 2009) (also see Chapter 3). Because these medications cause a generalized suppression of neuronal activity, they may also reduce the

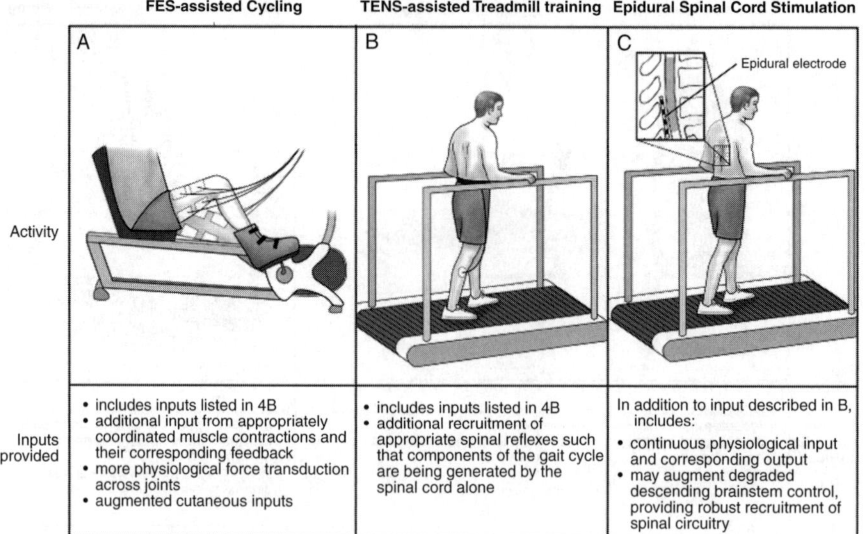

Figure 6–5 Enhancing peripheral inputs: incremental stimulation paradigms. In addition to manual manipulation and assistance, stimulation can add another layer of inputs that are interpreted in a useful manner by the spinal processor. If, instead of moving the legs passively in a cycling pattern as in Figure 6–4B, they are driven by appropriately timed muscular stimulation, an additional set of physiological inputs is provided that better approximates those seen in the healthy spinal cord (*A*). Gait training can be augmented similarly with direct muscular stimulation, or spinal reflexes can be harnessed for direct central contribution to the movement, as seen in this peroneal stimulation paradigm (*B*). Finally, by providing simultaneous stimulation of multiple levels of the spinal cord in a pattern similar to what this network would have otherwise been exposed to from above, the entirety of the gait cycle can be directly augmented (*C*). TENS = transcutaneous electrical neural stimulation, FES = functional electrical stimulation.

functional output of the injured nervous system, resulting in a pharmacologically induced apraxia (Elbasiouny et al., 2010). A deterioration of abilities, including gait, has been documented. Many would argue, though, that most of these patients generally lack significant motor control, making this irrelevant (Fiedler & Jeffrey, 2002).

Surgical placement of an epidural spinal cord stimulator (ESCS) has the potential to provide the most physiological input to the spinal cord (Dimitrijevic, 1985; Minassian et al., 2004). With proper lead positioning and adherence to stimulation specifications, it may be an effective modality. However, both technical inconsistencies and reports of long-term inefficacy have resulted in its falling into disfavor (Midha & Schmitt, 1998; Pinter et al., 2000). This modality is further discussed later in this chapter.

Ablative procedures

Ablative procedures for managing spasticity have included rhizotomies, myelotomies, and neurotomies (or lesions of the nerve roots, spinal cord, and peripheral nerves, respectively) (Smyth & Peacock, 2000; Burchiel & Hsu, 2001). Of these procedures, the only one that can reliably enhance active function in an appropriately selected patient is peripheral motor neurotomies. In these procedures, the majority of fascicles of a nerve contributing to specific muscle groups are cut. Generally this complement is compensated for by motor unit enlargement so that muscle fibers are rescued, but the complement of large afferent fibers providing feedback to the spinal cord from that particular muscle group is irreversibly reduced, reducing reflex activation. As a result, balance of muscular tone across a joint is restored as spasticity is reduced.

Although moving more proximally to interrupt the reflex through cutting the dorsal rootlets as they enter the cord (dorsal rhizotomies) demonstrates great efficacy in the immediate postoperative period, unfortunately a high rate of recurrence of spasticity has been reported (Smyth & Peacock, 2000). When a regional source of afferent input to the ILS is eliminated, the limited input to the lumbar spinal cord is further reduced. Initially this may result in effective spasticity reduction, similar to the initial "spinal shock" period following trauma; however, as occurs following any change in inputs to the nervous system, additional plasticity ensues with time. The "gain" within the ILS is thereby increased even more, and spasticity may ultimately recur based on amplification of the remaining inputs. Conversely, specific motor neurotomies maintain their efficacy, because they are focal and not regional. Therefore a generalized increase in gain would not re-create its over-activity in relation to that of its neighboring muscle groups.

An alternative method of rhizotomy for eliminating spasms, cutting the anterior rootlets exiting the spinal cord (anterior rhizotomy), was found to be both effective and lasting but induced severe atrophy. This often led to ulcerations and made care difficult because of a lack of some degree of useful tone.

Myelotomies have taken many forms over the years. The original Bischof myelotomy attempted to interrupt the reflex arc between the ventral and dorsal horns by dividing the distal spinal cord into dorsal and ventral halves. Although this was effective in relieving spasticity, the original series found recurrence in 25% of cases (Tonnis & Bischof, 1962). Additionally, residual function was eliminated. Eventually, this procedure was recommended only in cases of complete spinal cord injury. Later, to preserve motor and genitourinary function, this procedure was revised to what is now referred to as the *T-myelotomy* (Burchiel & Hsu, 2001). This lesion involves a dorsal midline incision, which is then extended laterally. Neuromonitoring techniques successfully identified the lowest safe extent of the lesion, preserving any residual bowel, bladder, and sexual function (Cusick et al., 1976). Motor function at the levels of the lesion, though, was still eliminated. Nonetheless, most patients could be weaned from their spasticity medications. Sindou modified the rhizotomy by dividing the afferent fibers as they enter the spinal cord in the dorsal root entry zone, making this a semimyelotomy (Sindou & Mertens, 2009). This lesion, 3 mm deep and directed at a 45-degree angle, is intended to disrupt myotactic fibers and the medial portion of Lissauer's tract, while sparing lemniscal fibers. This was effective in improving quality of life in 80% to 90% of patients by allowing them to sit and lie comfortably, but is not expected to improve volitional function.

Each of these modalities clearly has a role in the management of spasticity in specific clinical settings. Unfortunately, these modalities have often been administered in an effort to rid the patient of positive maladaptive spasticity instead of as part of a clinical program to transform spasticity into a more functional output.

6.2. Functional Augmentation: The Restorative Approach

Spasticity often represents the output of a healthy processor (the SLS) that is being presented an unhealthy input. Optimizing that input, through the reduction pathological inputs and augmentation of healthy inputs, may provide spasticity reduction as a by-product of the patient's functional augmentation (Figure 6–3). Our philosophy is presented in the following sections.

Reduction of pathological inputs

Reducing pathological input to the injured spinal cord begins by eliminating nociceptive stimuli. A thorough medical evaluation is always a critical first step in any intervention, and sources of pain must be identified and addressed. These may include urinary tract infections, bowel impaction, pressure sores, musculoskeletal pathology, deep venous thrombosis, hemorrhoids, or any sources of nociceptive input. In addition, it is essential to identify a "double lesion" should it exist. This is a phenomenon of coincident lumbosacral compromise below the level of injury, which may be a consequence of the same traumatic event. In one study such lesions were identified in approximately 20% of traumatic spinal cord injuries (Beric et al., 1987; Beric, 1993). Because of a lack of general awareness of this phenomenon, double lesions are rarely diagnosed. However, clinical examination may reveal delayed onset of lower extremity atrophy, urinary retention and/or attenuation of the expected hyperreflexia within the ILS, which can occur even years after the original injury. Urodynamics and electrodiagnostics, including lumbosacral evoked potentials, can be helpful in demonstrating the site and extent of the injury (Beric et al., 1987). Traumatic exacerbation of lumbar spondylosis accounts for a subset of these lesions. Post-traumatic arachnoiditis-induced nerve root clumping, spinal cord tethering, and compressive cysts account for others. In fact, in accordance with this, most appear to be compatible with a cauda equina distribution (Beric et al., 1987). Concordant findings of radiculopathy or severe denervation on electrodiagnostic investigation should prompt imaging, including magnetic resonance or myelography. If a surgical lesion is identified, an operation might be undertaken to eliminate the nociceptive input, to preserve the innervation to important muscle groups of this segment, and to prevent secondary consequences, including the development of syringomyelia or myelomalacia. Finally, any late change in a stabilized level of spasticity and/or function should prompt repetition of this evaluation (Calancie et al., 1994; Ramli et al., 2001). Thus, similar to the IM, the SLS may also benefit from late "optimization."

Optimization of physiological inputs

As noted previously, normal inputs to the infralesional segment of the spinal cord would include afferent input from the periphery and descending input from the supralesional segment. On a cellular level these inputs result in electrical and chemical changes. Therefore, two important methods for augmenting or replacing missing inputs are electrical stimulation and pharmacotherapy.

Epidural Spinal Cord Stimulation

Of therapeutic methods of nervous system stimulation, epidural spinal cord stimulation can provide the most physiological-appearing input to the ILS. In 2000, Pinter and coworkers demonstrated that the exact site of stimulation was critical for obtaining the desired effects with spinal cord stimulation (Pinter et al., 2000). This placement was determined not by the location of the injury, but by the site of the structures involved in direct afferent input and motor control of the lower extremities. A quadripolar electrode placed precisely posterior to the spinal cord at the T11–L1 vertebral levels with bipolar stimulation at 50 Hz to 100 Hz and 1 V to 10 V was found to effectively abolish spasticity. In this study investigating the use of epidural spinal cord stimulation for reduction of spasticity, six of the eight patients demonstrated a marked response, and two had a moderate response. In fact, all but one patient discontinued their antispasticity medications (Pinter et al., 2000).

Using a very similar paradigm, but at a different frequency, epidural stimulation can also elicit either stepping movements (Minassian et al., 2004) or lower limb extension in motor complete spinal cord injury patients (Jilge et al., 2004a). The type of motor output was apparently determined by the frequency of stimulation. The spinal processor could be alternatively activated to perform one of three tasks, based on the input received: from relaxation, to tonic extension, and finally to stepping (Jilge et al., 2004b). In 2002, Herman and coworkers tested the effects of superimposing the step-generating frequencies on the impaired motor control of an ASIA-C wheelchair-dependent patient with moderate spasticity. The patient underwent partial-weight-bearing therapy (PWBT) followed by SCS. PWBT led to improved stereotypic stepping patterns associated with markedly reduced spasticity, but was insufficient for overground walking. SCS with PWBT generated immediate improvement in the subject's gait rhythm, and overground walking was achieved. Over time the stimulation conferred no added benefit at short distances of ambulation, but it continued to enhance performance at longer distances (Herman et al., 2002). Whereas the site of activation appears to be through the dorsal roots, the spinal cord appears to interpret the signal as being similar to that of brain stem descending tonic input (Dimitrijevic et al., 1998). Further details of the neurophysiology of this technique are presented in Chapter 3.

Whether a patient might benefit from such epidural stimulation can be assessed with a transcutaneous version of the device in which electrodes are placed bilaterally over the paraspinous muscles at the T11–T12 level, with an indifferent electrode over the abdomen. This system is comprehensively discussed in Chapter 10. A patient may benefit from a period of therapy with this modality in conjunction with locomotor training, and graduate from requiring this augmentation. Alternatively, another may benefit from more long-term application via implantation of the epidural leads.

Should long-term placement be warranted, a quadripolar electrode may be inserted percutaneously, with local anesthesia, at the midline between T11 and L1 (Figure 6–6). The introducer needle is inserted into the epidural space, and the electrode is advanced through the needle until it comes to rest at about the T11 level. The position is confirmed using fluoroscopy. Additionally, electrophysiological confirmation of proper placement may be obtained with intraoperative stimulation using a pulse width of 210 microsec and frequency of 5 Hz. The recruitment order of muscle twitches is followed until the iliopsoas is reliably activated. This should place the first or second contact at the spinal cord segment corresponding with L2 function.

Migration of the electrode can be a problem. Tricks such as suturing it to the fascia with a suprafascial loop to avoid traction have been tried with anecdotal benefit, but surgical placement of a paddle electrode minimizes this risk and maximizes efficacy (Villavicencio et al., 2000; North et al., 2005) (Figure 6–7). This intervention improves

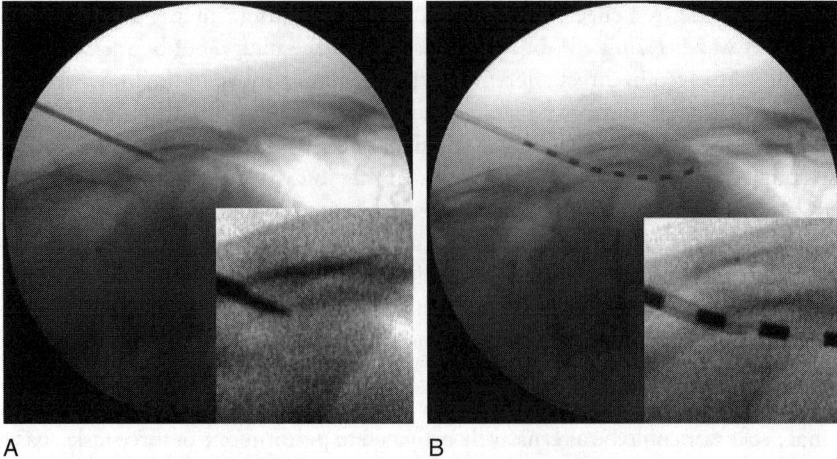

Figure 6–6 Transcutaneous placement of epidural electrode. The introducer needle must be placed at the appropriate angle and depth (*A*). Once this is achieved, fluoroscopy is used to confirm this position and guides the insertion of the electrode to the appropriate site (*B*). (From Zhu, J., Falco, F., Obi Onyewu, C., Josephson, Y., Vesga, R., Jari, R. "Alternative approach to needle placement in spinal cord stimulator trial/implantation." *Pain Physician* 14 (2011): 45–53.)

the efficacy as a result of providing a greater area of contact, having less room for migration, and allowing direct manipulation of the paddle and its associated wire in situ to ensure ideal placement. This is accomplished through an open approach by cutting down to the level of the lamina. The intralaminar ligamentum flavum is removed with Kerrison punches. The electrode is then inserted under direct

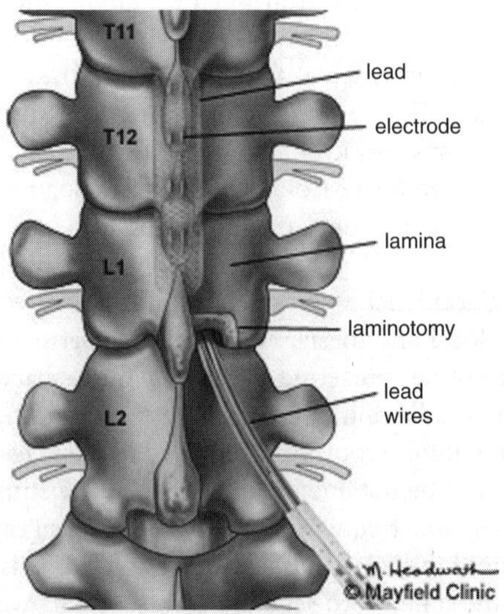

Figure 6–7 If migration of the wire is a problem, a small laminotomy is performed in the operating room, and the paddle is inserted into the epidural space and sutured to adjacent tissues. (Reprinted with permission from the Mayfield Clinic, Cincinnati, Ohio.)

visualization and its position confirmed using fluoroscopy and the same electrophysiological confirmation. Additionally, once the final position has been achieved, the paddle may be sutured to the dura or surrounding tissues (Figure 6-7).

When the effect has been demonstrated, a rehabilitation paradigm incorporating this augmentation is initiated. The patient is then slowly weaned from any pharmacological spasticity suppression until the the best functional state for the given patient is achieved.

Pharmacological Optimization

As discussed in the pharmacology section above, most agents used for spasticity suppression are inhibitory and can contribute to a pharmacological apraxia. In the short term, though, such agents may be useful in bringing spasticity under enough control that the patient becomes a candidate for some of the other modalities discussed.

Among the medications previously discussed, tizanidine stands alone in its potential to preserve strength while reducing spasticity (Fiedler & Jeffrey, 2002; Dimitrijevic 1995). Some have attributed this strength preservation to its inhibitory effect on polysynaptic excitation. Others have focused on a more "restorative" effect. This proposition is based on its potential to act on the receptors of missing noradrenergic descending fibers (Barbeau & Norman, 2003).

In addition to capitalizing on the reduced noradrenergic input, other studies have focused on the role of missing serotonergic fibers. Descending serotonergic fibers are believed to be involved in modifying the excitability of spinal neurons. Cyproheptadine, a serotonergic antagonist, has been administered orally and found to concomitantly reduce spasticity and enhance ambulation (Wainberg et al., 1990) (Figure 6–3). Combining clonidine, another noradrenergic agonist like tizanidine, with cyproheptadine also enhanced the response to locomotor training (Fung et al., 1990).

Unfortunately, significant side effects can limit the oral efficacy of some of these medications. For example, with clonidine and tizanidine, hypotension often limits its efficacy. As with baclofen, this concept has been further developed and hypotension avoided through intrathecal administration. Operative implantation of an intrathecal pump involves general anesthesia with the patient in the prone position. A longitudinal incision is made in the region of L2–L4, as this region is somewhat less mobile than L4–S1. At the level of the fascia just off midline, a Touhy needle is inserted rostrally to enter the dura one to two levels cephalad to the insertion site. The technique is similar to that used for placement of the epidural electrode, but must breech the dura (see Figure 6–6a). Fluoroscopy can be utilized to direct the placement. When CSF returns, the catheter is inserted to its final target, usually between T10 and T12 when lower-extremity spasticity is the indication. The catheter is anchored to the fascia and then tunneled to the abdomen where it is connected to the pump (Albright et al., 2006).

With the same restorative goal in mind, intrathecal clonidine has been found to not only reduce spasticity, but to enhance ambulation in a subpopulation of spinal cord injury patients, including the most severely impaired motor incomplete patients (Barbeau & Norman, 2003). This again demonstrates the concept that providing tonic input that resembles the lost descending control, or augments the residual control, will help transform dysfunctional movements or spasticity into a functional output.

The restorative approach: additional thoughts

Following the rule that the more physiologically "familiar" the input to the spinal cord, the more likely it is that the desired effect will be realized, it should be recognized that no healthy spinal cord runs a single monotonous motor program indefinitely. The spinal cord was designed to alternate among functional states and to habituate to continuous familiar stimuli. Unfortunately, this has not been considered in our interventions to date.

When a stimulator is implanted, it is most commonly set to a certain parameter, and left to run at that frequency continuously. Intrathecal medications are administered similarly, at constant, continuous doses. Typically these are only altered should the effect wane over time or complications arise. With so many available interventions, even within the same modality, this constraint can easily be alleviated. For example, baclofen can impair motor control during task performance; however, it provides excellent relaxation for avoiding sleep interruption from spasms. A double-chamber pump that provides baclofen at night and an augmentative alternative such as clonidine and/or cyproheptadine in the day is quite feasible. Similarly, given that epidural stimulation provides at least three functional states, allowing a means of toggling among these to suit the physical demands at hand is likely to allow greater extended efficacy. Finally, combining these modalities may be beneficial and potentially reduce the doses of pharmacotherapy required.

Therapeutic modalities such as those described above are tailored with the goal of achieving the most physiological output possible with the given constraints of the system. As this approach is pursued and maintained, plasticity will ensue and the best function for a given injury will be achieved. As functional improvement plateaus, specific muscle activation patterns within the extremity are investigated. Specific muscle imbalances across a joint are common. These limit the ultimate function achieved, and more focal interventions must be pursued. This will be further developed below.

7. FOCAL INTERVENTIONS FOR FUNCTION RECOVERY AND THE EXPANDING ROLE OF NERVE TRANSFERS

Unlike the patterned movements of the lower extremities, many of which can be accomplished by the processing capabilities of the lumbar spinal cord alone, most of the functional movements of the upper extremity require robust brain control. Therefore, once the condition of the IM has been optimized as described above, the next set of interventions to further improve upper extremity function may involve capitalizing on redundancy of the SLS via nerve or tendon transfers. Both nerve and tendon transfer procedures are used to address instances of paralysis of the arms and hands following nervous system injury and to bring cortically controlled supralesional nerves or muscles into a position to control lesional or infralesional muscle groups (Kozin, 2002; Brown & Mackinnon, 2008). Such interventions can be helpful for treating paralyzed muscle groups following both UMN and LMN injuries.

7.1. Tendon Transfer Surgery

Hand function is consistently rated as the most desired function for tetraplegic patients, above bowel and bladder function, sexual function, standing, and pain control (Snoek et al., 2004). Tendon transfers are the traditional approach for improving arm and hand function in individuals with tetraplegia. In this procedure, the distal end of a functional muscle is cut, moved, and reattached to the distal tendon of a nonfunctional muscle. The new configuration produces a new function approximating that of the muscle/tendon group to which the transferred tendon is attached (Figure 6–8, A and B).

Tendon transfers sacrifice a function at a lesser location to produce movement at a more important location. For example, when multiple muscles are present, each contributing to wrist extension in the absence of grip, one or more of these redundant muscle groups can be rearranged to pull on a finger- or thumb-flexing tendon to provide grasp to an otherwise paralyzed hand. These procedures have provided a certain amount of autonomy for people with tetraplegia.

Most activities of daily living (ADLs) are performed through lateral thumb pinch (key-pinch), grasp, and release. Restoration of these basic functions combined with reestablishment of elbow extension has been shown to increase independence, spontaneity, and function according to a variety of outcome measures (Hentz & Leclerq, 2002). Tendon transfers have been a useful method of accomplishing this goal.

Unfortunately, there are impediments to an ideal result following such interventions. Surgery should be performed early, prior to the development of hand contractures, which may interfere with the ability to create a useful pinch or grasp (Kozin, 2002). When this occurs, additional surgical procedures may be required. Muscle groups affected by LMN damage fibrose over time, leading to joint contractures. These contractures may develop in a delayed fashion and interfere with function of the reconstructed hand (Coulet et al., 2002). Additionally, there have been psychological barriers to appropriate candidates receiving these procedures, including fear of disfigurement when a "cure" may be on the horizon, perception of less than ideal results, and fear of the period of immobilization required following such procedures.

7.2. Nerve Transfer Surgery

Nerve transfers are a more recent addition to our armamentarium of procedures to restore function following spinal cord injury (Brown, 2011). Nerve transfers have most commonly been employed in paralyses resulting from peripheral nerve injury (LMN) (Narakas & Hentz, 1988; Tung et al., 2004; Midha, 2004). In a nerve transfer, a functional but expendable nerve or nerve branch (donor nerve) is cut, removing its connection to its original target. This cut proximal nerve stump is then sutured to the distal end of a different cut nerve corresponding to its new target, generally a critical but paralyzed muscle group (Figure 6–8, C and D). In time the axons from the cut donor nerve grow into the target muscle and restore contractility.

These procedures offer several advantages over tendon transfers. They preserve the natural biomechanics of the extremity, maintaining line-of-pull and excursion and avoiding scar-induced restrictions to movement. They do not require the extended periods of immobilization that are needed after tendon transfers. Nerve transfer operations provide options for many injuries that are not amenable to tendon transfers. Finally, they offer a greater functional gain for a given transfer (Brown, 2011). That is, the transferred axons, which originally provided innervation to a single muscle and thus a single function, can reinnervate multiple target muscles.

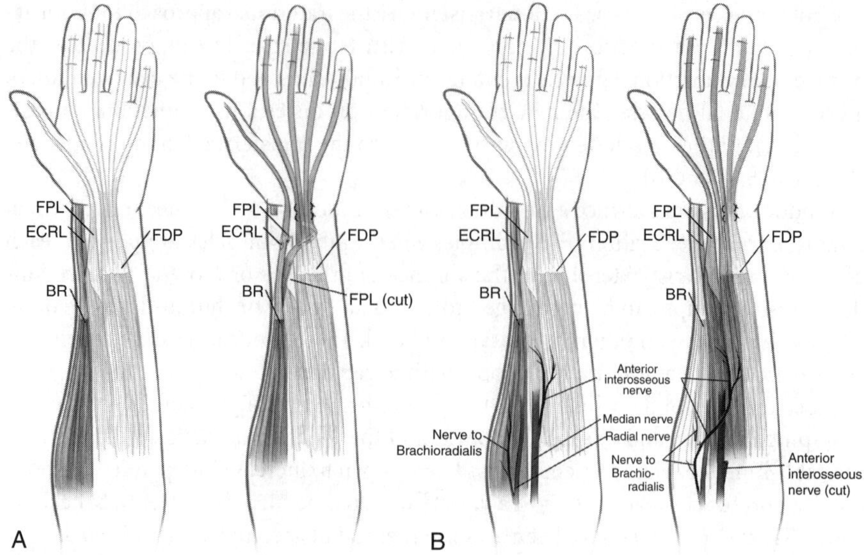

Figure 6–8 Comparison of nerve and tendon transfer procedures. (*A*) In a tendon transfer, the distal end of a functional muscle is cut, moved, and reattached to the distal tendon of a nonfunctional muscle—in this case the brachioradialis (BR) to the flexor pollicis longus (FPL) for thumb flexion, and the extensor carpi radialis longus (ECRL) to all four tendons of the flexor digitorum profundus (FDP) to flex digits 2–5. Muscle orientations are changed, the distances muscles move with contraction may vary, and only a single function is gained per muscle moved; however, function is present as soon as surgical casts are removed. (*B*) In a nerve transfer procedure, the donor nerve is transected and the proximal nerve stump is sutured to the distal end of another cut nerve that feeds a critical but paralyzed muscle group. In this case, transferred axons, which originally innervated a single muscle (BR) and thus contributed to a single function (elbow flexion), can reinnervate multiple target muscles—flexion of the thumb, index and middle fingers (FPL and radial half of the FDP), providing some independence to each. Muscle configurations are maintained and a larger repertoire of interventions may be available for a given deficit, but the time required for functional recovery can be substantial.

When this occurs, central plasticity ensues, often allowing independent activation of multiple functions. Each function is then driven by a subset of the same original axons. By contrast, with tendon transfers only one movement can generally be produced per muscle/tendon group transferred (Anastakis et al., 2008).

As discussed previously, the IM generally suffers a mixed upper and lower motor neuron injury, the latter resulting in part from central gray matter destruction (Kakulas, 2004) (Figure 6–1C). In addition, associated injuries to the nerve roots and brachial plexus are commonplace (Benzel & Larson, 1986; McGowin et al., 1989; Midha, 1997). A severe LMN injury involving a critical muscle group requires very different management than an UMN injury. With prolonged peripheral denervation, target muscles are not effectively reinnervated (Fu & Gordon, 1995; Brown et al., 2009). The distal nerve becomes progressively less permissive to regenerating axons due to collagenization of endoneurial tubes and Schwann cell loss (Bain et al., 2001) (Figure 6–10, C and D). Additionally, the target muscle undergoes severe atrophy and fibrosis (Carlson et al., 2002), which often contributes to the development of contractures (Coulet et al., 2002; Bryden et al., 2004; Thomas & Zijdewind, 2006).

In addition to the standard clinical assessment of the extremity, stimulating nerve trunks to elicit CMAPs and direct muscular stimulation are employed. In these evaluations stimulated manual muscle test (SMMT) assessments utilize the MRC 5-point grading scale to establish the effective peripheral innervation of UMN paralyzed muscle groups. Those muscles that when stimulated produce just enough contraction to be graded as a 1/5 or demonstrate no perceptible contraction are considered severely denervated and warrant early intervention, as is the case with a peripheral nerve injury (Peckham et al., 1976; Thomas & Zijdewind, 2006). The near-complete injuries (those graded 2–3/5) may be followed a bit longer. Waiting more than nine to 12 months in the setting of no improvement in SMMT grade is ill advised, because the success of reinnervation will be compromised.

When a patient presents within the window for effective reinnervation, a nerve transfer is the preferred intervention to restore function to a muscle group of the IM with a severe LMN injury (Figure 6–9B). Doing so will prevent atrophy, fibrosis, and contractures and can restore effective volitional function. When innervation must be restored but a supralesional donor is not available, an infralesional donor can be used (Krieger & Krieger, 2000) (Figure 6–9C). This has been found clinically useful in restoring phrenic nerve function when high spinal cord injury results in destruction of the motoneuron pool corresponding to respiration. In this case intercostal nerves from the ILS are used to reinnervate the phrenic nerve distally for later implementation of stimulation-based diaphragmatic pacing. When this strategy is applied to the hand, even without incorporating stimulation, this can prevent contractures and improve hand positioning. Additionally, it preserves musculature for the later implementation of an FES such as the Freehand™ system discussed in Chapter 3.

While the timing of nerve transfer interventions following a peripheral nerve injury or LMN injury resulting from gray matter destruction is critical, this is not the case when addressing a muscle group innervated by the ILS (affected by UMN injury) (Figure 6–9A). A nerve transfer can be effectively implemented even years after such an injury, provided the mechanical properties of the limb have not been irreversibly affected (Louie et al., 1987; Brunelli & Brunelli, 1999). This is because the peripheral axons for the most part remain intact. Therefore, the architecture of the nerve, its Schwann cells, and the target muscles are preserved, making this nerve an excellent conduit for regenerating axons (Figure 6–10, A and B). When a nerve transfer to such a nerve is undertaken, it is the first time this nerve has seen an injury. As a consequence of the transection of this nerve to accomplish the transfer, Wallerian degeneration takes place for the first time. Proliferation of Schwann cells and upregulation of neurotrophic factors and cell-adhesion molecules ensues. These events provide a powerful stimulus for drawing new axons into the distal nerve.

Nerve transfer interventions have been developed for restoring hand function in cervical spinal cord injury, as well as lower extremity function in low thoracic and lumber spinal cord injury. For the most part, such interventions are most successful when the nerve to a functional muscle group is in relative proximity to that of the intended target muscle, obviating the need for a graft. Additionally, it is important that the patient can easily conceptualize the reeducation design—that is, activating

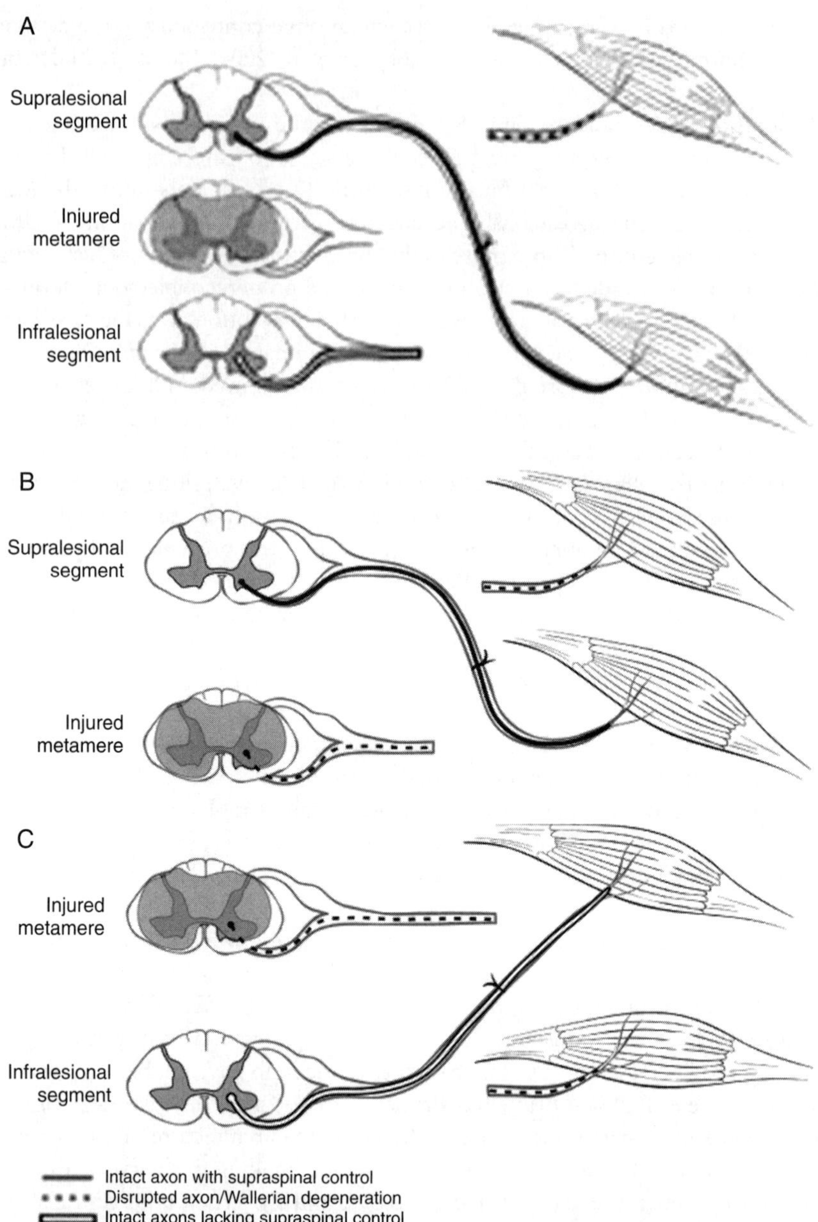

Figure 6–9 Types of nerve transfers available in SCI. (*A*) SLS to ILS: When a nerve originating in the SLS is expendable and can reach a critical muscle group of the ILS, dysfunctional spastic control can be replaced with volitional control even years after an injury. (*B*) SLS to IM: When the IM has a significant component of peripheral axon loss, this should be addressed in a timely manner with a transfer from the SLS to restore volitional control. (*C*) ILS to IM: If an SLS donor is not available, the architecture of the muscle associated with the IM can be preserved with a transfer from the ILS, but the same time constraints exist. Additionally, the latter transfer provides the possibility of later FES activation of this muscle group, as has been done with intercostal to phrenic nerve transfers followed by phrenic pacing.

the muscle transferred *from* in conjunction with that transferred *to*. A synergistic function is preferable, and antagonists are quite difficult to retrain. These interventions are a more recent addition to our surgical options for restoring function in patients with spinal cord injury; therefore, unlike tendon transfers, a standard set of nerve transfers has not yet emerged. Also, in cases amenable to either nerve or tendon transfers, the ultimate functional advantages of one strategy over another have not been fully elucidated.

Sensory deficits in critical regions of the extremity represent another important indication for nerve transfers (Brunelli, 2004) (Figure 6–11). Sensory input clearly enhances the functional results achieved with restoration of motor function (Moberg, 1983). It must be recognized that sensation gained as a result of these procedures is not "normal" and must be weighed in reference to any rudimentary sensation that may be present within the intended target region. Rules are similar to those guiding motor nerve transfers, with sensation gained appearing in its most rudimentary form at six or so months from the time of the intervention and improving over approximately two years.

7.3. Managing Focal Spasticity

Once general spasticity has been reduced and function enhanced via the restorative approach outlined previously, any residual focal spastic features that may persist should be addressed. Such features may occur in upper limbs, lower limbs, or both, and may interfere with function, cause pain, or complicate basic hygiene (Marciniak et al., 2008). There are three classifications of goals in the setting of this type of focal spasticity: *symptomatic improvement*, which pertains to the elimination of problematic spasms and secondary pain; enhancement of *passive function* to facilitate personal care and transfers; and finally, enhancement of *active function*, including grasp and ambulation (Esquenazi et al., 2010). Of note, in some individuals spasticity can actually be useful, substituting for absent volitional control in a muscle and providing rudimentary function (Waters et al., 1996). For example, spasticity in the thumb and/or finger flexors can facilitate lateral grasp.

When focal spasticity is a problem, proper assessment of all muscle groups contributing to spasticity across a joint is critical. It must be determined whether volitional control exists in any of the individual muscles, whether muscles respond synergistically or dyssynergically (e.g., with co-contraction) to an intended movement, whether muscles produce resistance to passive stretch, and whether a mechanical fixed-shortening exists (Esquenazi & Mayer, 2004; Esquenazi, 2007). These *phenomena of presence*, in combination with *phenomena of absence* (isolated weakness), contribute to an imbalance of forces across a joint, resulting in dysfunction (Esquenazi et al., 2010). These properties are best identified within specific muscle groups with the use of motion analysis in conjunction with dynamic EMG. This type of assessment helps determine which muscles are being activated at any time point within the cycle of movement and helps us understand whether selective control exists and whether a muscle's activation contributes to or resists the intended movement. A classification scheme has been developed to define the motor control in each muscle based on the dynamic EMG responses seen (Table 6–2) (Keenan et al., 1990).

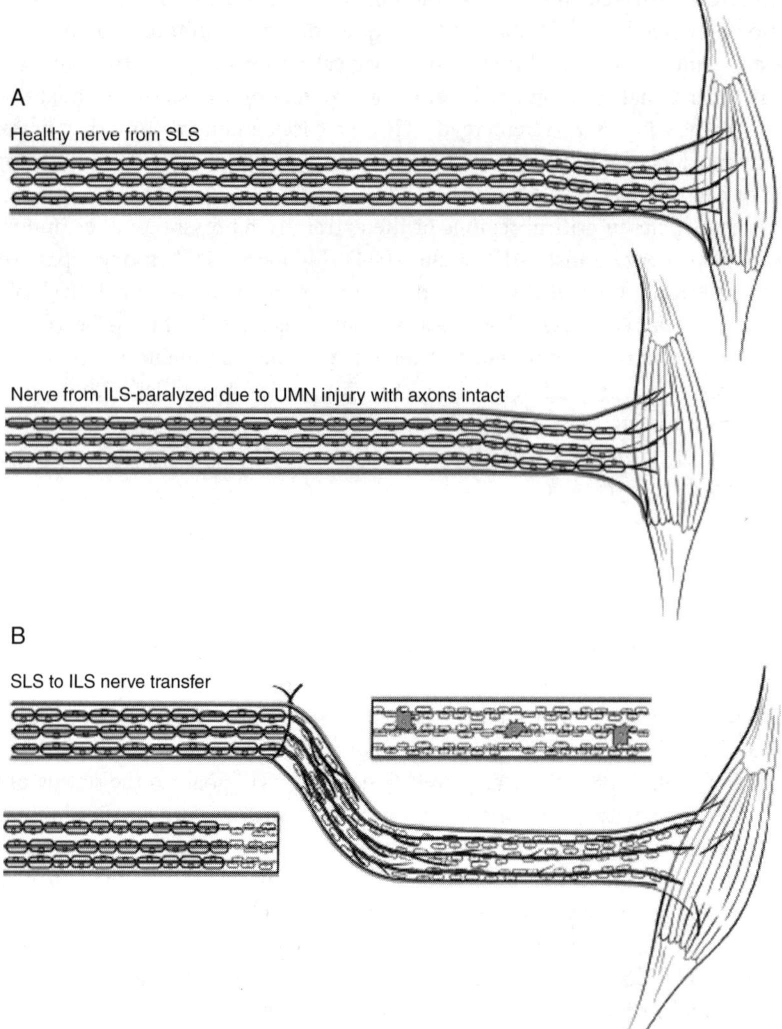

Figure 6–10 (*A*) Even years after a UMN injury, peripheral axons essentially remain intact. The architecture of the nerve, its Schwann cells, and the target muscles are preserved. (*B*) When this nerve is transected during a nerve transfer procedure, Schwann cells proliferate and neurotrophic factors and cell-adhesion molecules are upregulated, providing a powerful stimulus for drawing new axons into the distal nerve.

Neurolytic practices, including injection of alcohol or phenol, have, for the most part, been replaced by targeted injections of botulinum toxin (BTX) into the most problematic spastic muscles. BTX is an effective treatment for focal spasticity in patients with spinal cord injury (Marciniak et al., 2008). A 78% success rate in improving function has been cited with the application of BTX to specific muscle groups of the upper extremity, from the shoulder girdle to the finger flexors (Marciniak et al., 2008).

A number of surgical options also exist for enhancing function in this population. In the motor incomplete (ASIA-C or -D) patient, established interventions in the

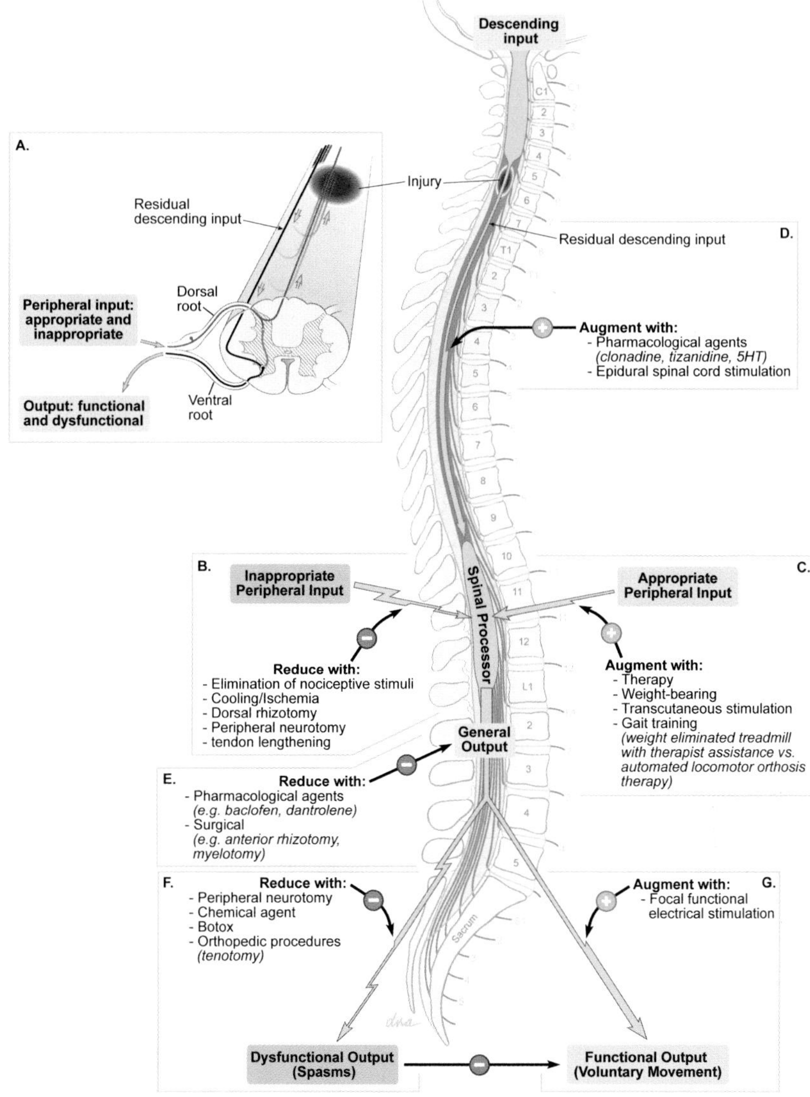

Figure 6–3 The infralesional segment of the spinal cord is typically a healthy processor whose outputs are often dysfunctional as a result of the altered inputs. While inputs are limited to those arriving from residual tracts that traverse the IM and those arriving via the dorsal roots, the latter provides a much greater influence than before injury; output through intact ventral roots remains essentially unaffected (*A*). A primary method of altering the output of the processor, therefore, is either reducing inappropriate inputs (*B*) or augmenting appropriate peripheral inputs (*C*). Advances are being made in providing input to the processor that either replaces lost descending neurotransmitters or mimics familiar descending electrical activity (*D*). Many of the spasticity treatments that are utilized today cause a general suppression of functional and dysfunctional output, reducing spasms and hindering potential ambulation (*E*). Alternatively, treatments are available that can specifically reduce dysfunctional output (*F*) or augment functional output (*G*).

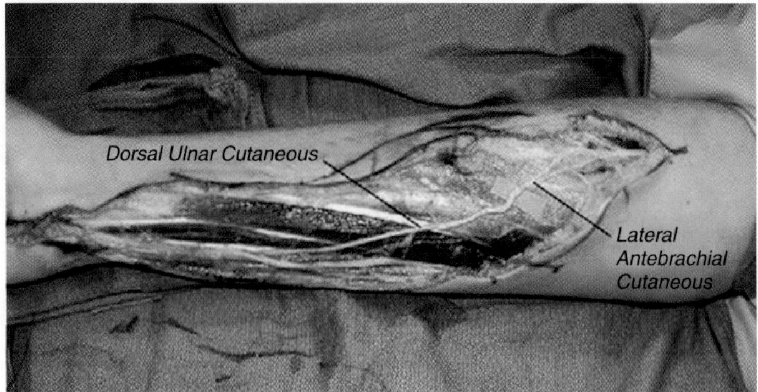

Figure 6–11 Sensory nerve transfers. When sensation is lacking from a critical region of the body, such as the digits, sensation can be transferred to this location from a neighboring nerve originating within the SLS, such as the sensory nerve to the lateral forearm. In this figure the lateral antebrachial cutaneous nerve is transferred to provide sensation to the ulnar distribution of the hand. (From Brown, J. M, Mackinnon, S. E. "Nerve transfers in the forearm and hand." *Hand Clinics* 24 (2008): 319–334.)

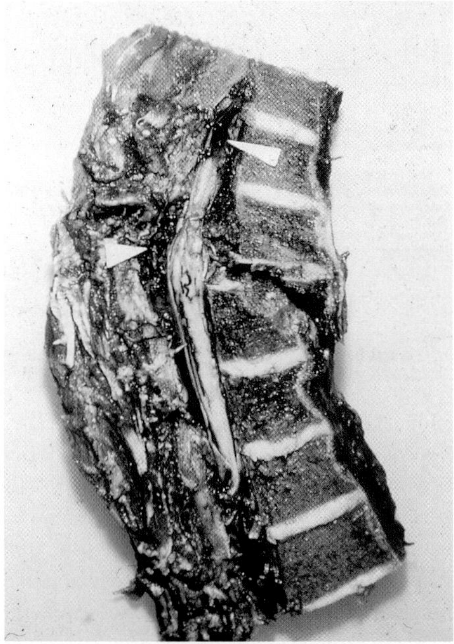

Figure 7–1 Vertical section of spinal cord and vertebral column three days after injury, showing forward dislocation at C5–C6. Note the extradural hemorrhages (*arrow*) and continuity of spinal cord tissue despite the severe trauma.

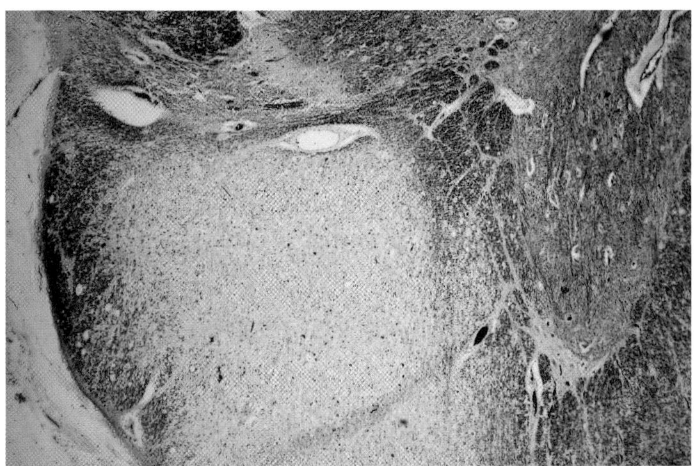

Figure 7–2 Cross-section of spinal cord at T6 several years post-injury, stained with the Loyez method for myelin (*black*) showing pallor of the lateral corticospinal tract indicating chronic Wallerian degeneration, which is a continuous process post-injury.

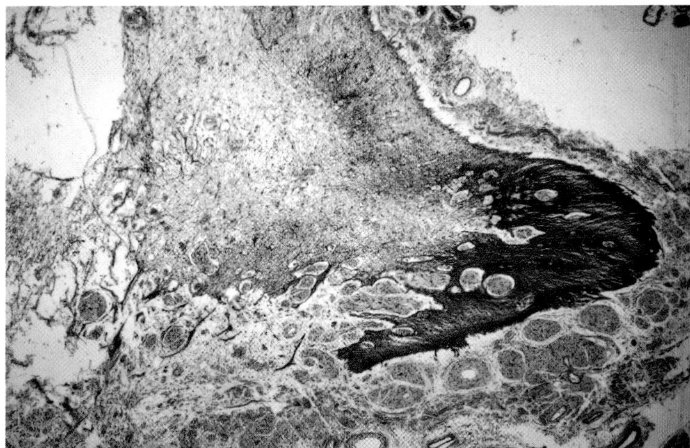

Figure 7–3 Spinal cord in cross-section at C5, many years after injury, stained with PTAH (*blue*, indicating advanced gliosis) with regenerated nerve roots inside and outside the cord (*red*). The regenerated nerve fibers arise from both anterior horn neurons and posterior root ganglia. They have no functional significance.

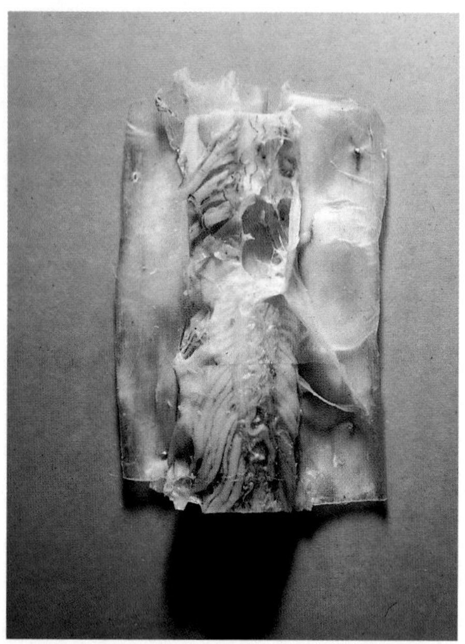

Figure 7–4 Spinal cord at C6 vertical and posterior longitudinal view showing the "end stage" lesion, many years post-injury. Removal of necrotic debris results in a multilocular cavity traversed by glio-vascular bundles. Note the preserved spinal cord tissue at left.

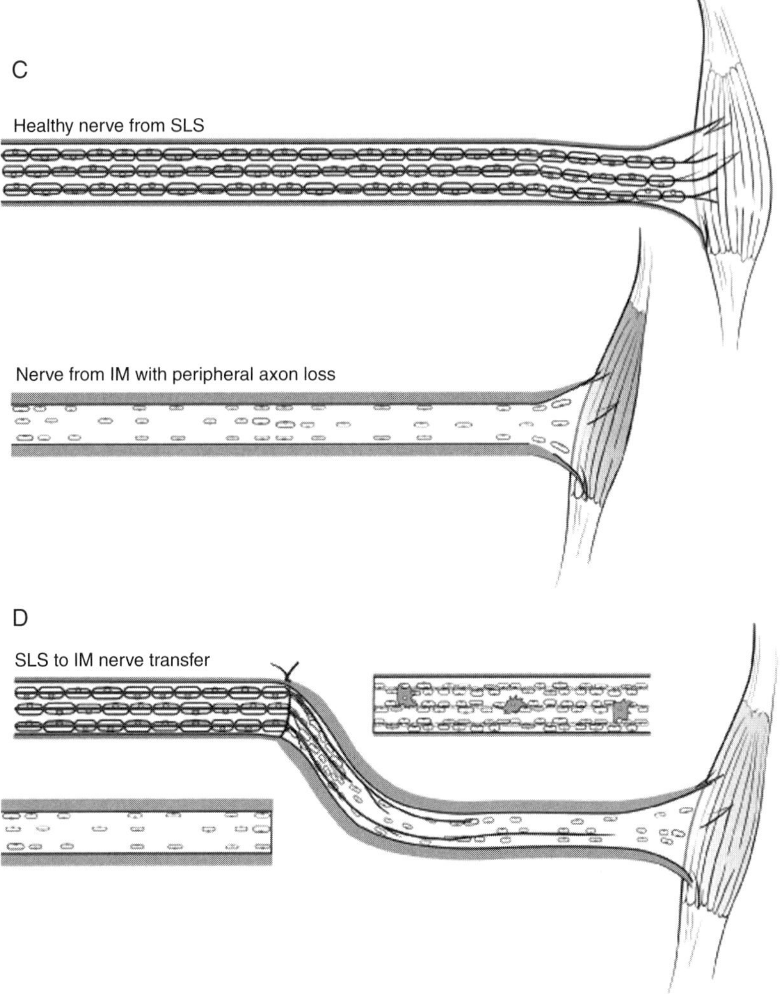

Figure 6–10 (*Cont'd.*)(*C*) Alternatively, in a LMN injury, axons are lost, and with time Schwann cells are fewer and provide less neurotrophic support, and connective tissue thickens, providing further mechanical barriers to axon regeneration. (*D*) While a nerve transfer provides a useful complement of newly regenerating axons, the environment of the recipient nerve is less favorable.

limbs include transecting the corresponding tendon (releases) for muscles with severe spasticity without phasic control. Spastic muscles with some degree of phasic control are treated with muscle-lengthening procedures or peripheral neurotomies, as described previously (Maarrawi et al., 2006; Keenan et al., 2003). Such interventions have even been demonstrated to reduce spasticity and enhance motor control within individual muscles of the spastic extremity (Keenan et al., 1990). In select cases tendon transfers are an important adjunct and can improve balance across a joint. When nerve transfers are added to the list of available procedures, goals can be

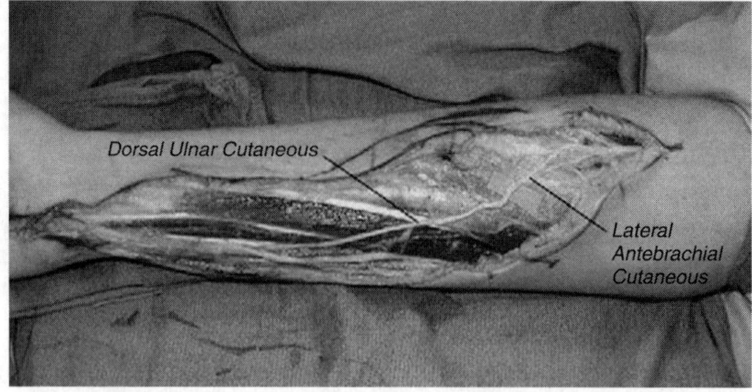

Figure 6–11 Sensory nerve transfers. When sensation is lacking from a critical region of the body, such as the digits, sensation can be transferred to this location from a neighboring nerve originating within the SLS, such as the sensory nerve to the lateral forearm. In this figure the intact lateral antebrachial cutaneous nerve (C5/6) is transferred to provide sensation to the insensate ulnar distribution of the hand (C8). (From Brown, J. M, Mackinnon, S. "Nerve transfers in the forearm and hand." *Hand Clinics* 24 (2008): 319–334.) (*See* color insert.)

expanded to potentially include what was previously considered unrealistic (Fuller, 2010), including restoring volitional control to specific muscles and increasing their muscle force generation.

In the motor complete patient with some preserved muscle groups within the SLS, as described previously, control can be brought to paralyzed muscles at and below the level of injury. When the target muscle is a spastic one (e.g., class IV), a nerve transfer will eliminate that spasticity and replace it with volitional, healthy control. In a patient with an incomplete injury, without a locally available SLS donor nerve, the nerve transfer is considered among the orthopedic options listed above. Nerve transfers in this scenario offer the possibility of exchanging function, replacing class IV–VI function with function-preserving class I–III function, class I and II being preferable. It may be even more critical when using infralesional donors to select a donor that is synergistic with the target function, because the degree of potential plasticity cannot be accurately anticipated. Therefore the functional consequences of potential failure to achieve independence of recipient from donor function must be carefully considered.

Table 6–2 Classification of EMG Activity

Class I	Normal phasic activity
Class II	Premature prolonged activity
Class III (a, b, c)	Phasic prolonged activity (mild, moderate, severe)
Class IV	Continuous activity
Class V	Stretch response activity
Class VI	Absent activity

From Keenen, M. A., Haider, T. T., Stone, L. R. 1990. "Dynamic electromyography to assess elbow spasticity." *Journal of Hand Surgery* (U.S.) 15, 4 (1990): 607–614.

Table 6–3 Current Reconstructive Neurosurgery Interventions in Spinal Cord Injury

Intervention	Objective
IM decompression/ optimization	Elimination of noxious input, reversal of neurapraxia;potential augmentation of residual function prevention of late deterioration
SLS decompression/ optimization	Elimination of noxious input; Preservation of LMN integrity
Epidural SCS	Augmentation of descending input to the SLS
Intrathecal drug delivery pumps	Augmentation of descending input via replacement of missing neurotransmitters within the SLS
Peripheral neurotomy	Reduction of pathological feedback by large afferents to the spinal cord
	Reduction of focal maladaptive outputs
Nerve transfer surgery	Redistribution of neural control to critical muscle groups
	Recovery of denervated muscle groups Restoration of sensation to critical regions

8. CONCLUSION

The injured spinal cord is most effectively managed by identifying the reversible and irreversible aspects of the injury, and then treating within the appropriate time frame. Neurophysiological evaluation helps make these determinations. Once a profile of the injury and surviving motor control has been determined, a clear treatment plan can be established. In this setting, reconstructive neurosurgery provides a number of interventions which are available today to restore function in the setting of spinal cord injury (Table 6–3).

References

Adams, M. M., Hicks, A. L. "Spasticity after spinal cord injury." *Spinal Cord* 43 (2005): 577–586.

Albright, A. L., Turner, M., Pattisapu, J. V. "Best-practice surgical techniques for intrathecal baclofen therapy." *Journal of Neurosurgery* 104 (4 Suppl) (2006): 233–239.

Anastakis, D. J., Malessy, M. J., Chen, R., Davis, K. D., Mikulis D. "Cortical plasticity following nerve transfer in the upper extremity." *Hand Clinics* 24 (2008): 425–444, vi–vii.

Anderson, P. A., Bohlman. H. H. "Anterior decompression and arthrodesis of the cervical spine: long-term motor improvement. Part II—Improvement in complete traumatic quadriplegia." *American Journal of Bone and Joint Surgery* 74 (1992): 683–692.

Azouvi, P., Mane, M., Thiebaut, J. B., Denys, P., Remy-Neris, O., Bussel, B. "Intrathecal baclofen administration for control of severe spinal spasticity: functional improvement and long-term follow-up." *Archives of Physical Medicine and Rehabilitation* 77 (1996): 35–39.

Bain, J. R., Veltri, K. L., Chamberlain, D., Fahnestock, M. "Improved functional recovery of denervated skeletal muscle after temporary sensory nerve innervation." *Neuroscience* 103 (2001): 503–510.

Barbeau, H., Nadeau, S., Garneau, C. "Physical determinants, emerging concepts, and training approaches in gait of individuals with spinal cord injury." *Journal of Neurotrauma* 23 (2006): 571–585.

Barbeau, H., Norman, K. E. "The effect of noradrenergic drugs on the recovery of walking after spinal cord injury." *Spinal Cord* 41 (2003): 137–143.

Benzel, E. C., Larson, S. J. "Recovery of nerve root function after complete quadriplegia from cervical spine fractures." *Neurosurgery* 19 (1986): 809–812.

Beric, A. "Central pain: 'new' syndromes and their evaluation." *Muscle Nerve* 16 (1993): 1017–1024.

Beric, A., Dimitrijevic, M. R., Light, J. K. "A clinical syndrome of rostral and caudal spinal injury: neurological, neurological, neurophysiological and urodynamic evidence for occult sacral lesion." *Journal of Neurology, Neurosurgery, and Psychiatry* 50 (1987): 600–606.

Bohlman, H. H., Anderson, P. A. "Anterior decompression and arthrodesis of the cervical spine: long-term motor improvement. Part I—Improvement in incomplete traumatic quadriparesis." *American Journal of Bone and Joint Surgery* 74 (1992): 671–682.

Bohlman, H. H., Kirkpatrick, J. S., Delamarter, R. B., Leventhal, M. "Anterior decompression for late pain and paralysis after fractures of the thoracolumbar spine." *Clinical Orthopaedics and Related Research* 300 (1994): 24–29.

Brodbelt, A. R., Stoodley, M. A. "Post-traumatic syringomyelia: a review." *Journal of Clinical Neuroscience* 10 (2003): 401–408.

Brown, J. M. "Nerve Transfers in Tetraplegia: Background and Technique." Surgical Neurology International (2011); 2:121.

Brown, J. M., Mackinnon, S. E. "Nerve transfers in the forearm and hand." *Hand Clinics* 24 (2008): 319–340.

Brown, J. M., Shah, M. N., Mackinnon, S. E. "Distal nerve transfers: a biology-based rationale." *Neurosurgical Focus* 26 (2009): E12.

Brunelli, G. A. "Sensory nerves transfers." *British Journal of Hand Surgery* 29 (2004): 557–562.

Brunelli, G. A., Brunelli, G. R. "Restoration of walking in paraplegia by transferring the ulnar nerve to the hip: a report on the first patient." *Microsurgery* 19 (1999): 223–226.

Bryden, A. M., Kilgore, K. L., Lind, B. B., Yu, D. T. "Triceps denervation as a predictor of elbow flexion contractures in C5 and C6 tetraplegia." *Archives of Physical and Medical Rehabilitation* 85 (2004): 1880–1885.

Burchiel KJ, Hsu FP. *Pain* and *spasticity after spinal cord injury: mechanisms* and *treatment*. Spine (Philadelphia, PA: 1976). 2001 Dec 15;26(24 Suppl): S146–160.

Cadotte, D. W., Singh, G., Fehlings, M. G. "The timing of surgical decompression for spinal cord injury." *F1000 Medicine Reports* 2 (2010): 67. PMCID: 2990468.

Calancie, B., Needham-Shropshire, B., Jacobs, P., Willer, K., Zych, G., Green, B. A. "Involuntary stepping after chronic spinal cord injury. Evidence for a central rhythm generator for locomotion in man." *Brain* 117 (1994): 1143–1159.

Carlson, B. M., Borisov, A. B., Dedkov, E. I., Dow, D., Kostrominova, T. Y. "The biology and restorative capacity of long-term denervated skeletal muscle." *Basic Applied Myology* 12 (2002): 247–254.

Carlstedt, T., Anand, P., Hallin, R., Misra, P. V., Noren, G., Seferlis, T. "Spinal nerve root repair and reimplantation of avulsed ventral roots into the spinal cord after brachial plexus injury." *Journal of Neurosurgery* 93 (2000): 237–247.

Carreon, L. Y., Dimar, J. R. "Early versus late stabilization of spine injuries: a systematic review." *Spine* (Philadelphia, PA: 1976): E727–E733 (2011).

Chiu, W.-T., Kao, M.-C., Hung, C.-C., Lin, S.-Z., Chen H.-J., Tang, S. F. T., et al., editors. *Reconstructive Neurosurgery.* Vienna: Springer-Verlag, 2008.

Coulet, B., Allier, Y., Chammas, M. "Injured metamere and functional surgery of the tetraplegic upper limb." *Hand Clinics* 18 (2002): 399–412, vi.

Cusick, J. F., Larson, S. J., Sances, S. "The effect of T-myelotomy on spasticity." *Surgical Neurology* 6 (1976): 289–292.

Dario, A., Tomei, G. "A benefit-risk assessment of baclofen in severe spinal spasticity." *Drug Safety* 27 (2004): 799–818.

Dietz, V. "Behavior of spinal neurons deprived of supraspinal input." *Nature Reviews. Neurology* 6 (2010): 167–174.

Dimitrijevic, M. R. "Motor control in the spinal cord." In *Recent Achievements in Restorative Neurology. 1. Upper Motor Neuron Functions and Dysfunctions,* edited by J. Eccles and M. R. Dimitrijevic, 150–162. Basel, Switzerland: Karger, 1985.

Dimitrijevic, M. R. "Evaluation and treatment of spasticity." *Journal of Neurologic Rehabilitation* 9 (1995): 97–110.

Dimitrijevic, M. R., Gerasimenko, Y., Pinter, M. M. Evidence for a spinal central pattern generator in humans. *Annals of the New York Academy of Science* 860 (1998): 360–376.

Dimitrijevic, M. R., Faganel, J., Lehmkuhl, D., Sherwood, A. "Motor control in man after partial or complete spinal cord injury." *Advances in Neurology* 39 (1983): 915–926.

Dimitrijevic, M. R., McKay, W. B., Sherwood, A. M. "Motor control physiology below spinal cord injury: residual volitional control of motor units in paretic and paralyzed muscles." *Advances in Neurology* 72 (1997): 335–345.

Doczi, T., Teasdale, G. "EANS Winter Meeting, February 7–9, 2003, Bonn, Germany: Functional and reconstructive neurosurgery." *Acta Neurochirurgica* (Vienna) 145 (2003): 327–330.

Elbasiouny, S. M., Moroz, D., Bakr, M. M., Mushahwar, V. K. "Management of spasticity after spinal cord injury: current techniques and future directions." *Neurorehabilitation and Neural Repair* 24 (2010): 23–33.

El Masry, W. S., Meerkotter, D. V. "Early decompression of the spinal cord following injury: arguments for and against." In *Spinal Cord Dysfunction: Intervention and Treatment,* edited by L. S. Illis, 7–27. New York; Oxford: Oxford University Press, 1992.

Esquenazi, A., Mayer, N. H. "Instrumented assessment of muscle overactivity and spasticity with dynamic polyelectromyographic and motion analysis for treatment planning." *American Journal of Physical and Medical Rehabilitation* 83 (2004): S19–S29.

Esquenazi, A. "Dynamic poly-EMG in gait analysis for the assessment of equinovarus foot." In *Foot and Ankle Motion Analysis: Clinical Treatment and Technology,* edited by R. M. Marks, G. F. Harris, P. A. Smith, 291–299. Boca Raton, FL: CRC Press, 2007.

Esquenazi, A., Cioni, M., Mayer, N. H. "Assessment of muscle overactivity and spasticity with dynamic polyelectromyography and motion analysis." *Open Rehabilitation Journal* 3 (2010): 143–148.

Falci, S. P., Indeck, C., Lammertse, D. P. "Post-traumatic spinal cord tethering and syringomyelia: surgical treatment and long-term outcome." *Journal of Neurosurgery. Spine* 11 (2009): 445–460.

Falcone, S., Quencer, R. M., Patchen, S. J., Post, M. J. "Progressive post-traumatic myelomalacic myelopathy: imaging and clinical features." *American Journal of Neuroradiology* 15 (1994): 747–754.

Fiedler, K., Jeffrey, D. R. "Spasticity in spinal cord injury: A clinician's approach." In *Clinical Evaluation and Management of Spasticity,* edited by D. A. Gelber, D. R. Jeffrey. Totowa, NJ: Humana Press, 2002. pp. 353–368.

Field-Fote, E. C., Tepavac, D. "Improved intralimb coordination in people with incomplete spinal cord injury following training with body weight support and electrical stimulation." *Physical Therapy* 82 (2002): 707–715.

Fu, S. Y., Gordon, T. "Contributing factors to poor functional recovery after delayed nerve repair: prolonged axotomy." *Journal of Neuroscience* 15 (1995): 3876–3885.

Fuller, D. A. "Surgery in the management of spasticity." In *Spasticity: diagnosis and Management,* edited by A. E. Brashear, E. P. Elovic, 243–270. New York: demos Medical, 2010.

Fung, J., Stewart, J. E., Barbeau, H. The combined effects of clonidine and cyproheptadine with interactive training on the modulation of locomotion in spinal cord injured subjects. *Journal of Neurological Sciences* 100 (1990): 85–93.

Gupta, R., Bathen, M. E., Smith, J. S., Levi, A. D., Bhatia, N. N., Steward, O. "Advances in the management of spinal cord injury." *Journal of the American Academy of Orthopedic Surgery* 18 (2010): 210–222.

Hall, E. D. "Acute treatment strategies for spinal cord injury: pharmacologic interventions, hypothermia, and surgical decompression." In *Spinal Cord Medicine: Principles and Practice,* edited by V. W. Lin. New York: demos Medical 2010. pp. 777–784.

Harkema, S. J., Hurley, S. L., Patel, U. K., Requejo, P. S., Dobkin, B. H., Edgerton, V. R. "Human lumbosacral spinal cord interprets loading during stepping." *Journal of Neurophysiology* 77 (1997): 797–811.

Hentz, V. R., and Leclerq, C. *Surgical Rehabilitation of the Upper Extremity in Tetraplegia.* London: W.B. Saunders, 2002.

Herman, R., He, J., D'Luzansky, S., Willis, W., Dilli, S. "Spinal cord stimulation facilitates functional walking in a chronic, incomplete spinal cord injured." *Spinal Cord* 40 (2002): 65–68.

Hesse, S., Werner, C., Bardeleben, A. "Electromechanical gait training with functional electrical stimulation: case studies in spinal cord injury." *Spinal Cord* 42 (2004): 346–352.

Holly, L. T., Johnson, J. P., Mascioppinto, J. E., Batzdorf, U. "Treatment of post-traumatic syringomyelia with extradural decompressive surgery." *Neurosurgical Focus* 8 (2000): E8.

Ishida, K., T. Tani, T. Ushida, V. Zinchk, H. Yamamoto. "Recovery of spinal cord conduction after surgical decompression for cervical spondylotic myelopathy: serial somatosensory evoked potential studies." *American Journal of Physical and Medical Rehabilitation* 82 (2003): 130–136.

Iskandar B. J., Nashold, B. S., Jr. "History of functional neurosurgery." *Neurosurgery Clinics of North America* 6 (1995): 1–25.

Jagatsinh, Y. "Intrathecal baclofen: its effect on symptoms and activities of daily living in severe spasticity due to spinal cord injuries: a pilot study." *Indian Journal of Orthopaedics* 43 (2009): 46–49. PMCID: 2739492.

Jilge, B., Minassian, K., Rattay, F., Pinter, M. M., Gerstenbrand, F., Binder H. "Initiating extension of the lower limbs in subjects with complete spinal cord injury by epidural lumbar cord stimulation." *Experimental Brain Research* 154 (2004a): 308–326.

Jilge B., Minassian, K., Rattay, F., Dimitrijevic, M. R. "Frequency-dependent selection of alternative spinal pathways with common periodic sensory input." *Biological Cybernetics* 91 (2004b): 359–376.

Kakulas, B. A.. Neuropathology: the foundation for new treatments in spinal cord injury. *Spinal Cord* 42, 10 (2004): 549–563.

Katayama, Y. "Activity Report". World Federation of Neurological Societies Neurorehabilitation and Reconstructive Neurosurgery Committee (2005–2009)." (2009).

Keenan, M. A., Haider, T. T., Stone, L. R. "Dynamic electromyography to assess elbow spasticity." *American Journal of Hand Surgery* 15 (4) (1990): 607–614.

Keenan, M. A., Fuller, D. A., Whyte, J., Mayer, N., Esquenazi, A., Fidler-Sheppard, R. "The influence of dynamic polyelectromyography in formulating a surgical plan in treatment of spastic elbow flexion deformity." *Archives of Physical and Medical Rehabilitation* 84 (2003): 291–296.

Kern, H., McKay, W. B., Dimitrijevic, M. M., Dimitrijevic, M. R. "Motor control in the human spinal cord and the repair of cord function." *Current Pharmaceutical Design* 11 (2005): 1429–1439.

Klekamp, J., Batzdorf, U., Samii, M., Bothe, H. W. "Treatment of syringomyelia associated with arachnoid scarring caused by arachnoiditis or trauma." *Journal of Neurosurgery* 86 (1997): 233–240.

Kliot, M., Smith, G. M., Siegel, J., Tyrrell, S., Silver, J. "Reconstructive neurosurgery: novel strategies promoting the regeneration of injured dorsal root sensory fibers into the adult mammalian spinal cord." In *Surgery of the Spinal Cord*, edited by R. N. Holtzman, B. M. Stein. New York: Springer-Verlag, 1992.

Kostyk, S. K., Popovich, P. G. "Mechanisms and natural history of spinal cord injury: morphological, cellular, and molecular features." In *Spinal Cord Medicine,* 2nd ed., edited by V. W. Lin, 871–882. 2010 New York: demos Medical

Kozin, S. H. "Tetraplegia." *Journal of the American Society for Surgery of the Hand* 2 (2002): 141–152.

Krause, P., Szecsi, J., Straube, A. "Changes in spastic muscle tone increase in patients with spinal cord injury using functional electrical stimulation and passive leg movements." *Clinical Rehabilitation* 22 (2008): 627–634.

Krieger, L. M., Krieger, J. "The intercostal to phrenic nerve transfer: an effective means of reanimating the diaphragm in patients with high cervical spine injury." *Plastic Reconstructive Surgery* 105 (2000): 1255–1261.

Lee, T. T., Arias, J. M., Andrus, H. L., Quencer, R. M., Falcone, S. F., Green, B. A. "Progressive post-traumatic myelomalacic myelopathy: treatment with untethering and expansive duraplasty." *Journal of Neurosurgery* 86 (1997): 624–628.

Loeser, J. D., Ward, A. A., Jr., White, L. E., Jr. "Chronic deafferentation of human spinal cord neurons." *Journal of Neurosurgery* 29 (1968): 48–50.

Louie, G., Mackinnon, S. E., Dellon, A. L., Patterson, G. A., Hunter, D. A. "Medial antebrachial cutaneous—lateral femoral cutaneous neurotization in restoration of sensation to pressure-bearing areas in a paraplegic: a four-year follow up." *Annals of Plastic Surgery* 19 (1987): 572–576.

Maarrawi, J., Mertens, P., Luaute, J., et al. "Long-term functional results of selective peripheral neurotomy for the treatment of spastic upper limb: prospective study in 31 patients." *Journal of Neurosurgery* 104(2) (2006): 215–225.

Marciniak, C., Rader, L., Gagnon, C. "The use of botulinum toxin for spasticity after spinal cord injury." *American Journal of Physical and Medical Rehabilitation* 87 (2008): 312–317; quiz, 8–20; 29.

Mazzocchio, R., Meunier, S., Ferrante, S., Molteni, F., Cohen, L. G. "Cycling, a tool for locomotor recovery after motor lesions?" *NeuroRehabilitation* 23 (2008): 67–80.

McCouch, G. P., Austin, G. M., Liu, C. N., Liu, C. Y. "Sprouting as a cause of spasticity." *Journal of Neurophysiology* 21 (1958): 205–216.

McAfee, P. C., Bohlman, H. H., Yuan, H. A. "Anterior decompression of traumatic thoracolumbar fractures with incomplete neurological deficit using a retroperitoneal approach." *American Journal of Bone and Joint Surgery* 67 (1985): 89–104.

McGowin, J. F., Schlitt, M., McCloskey, J. J. "Brachial plexus injuries associated with cervical spine fractures." *Journal of Spinal Disorders* 2 (1989): 104–108.

Midha, R. "Epidemiology of brachial plexus injuries in a multitrauma population." *Neurosurgery* 40 (1997): 1182–1188; discussion, 8–9.

Midha, R. "Nerve transfers for severe brachial plexus injuries: a review." *Neurosurgical Focus* 16 (2004): E5.

Midha, R., Schmitt, J. K. "Epidural spinal cord stimulation for the control of spasticity in spinal cord injury patients lacks long-term efficacy and is not cost-effective." *Spinal Cord* 36 (1998): 190–192.

Minassian, K., Jilge B., Rattay, F., Pinter, M. M., Binder, H., Gerstenbrand, F., et al. "Stepping-like movements in humans with complete spinal cord injury induced by epidural stimulation of the lumbar cord: electromyographic study of compound muscle action potentials." *Spinal Cord* 42 (2004): 401–416.

Moberg, E. "The role of cutaneous afferents in position sense, kinaesthesia, and motor function of the hand." *Brain* 106 (1983): 1–19.

Morikawa, T., Takami, T., Tsuyuguchi, N., Sakamoto, H., Ohata, K., Hara, M. "The role of spinal tissue scarring in the pathogenesis of progressive post-traumatic myelomalacia." *Neurological Research* 28 (2006): 802–806.

Muir, G. D., Steeves, J. D. "Sensorimotor stimulation to improve locomotor recovery after spinal cord injury." *Trends in Neuroscience* 20 (1997): 72–77.

Mulcahey, M. J., Smith, B. T., Betz, R. R. "Evaluation of the lower motor neuron integrity of upper extremity muscles in high level spinal cord injury." *Spinal Cord* 37 (1999): 585–591.

Narakas, A. "Brachial plexus surgery." *Orthopaedic Clinics of North America* 12 (1981): 303–323.

Narakas, A. O., Hentz, V. R. "Neurotization in brachial plexus injuries. Indication and results." *Clinical Orthopaedics and Related Research* 237 (1988): 43–56.

North, R. B., Kidd, D. H., Petrucci, L., Dorsi, M. J. "Spinal cord stimulation electrode design: a prospective, randomized, controlled trial comparing percutaneous with laminectomy electrodes: part II—clinical outcomes." *Neurosurgery* 57, 5 (2005): 990–996.

Peckham, P. H., Mortimer, J. T., Marsolais, E. B. "Upper and lower motor neuron lesions in the upper extremity muscles of tetraplegics." *Paraplegia* 14 (1976): 115–121.

Pinter, M. M., Gerstenbrand, F., Dimitrijevic, M. R. "Epidural electrical stimulation of posterior structures of the human lumbosacral cord: 3. Control of Spasticity." *Spinal Cord* 38 (2000): 524–531.

Polgar, S., Morris, M. E. "Reconstructive neurosurgery: progress towards a best practice treatment for people with Parkinson's disease." In *Parkinson's Disease: New Research*, edited by M. J. Willow, 41–68. New York: Nova Science Publishers, 2005.

Polgar, S., Morris, M. E., Reilly, S., Bilney, B., Sanberg, P. R. "Reconstructive neurosurgery for Parkinson's disease: a systematic review and preliminary meta-analysis." *Brain Research Bulletin* 60 (2003): 1–24.

Potter, S. E., Croce, E. J. "The treatment of peripheral nerve injuries complicated by skin and soft tissue defects." *Annals of Surgery* 125 (1947): 349–359.

Ramli, N., Merican, A. M., Lim, A., Kumar, G. "Post-traumatic arachnoiditis: an unusual cause of Brown-Sequard syndrome." *European Radiology* 11 (2001): 2011–2014.

Robinson, C. J., Kett, N. A., Bolam, J. M. "Spasticity in spinal cord injured patients: 2. Initial measures and long-term effects of surface electrical stimulation." *Archives of Physical and Medical Rehabilitation* 69 (1988): 862–868.

Shefner, J. M., Kothari, M., Logigian, E. L. "Does voluntary muscle contraction cause facilitation of peripherally evoked compound motor action potentials?" *Muscle Nerve* 18 (1995): 555–556.

Shibib, K., Brock, M., Muller, H., Gosztonyi, G. "Maximal regeneration distance. How far can a peripheral axon regenerate?" *Neurological Research* 7 (1985): 177–181.

Siddall, P. J. "Management of neuropathic pain following spinal cord injury: now and in the future." *Spinal Cord* 47 (2009): 352–359.

Sindou, M. P., Mertens, P. "Surgery in the dorsal root entry sone for spasticity." In *Textbook of Stereotactic and Functional Neurosurgery,* 2nd ed., edited by A. M. Lozano, P. L. Gildenberg, R. R. Tasker, 1959–1972. Berlin; Heidelberg: Springer-Verlag, 2009.

Sjolund, B. H. "Pain and rehabilitation after spinal cord injury: the case of sensory spasticity." *Brain Research Reviews* 40 (2002): 250–256.

Smyth, M. D., Peacock, W. J. "The surgical treatment of spasticity." *Muscle Nerve* 23 (2000): 153–163.

Snoek, G. J., Ljzerman, M. J., Hermens, H. J., Maxwell, D., Biering-Sorensen, F. "Survey of the needs of patients with spinal cord injury: impact and priority for improvement in hand function in tetraplegics." *Spinal Cord* 42 (2004): 526–532.

Stauffer, E. S. "Diagnosis and prognosis of acute cervical spinal cord injury." *Clinical Orthopaedics and Related Research* 112 (1975): 9–15.

Stevenson, V. L. "Rehabilitation in practice: spasticity management." *Clinical Rehabilitation* 24 (2010): 293–304.

Szecsi, J., Schiller, M. "FES-propelled cycling of SCI subjects with highly spastic leg musculature." *NeuroRehabilitation* 24 (2009): 243–253.

Tani, T., Yamamoto, H., Kimura, J. "Cervical spondylotic myelopathy in elderly people: a high incidence of conduction block at C3–4 or C4–5." *Journal of Neurology, Neurosurgery, and Psychiatry* 66 (1999): 456–464.

Taylor, B. V., Willison, H. J. "Multifocal motor neuropathy and conduction block." In *Peripheral Neuropathy*, edited by P. J. Dyck, P. K. Thomas. Philadelphia, PA: Elsevier Saunders, 2005. pp. 2277–2298.

Thomas, C. K., Grumbles, R. M. "Muscle atrophy after human spinal cord injury." *Biocybernetics and Biomedical Engineering* 25 (2005): 39–46.

Thomas, C. K., Zijdewind, I. "Fatigue of muscles weakened by death of motoneurons." *Muscle Nerve* 33 (2006): 21–41.

Tonnis, W., Bischof, W. "[Results of lumbar myelotomy by the Bischof technic.]" *Zentralblatt für Neurochirurgie* 23 (1962): 29–36.

Transfeldt, E. E., White, D., Bradford, D. S., Roche, B. "Delayed anterior decompression in patients with spinal cord and cauda equina injuries of the thoracolumbar spine." *Spine* (Philadelphia, PA: 1976) 15 (1990): 953–957.

Tung, T. H., Weber, R. V., Mackinnon, S. E. "Nerve transfers for the upper and lower extremities." *Operative Techniques in Orthopaedics* 14 (2004): 213–222.

Villavicencio, A. T., Leveque, J. C., Rubin, L., Bulsara, K., Gorecki, J. P. "Laminectomy versus percutaneous electrode placement for spinal cord stimulation." *Neurosurgery* 46(2) (2000): 399–405.

Wainberg, M., Barbeau, H., Gauthier, S. "The effects of cyproheptadine on locomotion and on spasticity in patients with spinal cord injuries." *Journal of Neurology, Neurosurgery, and Psychiatry* 53 (1990): 754–763.

Waters, R. L., Sie, I. H., Gellman, H., Tognella, M. "Functional hand surgery following tetraplegia." *Archives of Physical and Medical Rehabilitation* 77 (1996): 86–94.

Wright, F., Palmer, A. C. "Morphological changes caused by pressure on the spinal cord." *Pathologia Veterinaria* 6 (1969): 355–368.

Yablon, I. G., Palumbo, M., Spatz, E., Mortara, R., Reed, J., Ordia, J. "Nerve root recovery in complete injuries of the cervical spine." *Spine* (Philadelphia, PA: 1976) 16 (1991): S518–S521.

Zhu, H., Feng, Y. T., Young, W., You, S. W., Shen, X. F., Liu, Y. S., et al. "Early neurosurgical intervention of spinal cord contusion: an analysis of 30 cases." *Chinese Medical Journal* 121 (2008): 2473–2478.

7

Criteria for Biological Interventions for Spinal Cord Injury Repair

KEITH TANSEY AND BYRON A. KAKULAS

CONTENTS

1. Introduction
2. The Clinical Pathophysiology of Spinal Cord Injury
    2.1. The Acute SCI Lesion
    2.2. The Subacute Stage
    2.3. The Established Lesion
    2.4. Restorative Neurology
3. Biological Interventions in the Acute Phase
4. Biological Interventions in Established SCI
5. Clinical Application
6. Fictive
7. Conclusions and Recommendations
References

1. INTRODUCTION

In this chapter we review the pathophysiology of the spinal injured patient, establishing criteria for biological interventions and their application. As a preliminary, it should be emphasized that prior to introducing any method of intervention designed to improve the spinal cord injury (SCI) patient's neurological condition, the patient must be in an optimal clinical state. This includes mental and psychological factors in addition to the usual physical and medical aspects of rehabilitation and restoration. In the case of acute interventions, this requires that the patient receive excellent trauma care with integrated SCI-specific medical protocols. For interventions that may be given in the perioperative period, this means that the patient is receiving excellent surgical and intensive unit care. For interventions that would be applied in the subacute to chronic condition, the patient should be undergoing or have undergone SCI-specialized rehabilitation, including nursing, physical, and occupational therapy, as well as patient and family education that addresses not only the neurological disability, but also the complete spectrum of other organ system physiology that is affected by SCI. The patient must be free of infection, uncontrolled spasticity, contractures or heterotopic ossification, excessive pain (neuropathic or nociceptive), autonomic instability, respiratory compromise, poor bowel and bladder management, deep vein thrombosis, bedsores or unaddressed depression. It is only then that a biological intervention may be added to the management regime with the object of improving the patient's overall status and their neurophysiological functions in particular.

It is also necessary to be aware of the natural history of SCI pathophysiology and the extent of "natural" functional recovery over different time periods so that the planned intervention is appropriate to the given stage of the patient's SCI. This raises the issue of being able to detect whether an intervention has, in fact, had a greater impact than would have been seen within the expected range of "natural" recovery. While it is possible to detect that changes in patients receiving interventions may be statistically significantly different than in those not receiving interventions, it is also important to determine if those changes are biologically or functionally significant. Finally, it needs to be determined if the intervention's effect is of great enough magnitude to justify the financial cost of the intervention and the risk/benefit balance of the intervention in different groups of SCI patients. One needs to remember that SCI results not only in loss of function but also in "gain of function" with the development of so-called positive phenomena such as pain, spasticity, etc. An intervention that lessens the functional losses in SCI but exacerbates these positive phenomena would, of course, be of limited utility.

Obviously, there are limitations to both our neuropathological and physiological knowledge of SCI, which render any of the biological interventions, actual or theoretical, as being tentative at this point in time. There is a long history in translational neurology of promising interventions in the basic laboratory setting that failed in the clinical environment. This stems from a large number of issues, many of which are often overlooked before attempts at clinical application are begun. First, the typical observation in an animal model is that an intervention whose theoretical mechanism of action is, at best, modestly understood, results in some sort of functional benefit. What is not known is whether this intervention, via its theoretical mechanism of action, will work in human SCI.

This uncertainty comes from differences between humans and animal, usually rodent, models. For one thing, there is the issue of size. Regeneration of an axon over 0.5 cm in a rat or mouse might represent the potential to connect neural circuits over several spinal levels; whereas, in a human, this distance would represent only a within-spinal-level projection length; that is, less than one segment. There are so many differences in anatomy and physiology between animal models and humans. The relative weight of the spinal cord to the brain in rodents is approximately tenfold greater than in humans and suggests the relative amount of supraspinal versus spinal neural circuitry contributing to function may be different in the two species. The relative contribution of different pathways connecting the brain and spinal cord may also be different, as decorticate animals can function far better than humans with the same loss of neuroanatomy. There are also probably large differences in the number of neurons and axons in the larger spinal cord of humans, and it is unclear what the necessary and sufficient anatomical substrates are for different behaviors in humans versus rodents, not to mention how some of those behaviors differ (i.e., in bipedal vs. quadripedal locomotion). There are also differences between the animal models of

SCI and human SCI due to injury mechanisms, immune system differences, growth rates, and lifespans, to name but a few.

Critical to translating biological interventions for SCI from the basic science laboratory to clinical application is a careful "human neuroscience," which is necessary to understanding the neurobiological impact of that intervention in humans. Even then, we have only relatively limited methods with which to understand this neurobiology: namely, imaging (MRI, fMRI, diffusion tensor imaging), electrophysiology to test conduction (evoked potentials, electrical threshold perceptual testing) or processing (EMG patterns, reflex modulation), or behavioral testing (gait, balance, reaching/grasping, autonomic functions, etc.). Nevertheless, conducting in-depth investigations in a *small* cohort of individuals with SCI to try to understand the neurobiological mechanisms and effects of an intervention prior to the institution of *large* clinical trials is likely to increase the yield of those larger trials by filtering out interventions that are actually ineffective in humans, or by identifying which human SCI sub-populations are most likely to benefit from a given intervention. The following account should therefore be seen as reflecting the current state of our understanding of SCI and as only the beginning of realizing our hope for an eventual cure. Fundamentally, the criteria for biological interventions in SCI rest on a sound knowledge of the pathophysiology. For this reason, we begin with a description of the essential neuropathology as follows.

2. THE CLINICAL PATHOPHYSIOLOGY OF SPINAL CORD INJURY

It is important to recognize that the changes that occur in the spinal cord after injury are not static, but change continuously as time passes, and are represented at the bedside by a continuously evolving clinical picture. These manifestations are not confined to the nervous system alone, but indeed affect all bodily functions, and it is the patient as a whole who is being treated. In this context, it should also be appreciated that no two patients are exactly alike.

2.1. The Acute SCI Lesion

The immediate effect of trauma is tissue disruption associated with relatively little parenchymal and meningeal hemorrhages (Figure 7–1). Edema appears within minutes, and neutrophils may be found within 24 hours. Axonal disruptions are the first sign of nerve fiber damage, followed by end bulb formations and irregular, sausage-like swellings. The myelin sheaths of the disrupted axons are similarly fragmented. There is a release of excitatory neurotransmitters from injured cells that triggers excitotoxic injury to other cells, and the generation of reactive oxygen species that can induce apoptosis in both neurons and glia, occurring over hours to weeks following the injury.

In the next 72 hours, round cells (lymphocytes and macrophages) appear, and small blood vessels dilate. The macrophages begin to engulf the debris and continue to do so until the chronic stage is reached. It is in this reactive stage that secondary damage occurs in relationship to the inflammatory reaction. Astrocytes are first observed to lay down glial fibers within the lesion after about five days, and there is

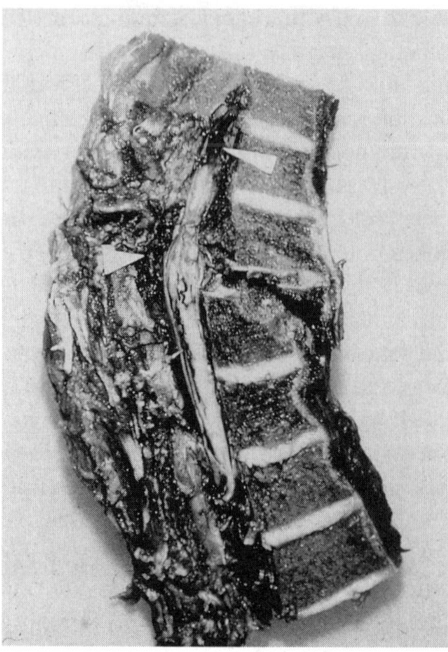

Figure 7–1 Vertical section of spinal cord and vertebral column three days after injury, showing forward dislocation at C5–C6. Note the extradural hemorrhages (*arrow*) and continuity of spinal cord tissue despite the severe trauma. (*See* color insert.)

a deposition of extracellular matrix proteins. These processes continue until a mature glial scar is formed (Kakulas 1999, 2004).

The clinical expression of major SCI in the acute stage is spinal shock, in which there are no voluntary neurological functions below the level of injury, and flaccid tetraplegia. This is thought to be due to hyperpolarization of spinal neurons, including motoneurons, because during this period it is often impossible to elicit F waves (the ability to antidromically excite the motoneuron cell soma to fire action potentials) on electrophysiological testing. Days later, this lower motoneuron effect will resolve and hyporeflexia will transition to hyperreflexia. This is thought to be due to afferent input to spinal circuits' no longer being under the supraspinal control they received before the SCI. Clinically, the reemergence of the bulbocavernosus reflex is considered to mark the beginning of recovery from spinal shock, and it is from this point forward that somatic motor hyperreflexia and even autonomic hypersensitivity can be seen. Once hyperreflexia can be found, other features of the "upper motoneuron syndrome" can be found, including hypertonia; flexor, extensor, or adductor spasms; dysynergias; and even contractures. The true neurological state can be established at the bedside by the experienced clinician, but the spectrum of the SCI "phenotype" is broad, not only in regard to the level and the completeness or incompleteness of the injury, but also in regard to the combination of sensory, motor, and autonomic findings, as well as the pattern of those findings. Therefore, characterizing SCI in individuals should probably go beyond categorical labels such as those of the American Spinal Injury Association (ASIA) and involve more complete assessments, including those that characterize the physiological state of neural circuitry below the level of injury, as can be done with the brain motor control assessment (BMCA; see Chapter 8). In incomplete SCI, various degrees of neurological recovery will thus be seen, the clinical features of which reflect the neuropathological lesion such that lost and retained functions show a strict clinical correlation with the anatomical lesion.

2.2. The Subacute Stage

In the weeks that follow, myelin and other debris are mopped up by macrophages, and glial scarring derived from astrocytes occurs within and around the site of injury. Injured axons retract, and Wallerian, that is, tract degeneration, begins distally in the descending motor and extrapyramidal pathways and proximally in the ascending sensory tracts. Again, there is a precise clinico-neurological correlation concerning neurological deficits due to the architecture of the spinal cord being segmental and stereotyped, but not so much so for function, which is more adaptable.

2.3. The Established Lesion

The cellular reaction continues to evolve until about the end of the first year after injury, after which it remains more or less stable, except for Wallerian degeneration of the myelinated pathways and nerve root regenerations arising from anterior horn cells and posterior ganglia, which is a continuous process (Figures 7–2 and 7–3).

Following removal of the necrotic debris, gliosis and a variable amount of collagenous fibrosis occurs so that what remains at the level of injury is a multilocular cavity traversed by glial-vascular bundles (Figure 7–4). A feature of human SCI is that, in almost every patient, a larger or lesser amount of white matter is usually

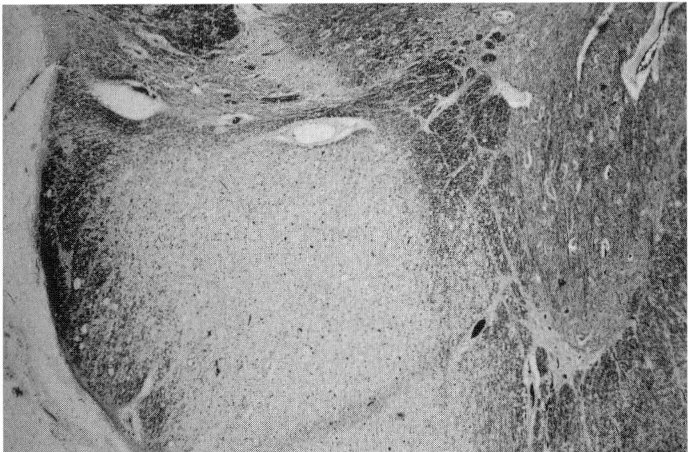

Figure 7–2 Cross-section of spinal cord at T6 several years post-injury, stained with the Loyez method for myelin (*black*) showing pallor of the lateral corticospinal tract indicating chronic Wallerian degeneration, which is a continuous process post-injury. (*See* color insert.)

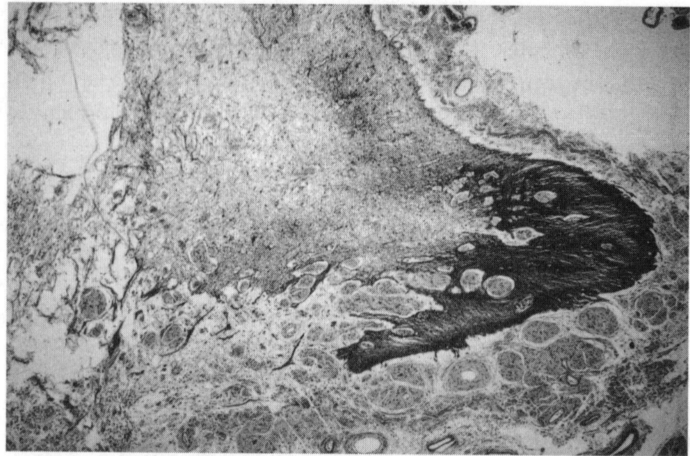

Figure 7–3 Spinal cord in cross-section at C5, many years after injury, stained with PTAH (indicating advanced gliosis) with regenerated nerve roots inside and outside the cord. The regenerated nerve fibers arise from both anterior horn neurons and posterior root ganglia. They have no functional significance. (*See* color insert.)

retained at the level of the lesion situated at the periphery of the cord. Since the myelinated nerves of the white matter are the conducting system, it is the functioning of this white matter that determines the neurological state of the patient, along with the minor contribution of residual gray matter at the segmental level. There is an approximate, but not exact, correlation between the amount of retained

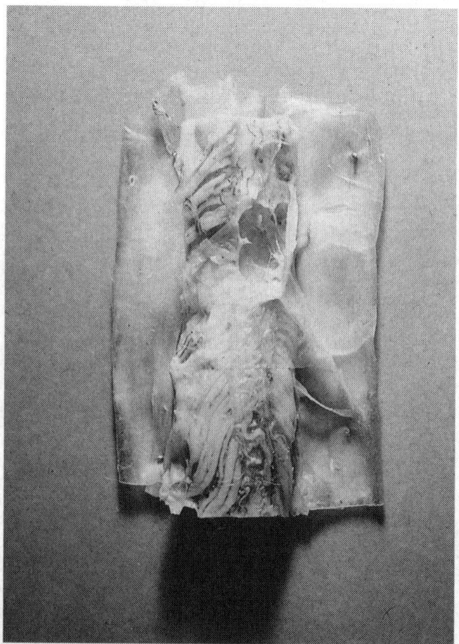

Figure 7–4 Spinal cord at C6 vertical and posterior longitudinal view showing the "end stage" lesion, many years post-injury. Removal of necrotic debris results in a multilocular cavity traversed by glio-vascular bundles. Note the preserved spinal cord tissue at left. (*See* color insert.)

white matter and the clinical picture in SCI, whether the injury is complete, discomplete, or incomplete (see Chapter 2 for definitions). It is also the quality, and not just the quantity or the anatomical position of this white matter, that is important in neural control and other physiological parameters. It is on this neuropathological basis that neuromonitoring depends, as described in Chapter 9.

In parallel with the changes in the spinal cord itself after SCI, both spinal and supraspinal neural circuitry undergoes anatomical and physiological alterations. There is evidence of anatomical neural plasticity in both spinal and supraspinal neural circuits, including sprouting of central pathways and of afferent inputs. Physiological neural plasticity at synapses also remains after SCI. These changes can include the activation of silent synapses, increases or decreases in synaptic strengths, or changed combinatorial effects of multiple synaptic inputs to specific neural populations. These processes are a product not only of the nervous system injury, but also of the medications and rehabilitation interventions that individuals receive.

Following SCI, the remaining nervous system is changed, and it is naïve to think that simple regeneration and anatomical reconnection of neural circuits disconnected by injury will result in the restoration of pre-injury physiology. It has been said that any neural repair strategy aimed at reconnection needs to acknowledge that it is a new nervous system that is being connected, one we know relatively little about.

There are two current theories of how functional recovery may occur, both of which are probably overly simplistic. The first theory could be called the "regenerate and they will come" theory. This theory assumes that if regeneration were possible, new inputs to neural circuitry above or below the injury would find "smart targets" that would guide these new connections to generate the most functionally appropriate behaviors. There is little evidence this occurs, even in animal models where some regeneration has been seen, and it flies in the face of neural development when a superfluous number of connections are made over time and space with specific molecular guidance, and then pruned and pared back by developmental programming and activity-dependent mechanisms to create the mature nervous system.

The second theory could be called the "smart spinal cord" theory, and this line of thinking suggests that many functions that were performed with a combination of brain and spinal cord circuits in the uninjured state may be recovered using only infra-injury spinal cord circuits. While this may be true for some behaviors in some animal models, locomotion in spinal cats for instance, there is little evidence so far that the human spinal cord in isolation or with minimal supraspinal input can execute pre-injury functions, at least with our current interventions.

On the other hand, little attention has been paid to some processes that could improve physiology with limited anatomical recovery. The major one of these is sprouting. If an SCI results in the loss of 70% of vestibulospinal connections, perhaps getting the remaining 30% to sprout to take over the vacant vestibulospinal synapses of their lost neighbors could be more feasible or effective than getting those 70% of lost connections to "realize" they no longer reach their targets, start them growing, get them to negotiate the glial scar and the inhospitable growth environment of the injured spinal cord, find appropriate targets, and reestablish their function.

Also, the attention on most neural plasticity following SCI has been focused in the spinal cord, but it is likely that as much or more plasticity is going on at supraspinal levels. Locomotor training in SCI, for instance, has resulted in supraspinal plasticity as measured by fMRI, and there is a correlation between the extent of gait recovery and of cerebellar activity following this training (Winchester et al., 2005). It is not surprising to think that the portion of the nervous system charged with comparing planned movements with executed ones is working overtime in a situation when descending motor commands are only partially getting through, and there has been a loss of some ascending feedback about the actual movements.

2.4. Restorative Neurology

Of great importance when considering the role of restorative neurology and the effect of interventions are the widespread and complicated properties of CNS plasticity. The function of the spinal cord is continuously under the influence of externally derived and internally generated neurological inputs. The effect of such stimulation may be detrimental; for example, causing unwanted reflexes, spasms, or pain; or helpful; for example, leading to recovered motor, sensory, or autonomic function. The biological interventions described below are designed to influence this plasticity for improved neurocontrol in the SCI patient. It is not an overstatement to suggest that function—that is, the neurophysiology—is subject to continuous change while the structure remains static, except perhaps at the microscopic synaptic level. The overall aim of the restorative neurologist is to beneficially influence neurocontrol of altered functions, especially voluntary motor activity, regardless of whether the lesion is complete, discomplete, or incomplete. The main issue is the optimal recovery of motor and sensory functions with some autonomic improvement toward normal.

3. BIOLOGICAL INTERVENTIONS IN THE ACUTE PHASE

It has been shown that conservative management with optimal care and rehabilitation will lead to complete or partial natural recovery in many SCI patients (El Masry 2006). It is against this background that the benefit of any interventions must be measured (see above). Many therapeutic agents have been administered in experimental animals in the acute phase that are designed to limit the extent of the lesion and salvage as many axons as possible. Some of these have been shown to be effective and have been introduced into the treatment regime of SCI. Notably, these are corticosteroids and 4 aminopyridine, which have been shown to provide some benefit in limiting the neurological effect of the injury (Hayes et al., 2003). However 4 aminopyridine, which chemically transiently overcomes demyelination by restoring saltatory axonal conduction, has been shown to have limited clinical efficacy in SCI in the human.

On the other hand, there are hundreds of agents that have had some theoretical basis for testing derived from animal model studies but have proven useless clinically. These include free-radical scavengers, cytokine blockers, trophic factors, white-matter-derived compounds, glutamate antagonists, and anti-apoptotic drugs, for example. A comprehensive account of experimental strategies to restore function after spinal cord injury is provided by Boulenguez and Vinay (2009). A promising line of approach on the horizon can be found in Martin Schwab's anti-Nogo experiments (Maier et al. 2009). This custom-made antibody blocks myelin compounds that are known to inhibit axonal regeneration. The anti-Nogo approach is currently under clinical trial in human SCI. There is also a clinical trial of Cethrin, a Rho kinase inhibitor to mimic neurotrophin effects, underway.

4. BIOLOGICAL INTERVENTIONS IN ESTABLISHED SCI

We now turn to a consideration of cellular transplant grafts and stem cells. Fetal grafts have been shown to be of no benefit, and while genetically engineered cells carrying trophic factors introduced into the lesion have benefits claimed the experimental animal, they have not yet been successful in humans. The same negative comment applies to Schwann cells introduced into the lesion. Peripheral nerve grafts are known to have produced dramatic effects when transplanted into the central visual pathways of animals. These experiments have stimulated a number of attempts in the human to produce central spinal cord regeneration. Homologous peripheral nerve grafts have been placed surgically into the lesion, but unfortunately with unconvincing clinical benefit. The same reserved judgment applies to the various types of stem cells that have been tried in humans. There are now a number of such attempts reported (Lima et al., 2006), but the best-conducted of these has given negative results even after three years of follow-up (Mackay-Sim 2005).

Several others claim benefits from stem cells in humans, but the outcome in these is uninterpretable; the reports of benefit are indistinguishable from the natural history of spontaneous recovery in SCI. The first FDA-approved stem cell trial is currently underway at several sites in the United States by the Geron Corporation, whose cellular product is embryonic stem cells guided down an oligodendrocyte-differentiation pathway. The FDA has only approved study of its safety in acute complete thoracic injury at this time.

5. CLINICAL APPLICATION

In the acute stage, scientifically established biological interventions are thus limited to steroids (Bracken et al., 1990), but it is now common practice to *not* use steroids, due to the clinical experience of limited benefit and the fear of side effects such as infection. Of great importance is physiological monitoring, including BMCA (see Chapter 8 and Appendix I). These physiological assessments allow intelligent application of proven methods of restorative neurology and reconstructive neurosurgery (see Chapters 3 and 6). These assessments will guide the use of pharmacological agents, such as intradural morphine in the control of unwanted reflex spasms, and other interventions.

Turning to physiological interventions, there is much that can be done without reference to the disordered anatomy, the intervention being purely empirical. Thus, careful neuromonitoring will reveal the deficits more accurately than bedside assessment, and can lay the groundwork for such interventions as direct spinal cord stimulation or mesh glove techniques, as well as extracranial magnetic stimulation. Magnetic stimulation drives the voluntary motor system, producing improved neurological functions by influencing centrally located plasticity modifying and recruiting new circuits and pathways.

6. FICTIVE

In the *chronic stage* post-injury, there are various types of grafts, transplants, and cellular implants which have potential value but that have not yet been established in a useful protocol. Despite the now many centers placing stem cells into a spinal injury, none of these has been demonstrated to be of unequivocal proven value. The shortcoming is the lack of a scientific approach, including untreated controls with double-blind evaluations. Provision for individual variation in the lesions and for natural recovery is paramount in any experimental design. Even more to the point is the fact that stem cells have not been properly tested in animal models of SCI. Not only is this a scientific necessity, but its delay is compromising the potential help that may come from stem cell treatment for human SCI. The single competent human trial of stem cells in SCI patients who were clinically complete at the start remained ASIA-A after three years observation (Mackay–Sim et al., 2008). Another cell transplantation trial, this time of activated macrophages (the Proneuron trial) also failed to show efficacy in a Phase II study, despite some hint of efficacy in its Phase I trial.

7. CONCLUSIONS AND RECOMMENDATIONS

Not to be neglected in recovery from SCI is the benefit to be derived from conventional rehabilitation complemented by task-specific occupational and physical therapy, and consequent neural plasticity with reorganized circuitry and similar treatments, which are important topics to be covered elsewhere. Future biological interventions depend on advances in the basic sciences and biomedical engineering. Investigation of the growth, development, and functioning of the CNS will provide more candidates for testing in the future that are worthy of experimental trial.

Other future avenues include the development of robotic devices and bionic implants. There is work in progress in this respect undertaken by Graham Clark (1990) of Melbourne, Australia, who has had great success with the bionic ear. There is a large body of research work and clinical experience with the first generation of rehabilitation robotics, but there remain fundamental questions, including: "What are optimal training programs?" "Should robotics provide assistance only or also resistance (perhaps later in training)?" and "How much error signaling should be provided by the robot to maximize neurological recovery?" It is not known what the necessary and sufficient features of robotics are to achieve specific outcomes, but predictive models are already published for the magnitude of effect based on initial clinical presentation and following a prescribed intervention program (Winchester et al., 2009).

In theory, the concept of biological or inorganic interventions is to reestablish lost central pathways and connections. This requires a knowledge of the exact neuropathological and neurophysiological condition so that the conducting systems may be rejoined by artificial or biological means. In order to restore lost functions, it is the white matter tracts that need to be regrown, rejoined, and reeducated. This basic principle has been given little thought in the myriad of experiments intended to "cure" SCI. The best that one may hope for in the present state of knowledge is the experimental development of a polysynaptic pathway from stem cells, but there is much to be done in animals before application to human SCI.

In all of the attempts to repair the spinal cord mentioned above, little or no consideration has been given to the complexity of the spinal cord. On one hand, there is the natural organization of the basic anatomy, in which as many as 100 million nerve fibers are arranged into voluntary and involuntary motor systems, sensory pathways, and local segmental connections, as well connections for the integration of autonomic and other systems. If this seems complex, a consideration of how they function is even more bewildering. Current knowledge of how it all comes together in growth, maintenance, repair, and learning is still primitive, so that our current interventions are necessarily limited, and we must go forward from here.

References

Boulenguez, P., Vinay, L. "Strategies to restore motor function after spinal cord injury." *Current Opinion in Neurology* 19 (2009): 587–600.

Bracken, M. B., Shepard, M. J., Collins, W. F., et al. "A randomized controlled trial of methylprednisolone or naloxone in the treatment of acute spinal cord injury." *New England Journal of Medicine* 322 (1990): 1405–1411.

Clark, G., Tong, Y. C., Patrick, J. F. *Cochlear Prosthesis*. Edinburgh, U.K.: Churchill Livingstone, 1990.

El Masry, W. S. "Traumatic spinal cord injury: The relationship between pathology and clinical features." *Trauma* 8 (2006): 29–46.

Hayes, K. C., Katz, M. A., Devane, J. G., Hsieh, T. C., Wolfe, D. L., Potter, P. J., Blight, A. R. "Pharmacokinetics of an immediate-release oral formulation of fampridine (4-aminopyridine) in normal subjects and patients with spinal cord injury." *Journal of Clinical Pharmacology* 43 (2003): 379–385.

Kakulas, B. A. "A review of the neuropathology of spinal cord injury with emphasis on special features." *The Journal of Spinal Cord Medicine* 22 (1999): 119–124.

Kakulas, B. A. "Neuropathology: the foundation for new treatments in spinal cord injury." *Spinal Cord* 42 (2004): 549–563.

Lima, C., Pratas-Vital, J., Escada, P., Hasse-Ferreira, A., Capucho, C., Peduzzi, J. D. "Olfactory mucosa autografts in human spinal cord injury." *Journal of Spinal Cord Medicine* 29 (2006): 191–203.

Mackay-Sim, A. "Olfactory ensheathing cells and spinal cord repair." *Keio Journal of Medicine* 54 (2005): 8–14.

Mackay-Sim, A., Feron, F., Cochrane, J., Bassingthwaighte, L., Bayliss, C., Davies, W., Fronek, P., Gray, C., Kerr, G., Licina, P., et al. "Autologous olfactory ensheathing cell transplantation in human paraplegia: A three-year clinical trial." *Brain* 131 (2008): 2376–2386.

Maier, I. C., Ichiyama, R. M., Courtine, G., et al. "Differential effects of anti-Nogo-A antibody treatment and treadmill training in rats with incomplete spinal cord injury." *Brain* 132 (2009): 1426–1440.

Winchester, P., McColl, R., Querry, R., Foreman, N., Mosby, J., Tansey, K., and Williamson, J., "Changes in Supraspinal Activation Patterns following Robotic

Locomotor Therapy in Subjects with Motor Incomplete Spinal Cord Injury." *Neurorehabilitation and Neural Repair* 19 (2005): 313–324.

Winchester, P., Smith, P., Proctor, E., Foreman, N., Mosby, J., Pacheco, F., Querry, R., and Tansey, KE. "A Prediction Model for Determining Over Ground Walking Speed following Locomotor Training in Persons with Motor Incomplete Spinal Cord Injury." *J. Spinal Cord Med.* 32 (2009): 26–34.

8

Neurophysiological Assessment of Human Motor Control and Changes Caused by Spinal Cord Injury

W. BARRY McKAY, ARTHUR M. SHERWOOD, AND SIMON F. T. TANG

CONTENTS

1. Introduction
2. Essentials of Measuring Motor Control Using Functional Electromyography (fEMG)
3. Characteristics of Non-Injured Motor Control
4. Characteristics Patterns of Motor Control in Chronic SCI
5. Selective Control of Voluntary Movement Disrupted by SCI
6. Data Analysis
7. Conclusions—Utilization of Results

References

1. INTRODUCTION

The control of movement provides us with the ability to manipulate and move about within our environment, to satisfy our survival needs and to interact with each other. Motor control is also the process by which we express our sameness and uniqueness within our society. Changes in motor control brought about by damage to our central nervous system, therefore, alter who we are in quite profound ways. This chapter will focus on the results of damage to the spinal cord and how output from the brain and brain stem to the spinal neural circuits, the motor neurons, and muscle fibers that they activate is altered.

In humans, spinal cord injury usually results in a diffuse distribution of axonal and interneuronal loss within the injury zone (Kakulas, 2004) (see Chapter 7). The injury zone "filters" or prevents some of the information from arriving at assigned spinal destinations within the required time. This filtering effect can be severe, eliminating most if not all communication between structures rostral and caudal to the lesion. Complete loss of transmission across the lesion is rare and the range of functional impairment brought by SCI is broad due to the diverse nature of the damage patterns experienced across the population of injured persons. This "filter" alters the mix of excitatory and inhibitory input from supraspinal, spinal, and peripheral sources that converges, largely through a preprocessing center, on the spinal motor neurons to "express" the intent of the brain to control movement.

Established during a process of early development and refined through practical use, these neural circuits determine efficient functional integration of the multiple, component sub-systems providing input to the pre-motor processor through which a "decision" to activate the motor unit is made (Eyre, 2003; 2007). Disruption of this integrative process that results from SCI has been and can only be studied in animal models. The loss of synaptic contacts on the spinal motor neurons themselves leave voids that either remain vacant or become occupied by outgrowths of nearby neurons (Illis, 1967) or are claimed by "sprouting" from peripheral nerve fibers (McGough et al., 1958) and surviving long-tract fibers (Hill et al., 2001; Fouad & Tse, 2008). However, these connections form without the benefit of the developmental guidance mentioned above, resulting in a "new anatomy," a highly individualized neural circuitry that often possesses very different processing characteristics and produces highly altered control of motor unit firing (Cioni et al., 1986; Dimitrijevic et al., 1997). Thus, in order to improve motor control, it is necessary to first develop a detailed description of the degree to which the lesion allows control over spinal motor output for the performance or attempted performance of single- and multi-joint movements. Surface electromyographic (sEMG) recording of motor unit firing allows the documentation of the functional organization that this "new anatomy" brings to the motor output of the central nervous system (CNS). The conditions under which certain patterns of motor unit firing can be seen offer information regarding the mechanisms by which they are produced.

2. ESSENTIALS OF MEASURING MOTOR CONTROL USING FUNCTIONAL ELECTROMYOGRAPHY (fEMG)

There are five essential principles that make it possible to use fEMG to quantitatively describe motor control. First, in order to accomplish a reliably repeatable assessment of motor function, *recording conditions must be carefully controlled*. Standards detailing proper recording control can be found in Appendix I of this book. The second principle is that output recorded in the form of *motor unit firing describes excitation of spinal motor nuclei and the distribution of excitation across the nuclei associated with the recorded muscles*. Third, *the distribution of this output across the recorded muscles is determined by the motor task presented to the nervous system and disrupted by the degree of damage*. For example, the distribution of motor unit firing to perform a requested voluntary movement will describe the functional organization accomplished for the performance of the task. Thus, processing altered by damage to the central nervous system will appear as reduced activation of motor units in the prime mover for the task, accompanied by differing degrees of motor unit activation in muscles antagonistic to or distant from the requested motor tasks. Furthermore, the processing of input from a peripheral nerve(s) into a reflex output will produce motor unit firing distributed across muscles, depending on the excitability of those motor units at the time of the arrival of that input. Fourth, *motor tasks are specifically selected to provide the most discrete and repeatable patterns of motor unit activity when performed by uninjured people.* Thus, the motor tasks that produce the most reliable results are those that are simple to instruct and perform. Fifth, *patterns of motor output in test subjects are compared to the expected patterns collected from neurologically intact subjects* using standardized methods to produce validity-tested parameter values.

3. CHARACTERISTICS OF NON-INJURED MOTOR CONTROL

This chapter deals with the measurement and analysis of motor unit firing recorded from selected muscles during specifically defined motor tasks under controlled conditions. The motor tasks selected for this assessment are those that, when performed by neurologically intact subjects, produce highly reproducible response patterns. For example, non-injured individuals are able to relax completely, producing no motor unit firing during a five-minute relaxation period (Sherwood et al., 1996). Reinforcement tasks such as deep breath and Jendrassik maneuvers do not elicit activation of lower-limb muscles (Sherwood et al., 1996). Passive movement of the limbs produces no motor unit firing under instructions to relax. Tendon taps may elicit no or low-amplitude responses and strong vibration most often brings slowly increasing motor unit firing within the muscle vibrated (Sherwood et al., 1993). Finally, withdrawal from plantar stimulation may or may not be present, but when present, the response can always be significantly volitionally suppressed under instructions to do so.

Voluntary movement tasks performed by non-injured people are characterized as: (1) having rapid recruitment of motor units in the prime mover muscle for the task; (2) being accompanied by only very low-amplitude motor unit activation in the antagonist muscle to provide joint compliance control; (3) activating only muscles specific to the task being performed (Figure 8–1) (McKay et al., 2011a). For example, a single-joint movement in the supine position, such as unilateral dorsiflexion of the ankle, characteristically brings rapid activation of motor units in the tibialis anterior muscle with very low-amplitude activation of the triceps surae and in some, very low-amplitude activation of the ipsilateral quadriceps muscle. However, there will be no activation of ipsilateral hip adductors or hamstrings muscles or of contralateral muscles. For the more complex multi-joint motor task of hip and knee flexion, the pattern produced by non-injured subjects includes the rapid activation of motor units in the quadriceps muscle with low-amplitude activation of hamstrings and hip adductors and rapid recruitment of motor units in the contralateral hamstrings to counter body rotation brought by the leg's weight being lifted from the bed. These patterns are highly repeatable within groups of non-injured subjects, making it possible to objectively quantify the degree to which they are disrupted by neurological injury such as SCI (Lee et al., 2004). However, with prolonged or fatiguing effort, co-activation of antagonistic and distant muscles will develop even in non-injured subjects as effort increases (Dimitrijevic et al., 1992).

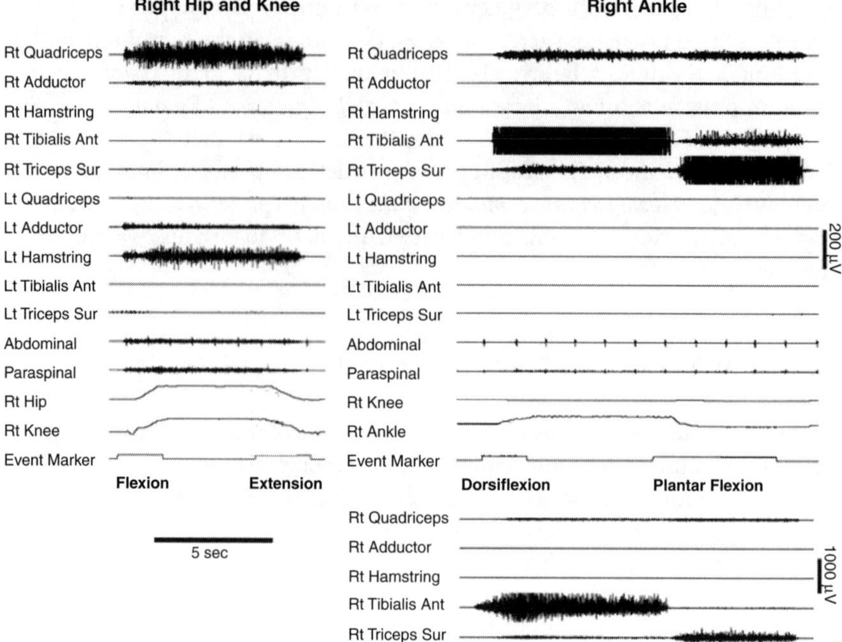

Figure 8–1 Distribution of motor unit activation across lower-limb muscles for voluntary hip and knee flexion and extension and ankle dorsi- and plantar flexion in a non-injured subject. The ankle task is shown repeated at a lesser display sensitivity (*below*) in order to show the relative amplitudes and envelope shape for the prime movers in the task because they over-range in the more sensitive display (*above*).

4. CHARACTERISTIC PATTERNS OF MOTOR CONTROL IN CHRONIC SCI

One motor characteristic and common complaint of persons after SCI is spasticity. For clinicians, spasticity is an increased responsiveness to muscle stretch that can be present in patients, whether paralyzed or clinically motor incomplete. They measure its severity using a 0 to 5 scale to describe the force that they perceive while passively manipulating selected joints (Ashworth, 1964). By simultaneously recording sEMG from multiple muscles, the responsiveness to passive movement can be specifically quantified along with the degree of concomitant activation of distant, even contralateral muscles, all of which often exhibit long-lasting, motor unit firing, whole-limb flexion and extension patterns and movements (Figure 8–2). This spread of excitability within the spinal cord neural circuitry illustrates the loss of descending control over inhibitory interneuronal circuitry. Furthermore, the degree of spreading of motor unit activation beyond the muscle stretched, the amount of activity elicited, and the duration of the response are quantifiable parameters that are useful in measuring changes that might be brought about through treatment.

Although the measurement of motor unit activation by passive stretch adds information to the current clinical description of "muscle tone," patient complaints of spasticity often refer to the frequency with which spasms occur and the degree to which they interfere with daily activities (Mahoney et al., 2007). Furthermore, such

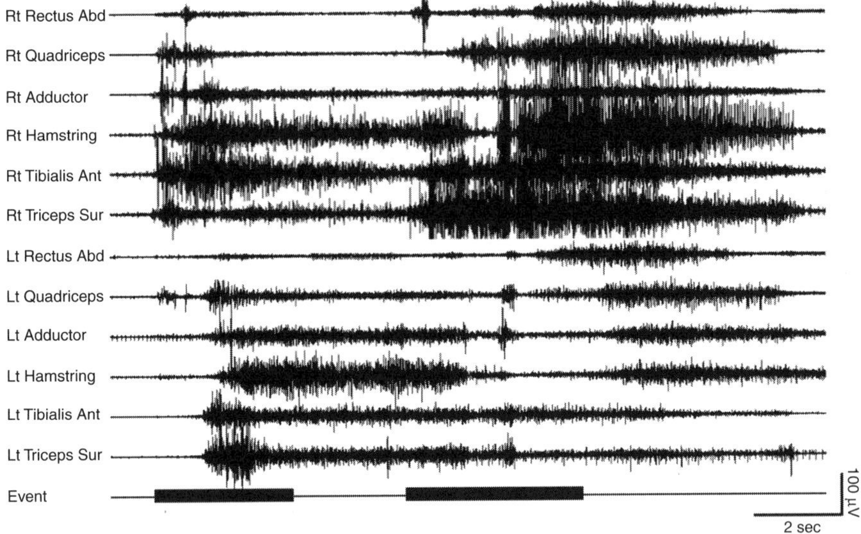

Figure 8–2 Passive stretch response to right hip and knee flexion and extension in the supine position. Note the activation not only of the muscle stretched but also others ipsilateral and contralateral to the stretch with the development of sequential activation leading to flexion–extension spasms in a person with a chronic C4, AIS-B SCI.

spasms often occur without the stretch of any muscle, but rather in response to such provocations as coughing (Figure 8–3) or touch (Figure 8–4). Furthermore, these events are indicators of the presence and form of surviving long-tract axons transiting the lesion (Dimitrijevic et al., 1989; Sherwood & McKay, 2006). In addition to spasms, long-duration motor unit activation may occur, bringing significant stiffness that competes with surviving volitional control (McKay et al., 2011b).

In persons whose SCI has left them unable to perform clinically recognizable voluntary movements below the level of the lesion, responsiveness to peripheral nerve input can be used to identify translesional connections. The ability of the spinal motor circuitry to reliably fire motor units in response to repeated input has been taken as an indication that excitatory support is present to prevent habituation. For example, in a decerebrate cat model, Matthews (1966) showed that vibration elicited a reflex response that continued unless the cat was additionally spinalized, indicating that, without support from the brain stem, the response from rapidly repeating muscle stretch disappears. In clinically paralyzed SCI patients, sustained responsiveness to vibration (Dimitrijevic et al., 1977; Sherwood et al., 1992) and sustained clonus (Dimitrijevic et al., 1980) were associated with neurophysiological or "subclinical" incompleteness. Some with clinically complete SCI can cause the activation of motor units caudal to the lesion through volitional effort to contract muscles rostral to the lesion (Dimitrijevic et al., 1984). The brain motor control assessment (BMCA) protocol asks subjects to perform reinforcement maneuvers, strong volitional contractions of non-paralyzed muscles, innervated from spinal segments rostral to the lesion, to cause activation of motor units caudal to the injury zone to indicate such neurophysiologically incomplete lesions (Figure 8–5). Together with the previously mentioned ability to sustain a response to repeated stretch induced by

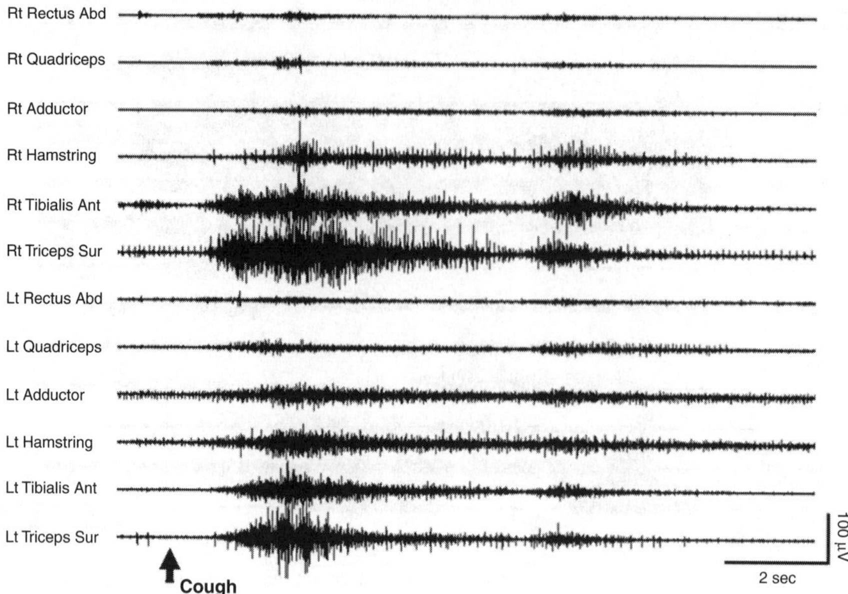

Figure 8–3 Spasm in lower limb muscles elicited by a cough in C5, AIS-B SCI.

vibration, this volitional "reinforcement" ability forms the excitatory criterion for the "discomplete" SCI syndrome (Dimitrijevic, 1988; Sherwood et al., 1996; McKay et al., 2005). The other neurophysiological measure used to determine the presence of this syndrome, illustrated in Figure 8–6, is the ability to, on command, volitionally suppress or inhibit responsiveness to cutaneous input from the plantar surface of the

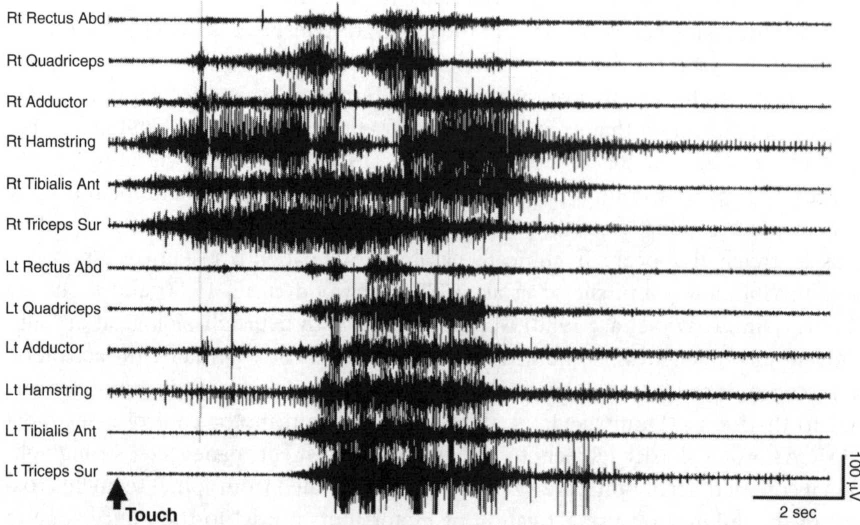

Figure 8–4 Touch of right lower extremity evokes considerable bilateral motor unit activation in the same subject appearing in Figure 8–3.

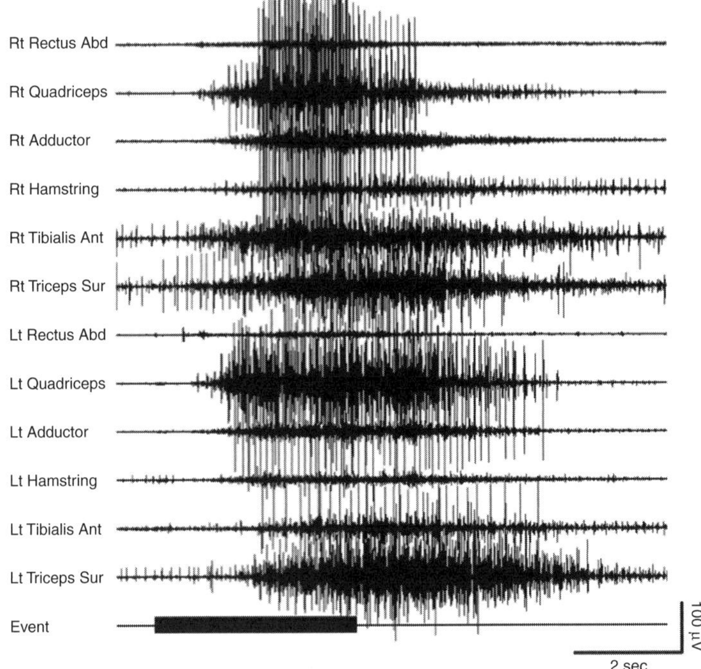

Figure 8–5 Example of a reinforcement response to a strong volitional activation of muscles innervated from above the spinal cord injury level in a person with C6 AIS-C SCI. The shoulder shrug task replaces the classic Jendrassik maneuver in persons with weakened grip.

foot (Cioni et al., 1986). Finally, it is possible to record voluntary activation of motor units in muscles that are paralyzed according to clinical examination (Figure 8–7).

5. SELECTIVE CONTROL OF VOLUNTARY MOVEMENT DISRUPTED BY SCI

An sEMG recording of the volitional activation of motor units within the primary mover—the muscle primarily responsible for developing the force needed to move a joint in a desired direction—measures the spatiotemporal distribution of motor unit firing within and across multiple muscles describing the functional organization developed within the CNS to produce the desired movement (Figure 8–8).

For example, after SCI, the attempt to perform a single-joint voluntary movement often results in full limb flexion with synergistic activation of motor units in multiple muscles, including those antagonistic to the movement and others distant and contralateral from the intended task. In fact, isolated contraction of the target muscle may not occur in the context of this single-joint task but may be accomplished only through the performance of a multi-joint movement task (Figure 8–9).

Furthermore, by simultaneously recording the activation of motor units from multiple muscles, a description of how the CNS has organized its motor output can

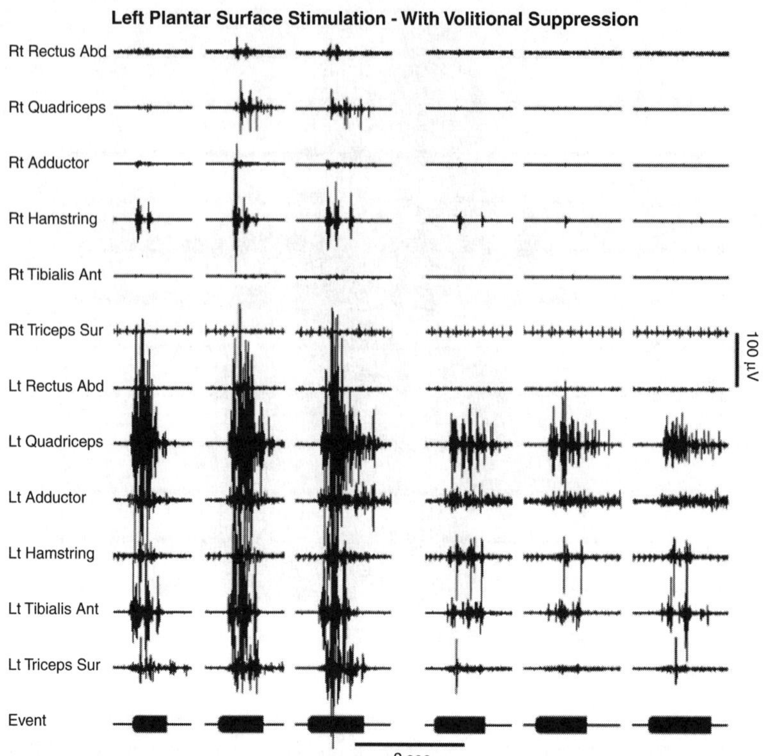

Figure 8–6 Left plantar surface stimulation (*left*) in a person with a C2, AIS-D injury elicits repeatable withdrawal responses from the muscles of both lower limbs. Note that volitional suppression (*right*) reliably reduces the response.

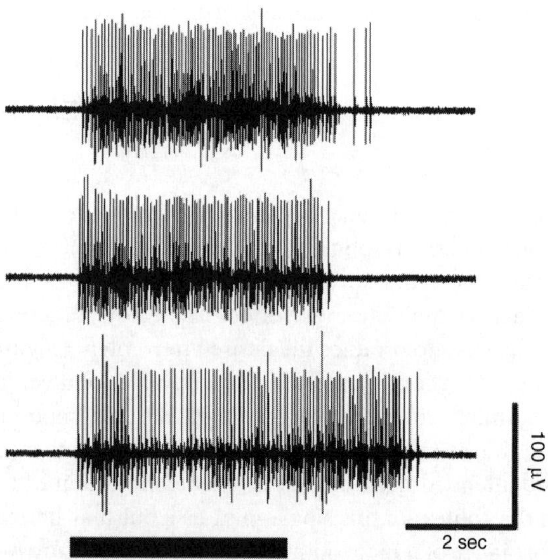

Figure 8–7 Left triceps surae activation during ankle plantar flexion attempt in a muscle scored as zero during the clinical AIS examination.

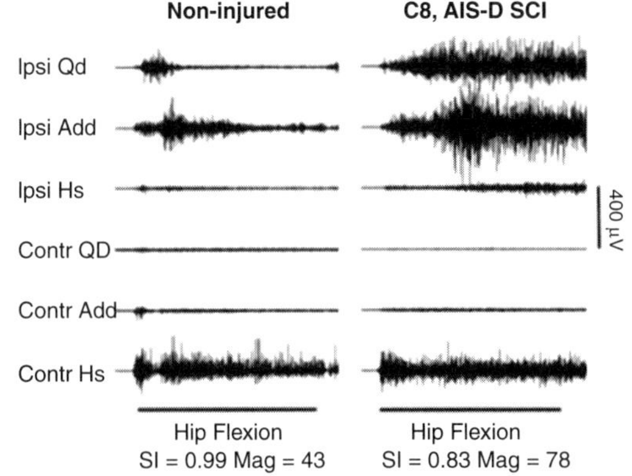

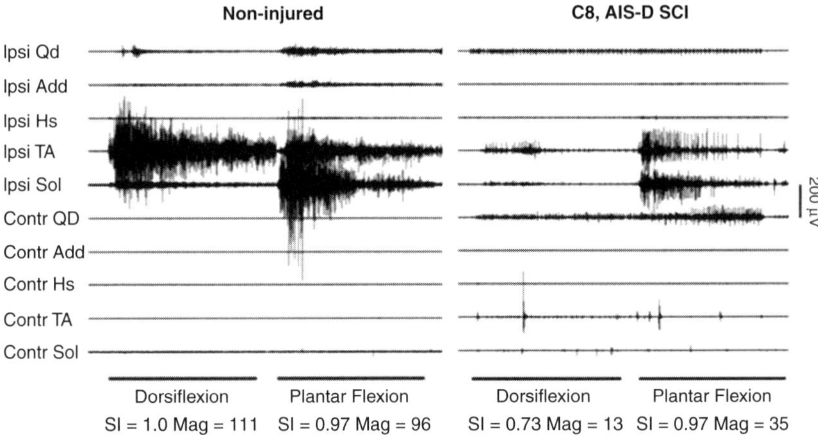

Figure 8–8 Examples of lower-limb volitional multi-joint (hip and knee flexion and extension) and single-joint (ankle dorsiflexion and plantar flexion) motor tasks in a non-injured individual and a person with C8, AIS-D SCI. Note the different distribution, amplitudes, and durations of motor unit activity in the two individuals for these tasks.

be obtained. By doing so, a map of the spatial distribution of CNS motor organization for whatever motor task is being attempted or successfully performed can be generated.

The voluntary motor task being performed by the CNS determines the spatiotemporal distribution of motor unit activation. Within the neurologically intact adult, processing neural circuitry has been refined during development to produce the most efficient performance of the desired task, whether that task is to move a limb, position the body, or relax completely while awake or asleep. By comparing the spatiotemporal characteristics of the motor output from persons with damaged CNS circuitry with that of neurologically intact persons, altered motor control can be objectively measured, and differences in control can be quantified, for use in comparing individuals within a selected population and tracking change that may be associated with disease progression, recovery, or effective treatment.

The repertoire of motor control patterns decreases with injury. In other words, injury-induced reduction of descending control results in a reduction in the range

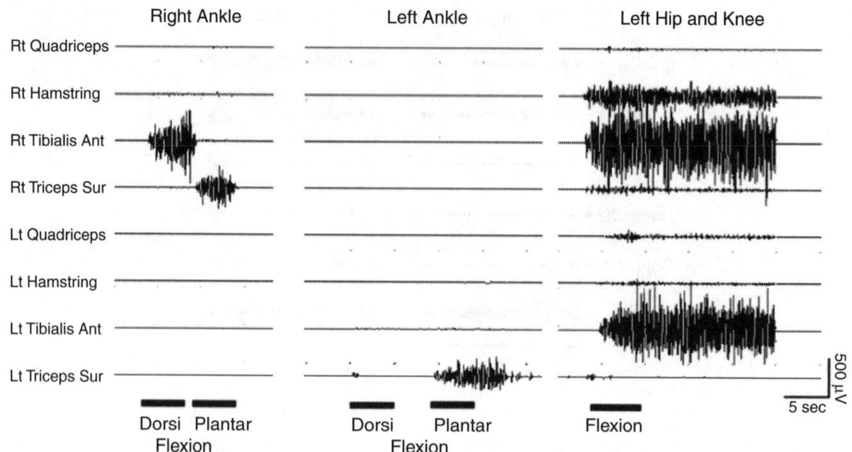

Figure 8–9 Voluntary movement attempts made by a person with C5, AIS-D SCI. Note that left tibialis anterior is activated during the multi-joint hip and knee flexion task but not during the single-joint left ankle dorsiflexion task.

and control of multi-muscle patterns available for motor task performance. The most severe damage results in an inability to volitionally activate motor units caudal to the SCI. Less severe is the discomplete syndrome (Dimitrijevic, 1988), in which no voluntary movement is possible but the ability to volitionally modulate generalized motor excitability caudal to the lesion is preserved to some extent. For example, strong volitional, postural, or respiratory activity rostral to the lesion can raise spinal motor excitability, increasing reflex responsiveness and even initiating broadly distributed activation of muscles caudal to the lesion (Dimitrijevic et al., 1984). However, the muscles activated and the sequence and relative amplitudes of their activation are often the same regardless of the task attempted (Figure 8–10).

Clinically incomplete SCI is recognized by the ability to voluntarily contract selected muscles caudal to the lesion that are relevant to a desired motor task. The selectivity and accuracy of this ability ranges broadly across the population of incomplete SCI and may be quite different within each individual, depending on which limb or body region is being examined.

SCI patients classified as being the same by the ASIA Impairment Scale (AIS) and with the same neurological motor level can have very different abilities to organize appropriate spinal motor output for simple voluntary movements (Figure 8–11). This is due to the great variety of SCI lesions and the fact that the AIS does not seek to examine the spatiotemporal distribution of spinal motor output control. However, such complexities of control are important for determining treatment planning and measuring its effects.

6. DATA ANALYSIS

The BMCA is always analyzed in two ways, first qualitatively and then quantitatively (Table 8–1). The qualitative review allows the recognition of *background conditions*

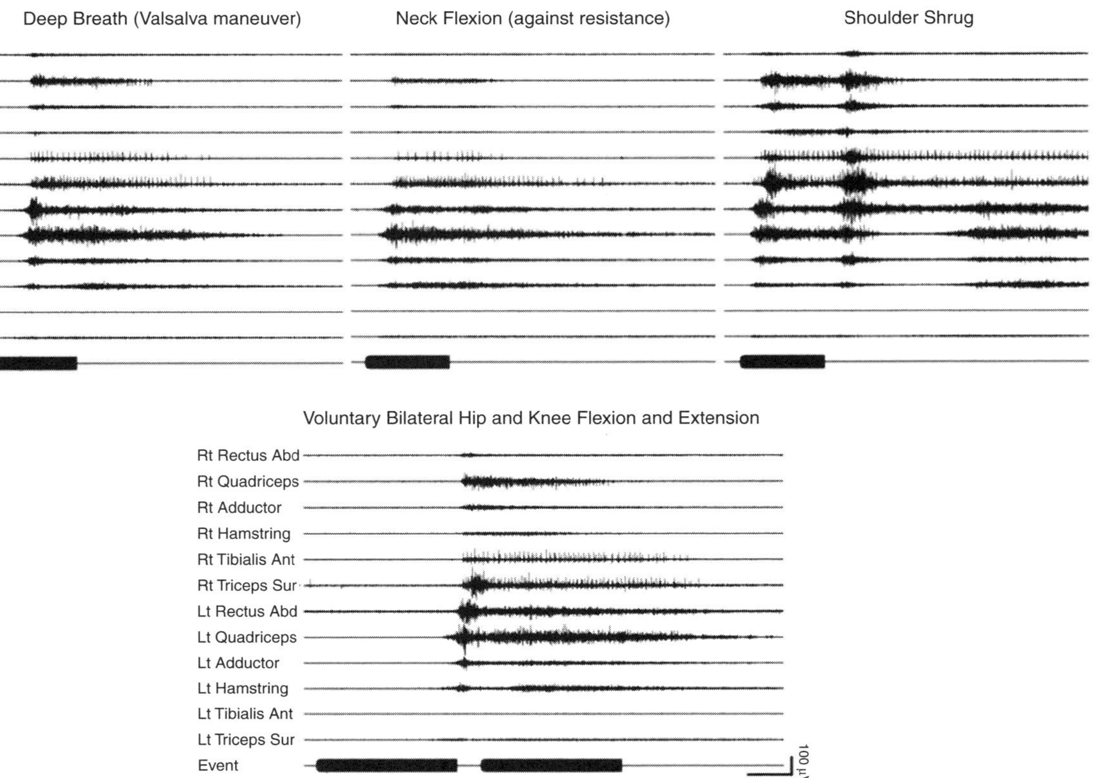

Figure 8–10 Stereotyped response to all volitional tasks in a subject with C5 AIS-C lesion.

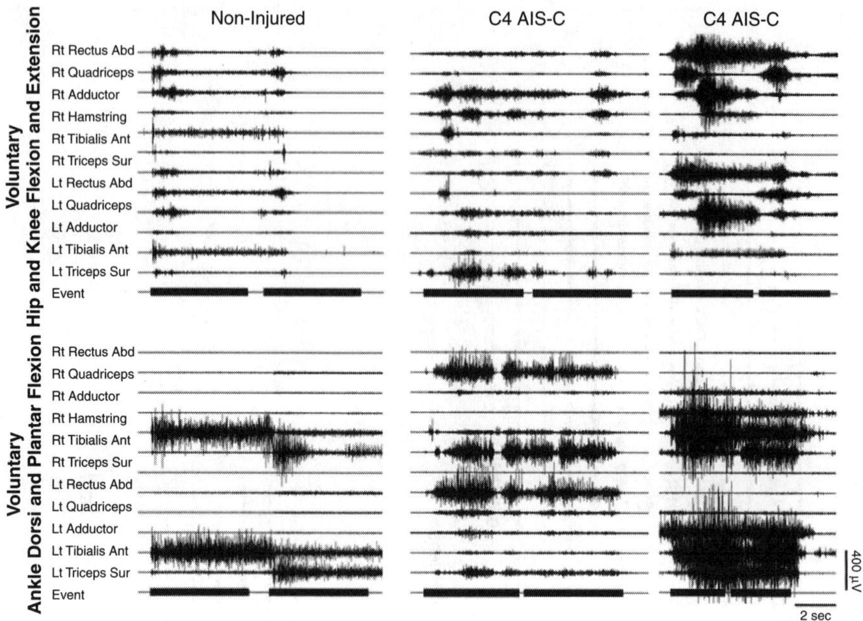

Figure 8–11 Multi-muscle patterns from two persons with AIS-C injuries at the C4 level compared to an example of the non-injured pattern for voluntary bilateral hip and knee flexion (*first event mark*) and extension (*second event mark*) and dorsal (*first event mark*) and plantar flexion (*second event mark*). Note the substantial differences between the patterns produced by the two persons identically classified as C4, AIS-C SCI.

such as the presence of long-lasting or continuous activation, tremor, spasms triggered by extra-protocol events, and unresolved artifacts. Also, when responses are at their very minimum amplitude—when single or few motor units are fired during volitional tasks, for example—they may be lost in the data reduction step of the quantification process described later in this chapter. *Repeatability* or consistency across repeated trials for each task is useful for recognizing decreasing responsiveness (habituation), or contamination by events unrelated to the tested motor tasks. For example, a recurring spasm identified during relaxation can occur within the time window of a volitional task and be inappropriately identified as a response contaminating the quantification phase of data reduction. Otherwise, the BMCA can be reduced to numbers, raw amplitudes, and index values based on the amplitudes that serve as the parameters with which to profile motor control and track changes related to treatment.

Quantification of sEMG activity can be carried out using a number of methods and depends on the type of motor task being quantified (Table 8–1). For all but the five-minute relaxation period that begins the BMCA, quantification is performed in a time window of standard duration: eight seconds for reinforcement maneuvers and five seconds for all others. The window begins with the event mark that cues the test subject to begin the task or marks the beginning of a passive movement or other stimulus. In addition, a one-second window that precedes the event mark is used to measure background noise or pre-task activity to be subtracted from the values obtained during task performance. Any process that converts the signal to positive

Table 8-1 Qualitative and Quantitative Analysis of Results

	Analysis Method	
	Qualitative	**Quantitative**
Relaxation	Complete sEMG silence; random single motor units firing; episodic bursts; long-lasting or continuous activation	Number of events in five minutes; number of muscles involved; duration; total amplitude (μVRMS)
Reinforcement	Symmetry; repeatability; first muscle responding; most prominent muscle responding	How many muscles respond; onset delay; duration (average for three trials); average amplitude (μVRMS)
Voluntary	Repeatability	Agonist onset-to-peak time; magnitude; similarity index
Passive stretch	Presence or absence of response to initial touch; Repeatability; first muscle responding; most prominent muscle responding	How many muscles respond; onset delay; duration (average for three trials); average amplitude (μVRMS)
Tendon-tap	Response presence in muscle tapped; tonic or clonic after-discharge; spread to other ipsilateral and contralateral muscles	Peak-to-peak amplitudes (average for 10 taps); latency can be measured if event mark is reliable
Clonus	Presence or absence of response; spread to other muscles	Duration (average for three trials); average beat frequency
Vibration	Presence or absence of response in muscle vibrated; tonic, clonic or mixed quality; spasms triggered; other muscles activated	Duration; amplitude in muscle vibrated
Plantar Stimulation	Repeatability; unilateral or bilateral distribution	Average amplitude in flexor (ankle) muscle; average overall amplitude; change with suppression attempt

values and then calculates the area under the curve produced can be used. The method most often appearing in the literature is to use the root mean square (RMS) algorithm. Thus, a value is acquired for each muscle that is the average RMS (or other) amplitude in μV/second that has had the average pre-task activity amplitude subtracted. These are the values used to quantify the amplitude of responses and calculate the indices described below.

Across individuals with SCI, the disruption of voluntary control of muscles caudal to the lesion is highly individualized. In fact, the degree of disruption determines their functional independence, specifically the degree and type of support needed to perform activities of daily living such as ambulation. Tang and coworkers (1994) showed that the distribution of motor activity across muscles of the legs during voluntary hip and knee flexion and extension in the supine position predicted the degree and type of support that was needed for ambulation. They categorized patterns from 36 motor-incomplete SCI subjects on the basis of the amount of sEMG, and its distribution and timing across muscles. They showed that patients with patterns from this supine task that resembled those of non-injured subjects were able to ambulate without external support. Those whose patterns showed clear differentiation between flexion and extension phases would require canes or walkers to ambulate, and those in whom only low-amplitude sEMG was elicited or there was only diffuse activation of agonist and antagonist muscles, were wheelchair-bound.

In non-injured individuals, overall sEMG amplitudes produced for voluntary movements can vary from subject to subject. However, the distribution of activity across muscles remains proportionately the same for the simple tasks performed during the BMCA (Lee et al., 2004). Therefore, it is possible to calculate indices that describe how different the distribution pattern of motor unit firing in the set of muscles determined to be appropriate for the task being evaluated in a test subject with neurological damage is from a prototypical pattern recorded from a group of non-injured control subjects. To address the quantification of voluntary motor activity, Lee and coworkers (2004) created the voluntary response index (VRI) as a measure of "goodness" of voluntary motor control. This is based on the fact that the voluntary tasks included in the protocol are conceptually simple and are executed in the same way, with the same multi-muscle distribution of activity, by a group of neurologically intact subjects. In its present form, the VRI is composed of two components, the magnitude and the similarity index (SI). The magnitude is an expression of the total amount of EMG activity across muscles, expressed in terms of the length or magnitude of the vector formed from the EMG amplitudes in the various muscles composing the elements of the vector. Likewise, the SI is formed by measuring the angle between the vector representing the multi-muscle pattern from the subject in question (response vector—RV), and a composite vector formed from a group of neurologically healthy subjects' responses to the same motor task (prototype response vector—PRV). The SI is then expressed as the cosine of the angle between the RV and the PRV. When the angle is zero, multi-muscle distributions are equal and the cosine is 1. As the distribution within the RV changes from that of the PRV, the angle between the two vectors increases and its cosine, or SI value, decreases. The validity of this method has been extensively tested showing it has a high sensitivity to lesion severity in relationship to the ASIA Impairment Scale (Lim et al., 2005), has good internal and test-retest reliability (Lim & Sherwood, 2005), is sensitive to minimal motor control unrecognized by clinical examination (McKay et al., 2004) and can quantitatively track recovery (McKay et al., 2011a). However, this index value offers only a measure of how different motor control is in a test subject from that of a non-injured group but does not describe in what way(s) it is different. Additional parameters need to be identified and validity-tested, such as the rate of motor unit recruitment in the prime mover muscle (McKay et al., 2011a) or the use of agonist-to-antagonist muscle ratios and others that can be derived directly from the sEMG signals.

7. CONCLUSIONS—UTILIZATION OF RESULTS

The BMCA tests the ways in which spinal motor neurons can be excited, inhibited, and combined in response to peripheral input, "non-specific" increases and decreases in the central state of spinal excitability, and to perform purposeful movement. Thus, it is designed to provide a neurophysiological profile of motor control that covers the spectrum from paralysis to full volitional function. In paralyzed persons, discomplete markers demonstrate the degree to which surviving structures in the spinal cord can be used to modify spinal motor excitability caudal to the injury that are subclinical, providing evidence of neural function not measured by clinical examination. Within the wide range of function seen in motor-incomplete lesions, the rate of motor unit recruitment of the prime mover and the voluntary response index parameters characterize the condition of volitional control. Furthermore, the interplay between the markers of excitability modulation and volitional control creates a continuum of control across which any person with SCI can be placed and from which changes can be tracked. For example, using a group of 25 motor-incomplete SCI subjects, it was possible to plot the presence, as prevalence, of full relaxation, reinforcement activation, vibration response, passive stretch response, and the ability to suppress plantar surface-stimulation withdrawal against increasing VRI similarity index values (McKay et al., unpublished data) (Figure 8–12). This plot illustrates the point that appropriate control over motor unit firing requires both excitatory and inhibitory neural function. Thus, SCI lesions that support or allow the initiation of excitation of motor units caudal to the lesion can produce part of the distribution pattern needed to perform voluntary movement. Such excitatory ability alone produces distribution patterns with SI values reaching approximately 0.75. However, the abilities to fully relax in the supine position and to volitionally suppress the cutaneomuscular reflex response are closely associated with the ability to inhibit the co-activation of motor units in antagonistic and distant muscles and produce SI values that approach those of non-injured subjects. These findings agree with those published by Chou and coworkers (2005) in a study that used a qualitative evaluation of the sEMG patterns.

The ability to fully relax while awake is well within the capabilities of the neurologically healthy central nervous system. Thus, the long-lasting, continuous or episodic activation of motor units under the conditions of BMCA recording is indicative of an excitatory bias at the spinal motor neuron. For example, a loss of descending long-tract fibers ending on inhibitory interneurons or of those interneurons themselves might be indicated by the long-lasting activity (Gelfan & Tarlov, 1959). The presence of episodic events might indicate translesional excitation (Dimitrijevic et al., 1984), irritative lesions within the spinal cord (Nogues et al., 1999; Nogues &

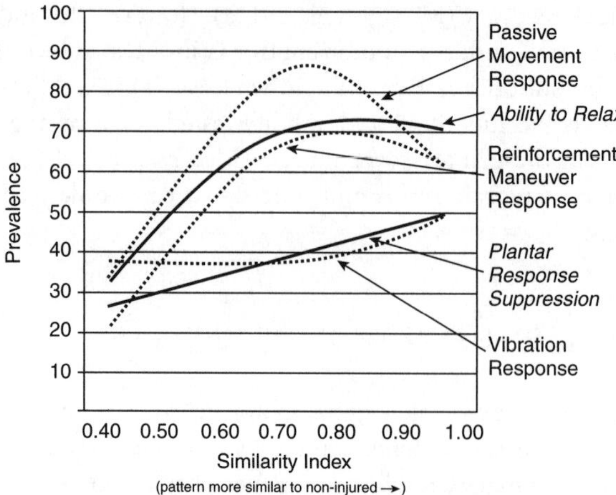

Figure 8–12 Trend lines (second-order polynomial) for prevalence of the ability to relax completely and suppress plantar surface stimulation withdrawal response (*solid lines*) and the responses to passive movement, reinforcement maneuvers, and vibration (*dotted lines*) plotted against how similar sEMG patterns in SCI subjects are to those recorded from non-injured subjects. Notice that responses to passive stretch and reinforcement maneuvers peak at similarity index values around 0.75 and then decrease while the ability to relax completely and volitionally suppress withdrawal increases with improving voluntary control.

Stalberg, 1999), or unperceived noxious input to the spinal cord from peripheral sources (Calancie, 2004; 2006). Each of these findings suggests different neural mechanisms that could be targeted for treatment of what patients will describe as spasticity or to develop gross but useful volitional control. Moreover, they offer quantifiable parameters with which to track treatment effects. The support for spinal motor excitability that provides continued responsiveness to repetitive input without the development of habituation indicates weak and diffuse but present long-tract conduction across the lesion (Dimtrijevic et al., 1977; Sherwood et al., 1992). The ability to volitionally increase spinal motor excitability caudal to the lesion in the absence of the ability to perform voluntary movement (Dimitrijevic et al., 1984) could be trained to aid in activities of daily living. The ability to volitionally suppress the plantar withdrawal reflex (Cioni et al., 1986) offers a target for training that could aid in the control of spasticity. The combination of these translesional capabilities both provides opportunities for treatment and contaminates the effects and evaluation of treatment when it goes unrecognized. Finally, the neurophysiological characterization of voluntary control over the motor units of the many muscles of the body to efficiently perform goal-directed movement provides a measure that can not only be used to quantify improvement with recovery or treatment, but also indicates the likelihood that treatment will be successful and how long improvement will take, and provides detailed information that will be useful in tailoring treatment to the individual needs of the patient. However, clinical use and an increased array of interventions to test and use will be needed to develop the standards by which this neurophysiological tool can provide such information.

Until now, systemic medical treatment of motor dysfunction has been fraught with problems, causing considerable cognitive dysfunction and damaging other body systems. Focal application of substances has reduced collateral side effects but still results in generalized suppression of motor activity. Neuromodulation through electrical stimulation, whether to the muscles, peripheral nerves, or spinal cord, is a powerful tool that improves muscle bulk and autonomic function, but criteria for patient selection, application, or evaluation of effects need further development. Repetitive-use and restricted-use therapies that target the inherent plasticity of the nervous system also hold great promise for improving residual neural function after SCI. The information provided by the method presented here and detailed in the accompanying appendix can already be used to detail the selection of appropriate candidates for therapies that are currently in use. For example, the patient who complains of spasms but shows the ability to volitionally suppress the cutaneo-muscular reflex could be trained to suppress other triggered events by volitionally lowering their spinal motor excitability in a generalized fashion. They and others with long-lasting or continuous sEMG firing might benefit from spinal cord stimulation. Those with the ability to volitionally activate a whole-limb extension would probably benefit from standing, and those who can also perform gross flexion on command might do well with weight-supported treadmill training. Others with some selectivity of control in which they can volitionally differentiate between antagonistic muscles might benefit from selective task training, possibly with added botulinum toxin injections to temporarily reduce the power of overactive muscles while weakened control is strengthened through use. The simple truth is that if treatment of SCI-altered motor control is to be effective, a detailed knowledge of what form that altered control takes after injury will be necessary. In addition, the selection of strategies to be used will need to be highly individualized based on this detailed knowledge, and effects will need to be tracked sensitively. Thus, a new philosophy of treatment involving a more detailed, subclinical view of neural processing is needed to properly select and apply existing treatments and investigate new intervention methods.

References

Ashworth, B. "Preliminary trial of carisoprodal in multiple sclerosis." *Practitioner* 192 (1964): 540–542.

Calancie, B., Needham-Shropshire, B., Jacobs, P., Willer, K., Zych, G., Green, B. A. "Involuntary stepping after chronic spinal cord injury. Evidence for a central rhythm generator for locomotion in man." *Brain* 117 (1994): 1143–1159.

Calancie, B. "Spinal myoclonus after spinal cord injury." *Journal of Spinal Cord Medicine* 29 (2006): 413–424.

Chou, S. W., Pei, Y. C., Lai, C. H., Kuo, C. H., Fu, T. C., Hong, W. H. "Motor control in patients with incomplete spinal cord injuries and various voluntary movement capabilities." *Chang Gung Medical Journal* 28 (2005): 349–356.

Cioni, B., Dimitrijevic, M. R., McKay, W. B., Sherwood, A. M. "Voluntary supraspinal suppression of spinal reflex activity in paralyzed muscles of spinal cord injury patients." *Experimental Neurology* 93 (1986): 574–583.

Dimitrijevic, M. M., Dimitrijevic, M. R., Sherwood, A. M., Van der Linden, C. "Clinical neurophysiological techniques in the assessment of spasticity." In *Physical*

Medicine & Rehabilitation: State of the Art Reviews vol. 3(2) 64–83. Philadelphia, PA: Hanley & Belfus, 1989.

Dimitrijevic, M. R., McKay, W. B., Sarjanovic, I., Sherwood, A. M., Svirtlih, L., Vrbova, G. "Co-activation of ipsi- and contralateral muscle groups during contraction of ankle dorsiflexors." *Journal of Neurological Science* 109 (1992): 49–55.

Dimitrijevic, M. R., McKay, W. B., Sherwood, A. M. "Motor control physiology below spinal cord injury: Residual volitional control of motor units in paretic and paralyzed muscles." In *Advances in Neurology, Vol. 72: Neuronal Regeneration, Reorganization, and Repair,* edited by F. J. Seil, 335–346. Philadelphia, PA: Lippincott-Raven Publishers, 1997.

Dimitrijevic, M. R., Dimitrijevic, M. M., Faganel, J., Sherwood, A. M. "Suprasegmentally induced motor unit activity in paralyzed muscles of patients with established spinal cord injury." *Annuls of Neurology* 16 (1984): 216–221.

Dimitrijevic, M. R., Nathan, P. W., Sherwood, A. M. "Clonus: The role of central mechanisms." *Journal of Neurology Neurosurgery & Psychiatry* 43 (1980): 321–332.

Dimitrijevic, M. R., Spencer, W. A., Trontelj, J. V., Dimitrijevic, M. M. "Reflex effects of vibration in patients with spinal cord lesions." *Neurology* 27 (1977): 1078–1086.

Dimitrijevic, M. R. "Residual motor functions in spinal cord injury." *Advances in Neurology* 47 (1988): 138–155.

Eyre, J. A. "Development and plasticity of the corticospinal system in man." *Neural Plasticity* 10 (2003): 93–106.

Eyre, J. A. "Corticospinal tract development and its plasticity after perinatal injury." *Neuroscience & Biobehavior Review* 31 (2007): 1136–1149.

Fouad, K., Tse, A. "Adaptive changes in the injured spinal cord and their role in promoting functional recovery." *Neurological Research* 30 (2008): 17–27.

Gelfan, S., Tarlov, I. M. "Interneurones and rigidity of spinal origin." *Journal of Physiology* 46 (1959): 594–617.

Hill, C. E., Beattie, M. S., Bresnahan, J. C. "Degeneration and sprouting of identified descending supraspinal axons after contusive spinal cord injury in the rat." *Experimental Neurology* 171 (2001): 153–169.

Illis, L. "The motor neuron surface and spinal shock." In *Modern Trends in Neurology,* Vol. 4, edited by D. Williams, 53–68. New York: Appleton-Century-Crofts, 1967.

Kakulas, B. A. "Neuropathology: The foundation for new treatments in spinal cord injury. (Sir Ludwig Guttman Lecture)." *Spinal Cord* 42 (2004): 549–563.

Lee, D. C., Lim, H. K., McKay, W. B., Priebe, M. M., Holmes, S. A., Sherwood, A. M. "Toward an objective interpretation of surface EMG patterns: A voluntary response index (VRI)." *Journal of Electromyography & Kinesiology* 14 (2004): 379–388.

Lim, H. K., Lee, D. C., McKay, W. B., Priebe, M. M., Holmes, S. A., Sherwood, A. M. "Neurophysiological assessment of lower-limb voluntary control in incomplete spinal cord injury." *Spinal Cord* 43 (2005): 283–290.

Lim, H. K., Sherwood, A. M. "Reliability of surface electromyographic measurements from subjects with spinal cord injury during voluntary motor tasks." *Journal of Rehabilitation Research & Development* 42 (2005): 413–422.

Mahoney, J. S., Engebretson, J. C., Cook, K. F., Hart, K. A., Robinson-Whelen, S., Sherwood, A. M. "Spasticity experience domains in persons with spinal cord injury." *Archives of Physical Medicine & Rehabilitation* 88 (2007): 287–294.

Matthews, P. B. C. "The reflex excitation of the soleus muscle of the decerebrate cat caused by vibration applied to its tendon." *Journal of Physiology* 184 (1996): 450–472.

McCouch, G. P., Austin, G. M., Liu, C. N., Liu, C. Y. "Sprouting as a cause of spasticity." *Journal of Neurophysiology* 21 (1958): 205–216.

McKay, W. B., Lim, H. K., Priebe, M. M., Stokic, D. S., Sherwood, A. M. "Clinical neurophysiological assessment of residual motor control in post-spinal cord injury paralysis." *Neurorehabilitation & Neural Repair* 18 (2004): 144–153.

McKay, W. B., Ovechkin, A. V., Vitaz, T. W., Terson de Paleville, D. G. L., Harkema, S. J. "Neurophysiological characterization of motor recovery in acute spinal cord injury." *Spinal Cord*; 49(2011a): 421–429.

McKay, W. B., Ovechkin, A. V., Vitaz, T. W., Terson de Paleville, D. G. L., Harkema, S. J. Long-lasting involuntary motor activity after spinal cord injury. *Spinal Cord* 49 (2011b): 87–93.

Nogués, M. A., Leiguarda, R. C., Rivero, A. D., Salvat, F., Manes, F. "Involuntary movements and abnormal spontaneous EMG activity in syringomyelia and syringobulbia." *Neurology* 52 (1999): 823–834.

Nogués N. A., Stalberg, E. "Electrodiagnostic findings in syringomyelia." *Muscle & Nerve* 22 (1999): 1653–1659.

Sherwood, A. M., Dimitrijevic, M. R., Bacia, T., McKay, W. B. "Characteristics of the vibratory reflex in humans with reduced suprasegmental influence due to spinal cord injury." *Restorative Neurology & Neuroscience* 5 (1993): 119–129.

Sherwood, A. M., McKay, W. B. "Assessment of spasticity and upper motor neuron dysfunction." In *Wiley Encyclopedia of Biomedical Engineering,* Vol. 5, edited by M. Akay, 3306–3315. New York: John Wiley & Sons, 2006.

Sherwood, A. M., McKay, W. B., Dimitrijevic, M. R. "Motor control after spinal cord injury: Assessment using surface EMG." *Muscle & Nerve* 19 (1996): 966–979.

Tang, S. F., Tuel, S. M., McKay, W. B., Dimitrijevic, M. R. "Correlation of motor control in the supine position and assistive device used for ambulation in chronic incomplete spinal cord–injured persons." *American Journal of Physical Medicine & Rehabilitation* 73 (1994): 268–274.

9

Neurophysiological Monitoring of the Human Spinal Cord Functional Integrity during Surgical Interventions

VEDRAN DELETIS, FRANCESCO SALA, AND PAOLO COSTA

CONTENTS

1. Methodology for Monitoring Fast Neurons of the Corticospinal Tract
   1.1. D Wave Recording Technique Through an Epidurally or Subdurally Inserted Electrode
   1.2. Electrode Montage for Eliciting Single and Multipulse Stimulation Techniques
2. Neurophysiological Markers for Transient and Permanent Paraplegia
3. Intraoperative Neurophysiology of Acute Traumatic Spinal Cord Injured Patients
   3.1. Protocol: Materials and Methods
   3.2. Results
   3.3. Discussion
      — Epidural motor evoked potentials
      — Muscle motor evoked potentials.
      — Epidural somatosensory evoked potentials
      — Cortical SEPs
      — Safety
4. Neurophysiological Determination of the Spinal Cord Injury Site: The Killed-End Potential
5. Conclusions
References

1. METHODOLOGY FOR MONITORING FAST NEURONS OF THE CORTICOSPINAL TRACT

1.1. D Wave Recording Technique Through an Epidurally or Subdurally Inserted Electrode

This method is a direct clinical application of Patton and Amassian's discovery in the 1950s that electrically stimulated motor cortex in monkeys generates a series of well-synchronized descending volleys in the pyramidal tract. This knowledge of corticospinal tract (CT) neurophysiology, which was collected in primates, can be applied to humans in most cases.

1.2. Electrode Montage for Eliciting for Single and Multipulse Stimulation Techniques

The electrode placement on the skull is based on the international 10/20 EEG system (Figure 9–1). For transcranial stimulation, corkscrew-like electrodes (CS electrodes; Neuromedical Inc., Herndon, Virginia) are preferable due to their secure placement and low impedance (usually 1 KΩ). Alternatively, an EEG needle electrode may be used. We do not recommend the use of EEG cup electrodes fixed with collodion, because they are impractical and their placement is time-consuming. The only exception is for young children in whom the fontanel still exists. Since the CS electrodes could penetrate the fontanel during placement, the use of EEG cup electrodes is suggested. The skull presents a barrier of high impedance to the electrode current applied transcranially, therefore we can not completely control the spread of electrical current when it is applied. Therefore, various combinations of electrode montages may need to be explored to obtain an optimal response. The standard montage is C3/C4 for eliciting MEPs in the upper extremities and C1/C2 for eliciting MEPs in the lower extremities. With sufficient intensity of stimulation, C1/C2 preferentially elicits MEPs on the right limb muscles, while C2/C1 elicits MEPs in the left limb muscles. For eliciting the "D wave," a single-pulse stimulation technique applied transcranially or over the exposed motor cortex should be used while the descending volley in the CT is being recorded over the spinal cord as a direct wave. By using a short train of five to seven electrical stimuli applied transcranially or over the exposed motor cortex while muscle motor-evoked potentials (mMEPs) from limb muscles are recorded (Figure 9–1).

2. NEUROPHYSIOLOGICAL MARKERS FOR TRANSIENT AND PERMANENT PARAPLEGIA

During surgery for intramedullary spinal cord tumors in the thoracic region, MEPs in the tibial anterior (TA) muscles will frequently disappear while the D wave remains unaffected. All patients demonstrating this finding during surgery wake up paraplegic (or monoplegic if the TA mMEPs disappear in one leg). In patients in whom we have observed this phenomenon, motor strength is typically recovered in a few hours

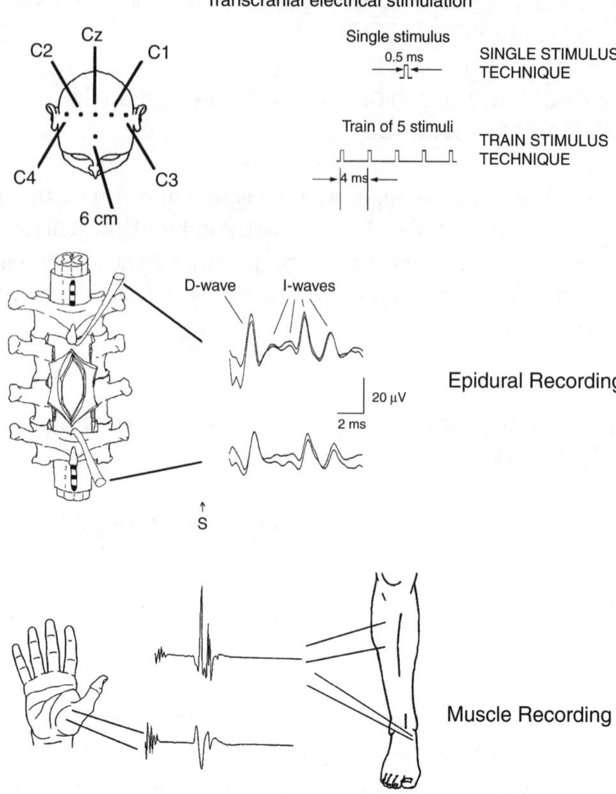

Figure 9–1 *Top*: Schematic illustration of electrode positions for transcranial electrical stimulation of the motor cortex according to the International 10–20 EEG system. The site labeled "6 cm" is 6 cm anterior to CZ. *Middle*: Schematic diagram of the positions of the catheter electrodes (each with three recording cylinders) placed cranial (control electrode) and caudal to the lesion site, to monitor the descending signal after passing through the site of lesion. To the right are D and I waves recorded rostral and caudal to the lesion site. *Bottom*: Recording of muscle motor evoked potentials from the thenar and tibial anterior muscles after eliciting them with multipulse stimuli applied either transcranially or over the exposed motor cortex.

to a few days following surgery. No permanent motor deficits have been observed (Kothbauer et al., 1998, Deletis & Kothbauer, 1998) (Figure 9–2).

3. INTRAOPERATIVE NEUROPHYSIOLOGY OF ACUTE TRAUMATIC SPINAL CORD INJURED PATIENTS

Spinal cord injury (SCI) has been reported to occur in developed countries with an annual incidence of 11.5 to 53.4 cases per million and a prevalence of between 721 and 906 per million people (Kraus et al., 1996; Sekhon & Fehlings, 2001; National Cord Injury Database in the United States—www.spinalcord.uab.edu). The direct

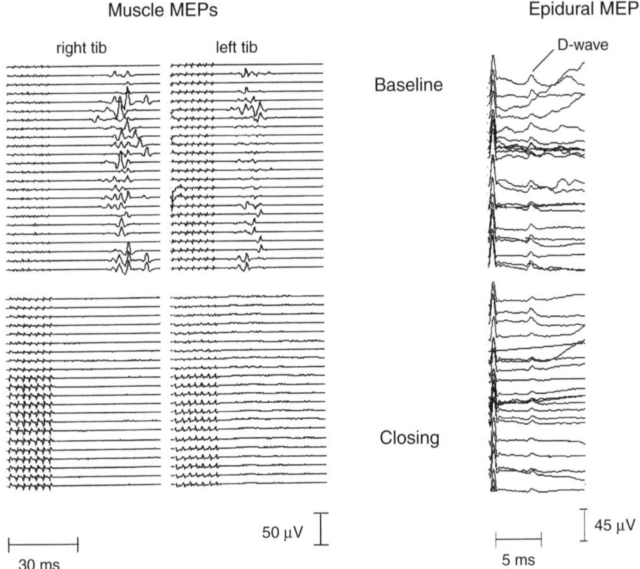

Figure 9–2 Muscle MEPs recorded from right and left TA muscle (*left*) and D wave recorded epidurally over the lower cervical spinal cord (*right*). During surgery, muscle MEPs completely disappeared, while the D wave decreased in amplitude (less than 50%), resulting in transient paraplegia for this patient during surgery for an intramedullary spinal cord tumor. The patient completely recovered within a week.

monetary costs are enormous (Stripling, 1990; Sekhon & Fehlings, 2001): the cost of human suffering related to disability in terms of impaired ambulation, sensation, and sphincters functions are not quantifiable.

A correct and timely prognosis is of paramount importance not only for decision making in the acute phase of SCI, but also to guide the rehabilitation strategy and help evaluate the effectiveness of therapeutic interventions. Nowadays, the prognosis of spinal cord injury is made on a clinical basis within 72 hours to one month post-trauma, and the magnitude of expected recovery is based on physical examination (Kirshblum & O'Connor, 1998; Burns & Ditunno, 2001). Neurophysiological techniques are considered helpful in determining outcome only when used in association with the clinical examination (Kirshblum & O'Connor, 1998). However, the last few years have been testimony to the increasing application of intraoperative monitoring with cortical and epidural somatosensory evoked potentials (SEPs) and transcranial, electrically elicited, muscle and epidural motor evoked potentials (MEPs). All of these have shown evidence of being reliable in the assessment of the spinal cord function during the removal of spinal cord tumors, correction of scoliosis, and cervical spine surgery (Jones et al., 1985; Burke et al., 1992; Nuwer et al., 1995; Kothbauer et al., 1997;1998; Morota et al., 1997; Jones et al., 1996; Pelosi et al., 2002; MacDonald et al., 2003; DiCindio et al.,2003; Hilibrand et al., 2003; Quiñones-Hinojosa et al., 2005; Costa et al., 2007).

Various animal models of experimental spinal cord injury in non-primates and primates have shown that epidural MEPs and SEPs are a sensitive measure of post-injury motor performance (Sudo, 1980a; Levy, 1983; Levy et al., 1984; 1987; Baskin & Simpson, 1987; Fehlings et al., 1987; Shiau et al., 1992; Jou, 2000; Arunkumar et al., 2001; Fukaya et al., 2003). However, there are only a few reports on SEPs that promote their possible utility as a tool to neurophysiologically test SCI patients (Sudo, 1980b; Halter et al., 1989; Stetkarova et al., 1993; Tsirikos et al., 2004).

The primary scope of this study was to predict the motor and sensory outcome following SCI by comparing intraoperative recording of muscle MEPs (mMEPS) , epidural MEPs (eMEPs) as well as cortical (cSEPs) and epidural SEPs (eSEPs) during posterior stabilization in neurologically uncompromised and in complete SCI patients. The second goal was to determine possible benefits from the continuous monitoring during surgery of electrical activity in the motor and sensory pathways in uncompromised or incomplete SCI patients.

3.1. Protocol: Materials and Methods

Intraoperative recording of mMEPs and eMEPs along with cSEPs and eSEPs was attempted in 41 patients (19 with a complete SCI, 10 incomplete -5 of them with central cord syndrome, one patient with central cord plus Brown Sequard syndrome, and 12 patients neurologically uncompromised during posterior stabilization for spine due to the spinal cord injury. All patients gave informed consent after being told that potential risks included: seizures, skin burns from stimulating electrodes, tongue bites, cardiac arrhythmias, inadvertent injury caused by TES-induced movement, epidural bleeding, or infections. Patients with implanted heart pacemakers or brain stimulators and subjects with SCI distal to the bony level T10 were excluded from the study. Patients were assessed clinically, by the ASIA and McCormick scales preoperatively, within 12 hours after surgery, seven days after surgery, and three, six, and 12 months after surgery.

The anesthetic protocol during surgery included a combination of the two drugs, Remifentanil and Propofol, with total intravenous anesthesia (TIVA). No muscle relaxants were used after patient's induction and intubation. Two flexible epidural electrodes with three contacts (CEDL-3PIDINX, Ad-Tech Medical instruments Corp., Racine, WI) were inserted cranially and caudally to the injured site through a small laminectomy or flavectomy, to monitor both epidural motor and somatosensory evoked potentials during surgery. A commercially available neurophysiologically evoked potential machine (Nicolet Endeavour; Nicolet Biomedical, Madison, WI) was used for SEPs stimulation and recording.

SEPs were elicited by 100 μs or 200 μs square-wave electrical pulses presented sequentially to the median or ulnar nerve at the wrist and to the posterior tibial nerve at the ankle (rate 4.1–7.1/sec., stimulus intensity adjusted individually from 14 mA to 40 mA). In order to optimize the montage, needle electrodes were placed at Cz,' C3,' C4' and Fz (international 10–20 EEG system) and the best traces among Cz'-Fz, C3'-Fz, C4'-Fz, C3'-C4, C4'-C3 were used for monitoring. Filtering was typically 20 Hz –30 Hz to 300 Hz –500 Hz, with a 100 ms analysis time; averaging was stopped manually when SEPs were clearly reproducible. Similar stimulation and filtering parameters were used for eSEPs: the recording montage was electrode 3 to 1 (active to reference) for the rostral electrode and 1 to 3 for the caudal electrode in regard to the lesion site.

mMEPs were elicited transcranially with applied trains of 3 to 7 anodal electrical pulses, with interpulse interval of 2 to 4 ms) (N = 3–7, ISI 2 ms–4 ms), delivered via two corkscrew-type electrodes inserted over the motor cortex regions at C1, C2, C3, and C4 (international 10–20 EEG system). A C1–C2 or C3–C4 montages was used to elicit right mMEPs, and vice versa. Stimuli were delivered through commercially available constant-voltage stimulators (D185; Digitimer, Welwyn Garden City, United Kingdom) (pulse width = 50 μs, voltage 200 V–700 V) or a constant-currentstimulator (CROSTIM 2, Inomed, Tenningen, Germany; pulse width = 500 μs, current 80 mA–200 mA). Responses were recorded on commercially available neurophysiology instrumentation (Nicolet Endeavour; Nicolet Biomedical, Madison, WI).

mMEPs were recorded with a needle electrode placed in the muscle with a belly-tendon montage from the abductor pollicis brevis for the upper extremities and both tibialis anterior and abductor hallucis muscles for the lower extremities. The time base was 100 ms–200 ms and the filter band pass 30–150 Hz/500–3000 Hz. A bite block consisting of rolled gauze was used after induction of anesthesia to avoid lip or tongue bites.

In order to record eMEPs (D wave), a two flexible three-contact platinum epidural electrodes (CEDL-3PIDINX, Ad-Tech Medical Instruments Corp., Racine, WI) were inserted by the surgeon cranially and caudally to the site of surgery. D waves were elicited by a single anodal stimulus delivered with the same stimulators as were used for mMEPs, and recorded with electrodes used for sSEPs. Filters were typically set to 200 Hz/500–3000 Hz. Time base was 10 ms–20 ms; in some cases an averaging of 4–10 responses was necessary to improve signal-to-noise ratio. The recording montage was electrode 1 to 2 (active to reference) and/or 2 to 3 for the rostral electrode, and 2 to 1 and/or 3 to 2 for the caudal electrode, so as to obtain the same response polarity from both electrodes montage.

3.2. Results

All uncompromised patients had recordings of the motor and sensory evoked potentials from the upper and lower extremities within normal limits (Figure 9–3). No significant evoked potentials changes were observed in any case, and none of the subjects presented postoperative neurological deficits.

Neurologically complete SCI patients: In all patients the intraoperative neurophysiological profile was characterized by absence of both mMEPs and D wave caudal to the lesion site associated with the lack of cSEPs and eSEPs cranially to the lesion site (Figure 9–4). None of these patients neurologically recovered (Table 9–1).

In one subject, with an ASIA-A, and C5 spinal cord injury level, the presence of mMEPs recorded from the abductor pollicis brevis correctly predicted the recovery of hand but not leg function (Figure 9–5).

The intraoperative pattern of neurologically incomplete SCI patients generally mirrored the clinical presentation, but a clear caudal D wave, even if with low amplitude values, was recordable in all subjects. In particular, in central cord syndrome the neurophysiological profile was characterized by low voltage mMEPs from hand muscle (Figure 9-6).

One out of nine neurologically incomplete patients with absent mMEPs and D wave (recorded caudal to the spinal cord lesion) neurologically significantly

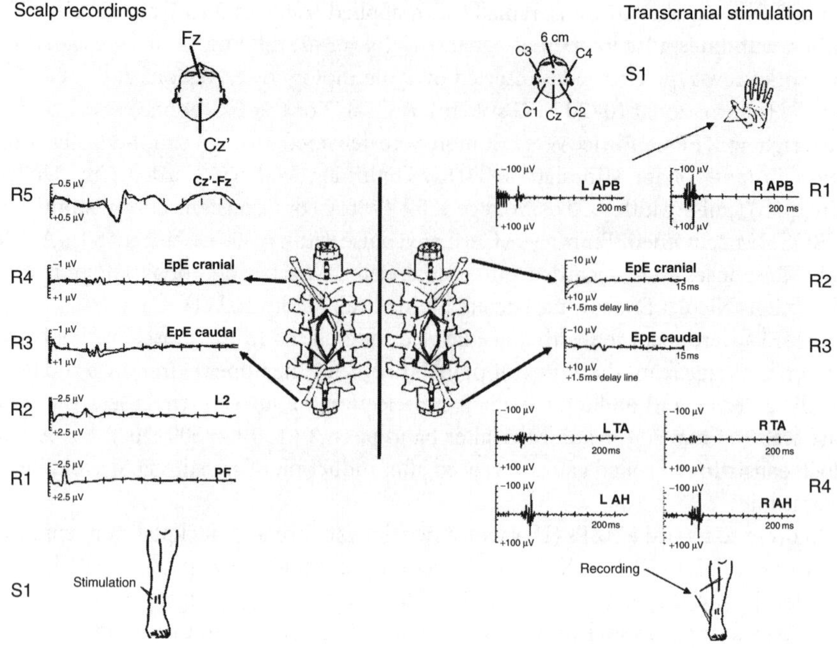

Figure 9–3 Neurophysiological profile of neurologically intact SCI patient. To the left: Spinal SEPs (R1 to R4) after stimulation of the tibial nerve at the ankle (S1) recorded caudally (R3, EpE caudal) and cranially to the lesion site (R4, EpE cranial). PF = tibial nerve neurogram from the popliteal fossa. L2 = spinal SEPs over L1 vertebral level. R5: cortical SEPs. To the right: D wave recorded cranially (R2, EpE cranial) and caudally (R3, EpE caudal) to the lesion site, and elicited by transcranial electrical stimulation (TES, S1). Muscle motor evoked potentials recorded from the upper (R1) and lower extremities muscles (R4). RAPB, LAPB = right and left abductor pollicis brevis mm. RTA, LTA = right and left tibial anterior mm. RAH, LAH = right and left abductor hallucis brevis mm.

recovered. One 69-year-old male (Table 9–2, patient no.2), had history of liver cirrhosis and diabetes. On May, 4, 2006, he had minor brain trauma due to a fall (brain CT and cervical X-ray were normal). Twenty-four hours later he developed a rapidly evolving tetraplegia (in a matter of hours he could move only the big toe bilaterally). On May 7, a cervical decompression with a posterior approach was performed. Although intraoperative mMEPs recorded from upper and lower extremities were absent, D wave recorded at the upper thoracic spinal cord was present with low amplitude and delayed latency of 10 ms (Figure 9–7).

The patient quickly improved in term of days (lower extremities muscle strength was 4/5, and he was able to walk with a cane in a couple of weeks).

In one out of ten neurologically incomplete SCI patients (Table 9–2, patient no. 7) during surgical maneuver for decompression-traction for spine alignment, deterioration of mMEPs and reduction in amplitude of the D wave occurred. mMEPs and D wave returned to the baseline after stopping of the maneuver (Figure 9–8).

Another one of ten incomplete SCI patients (Table 9–2, patient no. 10) with spinal cord hyperintensity at C2 level, significantly improved. This subject had a clinical presentation of bilateral upper limb and left lower limb deep paresis associated with

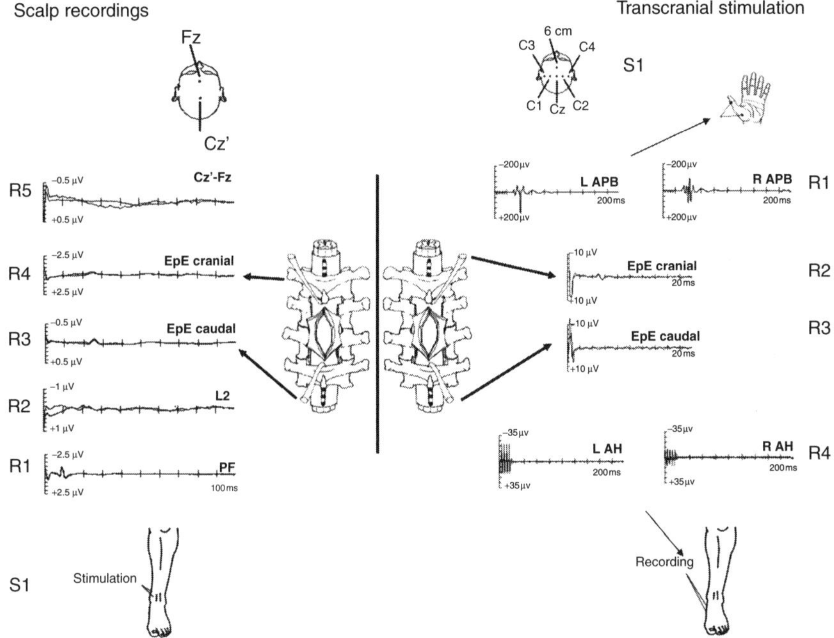

Figure 9–4 An example of typical neurophysiological profile of patient with neurological complete spinal cord injury at the upper thoracic level. *To the left*: Absence of cortical (R5) and epidurally recorded spinal SEPs (R4). *To the right*: Presence of mMEPs from upper (R1) and absence from lower extremities (R4), together with presence of the D wave cranially (R2) and absence caudal to the lesion site (R3).

right hemihypoesthesia: the intraoperative profile was characterized by absent mMEPs from upper limbs and from right lower limb associated with absent right limbs SEPs. However, the caudal D wave was clearly recordable, even if of lower amplitude than expected, with recordings at this spinal cord level. The patient recovered in two months (Figure 9-9).

3.3. Discussion

Recent progress in understanding basic mechanisms, the rapid evolution of diagnostic technologies, and the development of surgical and post-surgical protocols have significantly ameliorated the prognosis of traumatic SCI. Actually the assessment and prognosis of SCI patients is still dominated by the clinical findings associated with neuroimaging; however, even the most sophisticated imaging techniques mainly provide information about *anatomy* and not *functional integrity* of the spine and spinal cord.

A precise neurophysiological assessment of spinal cord functional integrity should be able to provide significant data both to correctly plan the rehabilitative strategies (Kirshblum & O'Connor, 1998; Burns & Ditunno, 2001) and to evaluate the new therapeutic opportunities that are potentially beneficial to the injured spinal cord (Bridwell et al., 2004; Hawryluk et al., 2008).

Table 9–1 Results of Clinically Complete SCI Patients at Time of Diagnosis

				SEPs			MEPs			
Nr.	Pt.	Level	Pre-op ASIA	Caudal epidural	Cranial epidural	Scalp	Cranial D Wave	Caudal D Wave	Caudal mMEPs	ASIA at discharge or FU
1	NA, m, 34	T6	A	+	-	-	+	-	-	A
2	DP, m, 20	T3	A	+	-	-	+	-	-	A
3	MAF, m, 21	C4–C7	A	+	-	-	+	-	-	A
4	BR, m, 74	T4	A	+	-	-	+	-	-	Deceased in ICU
5	SP, m, 45	T6	A	+	-	-	+	-	-	A
6	RG, m, 66	T9	A	+	-	-	+	-	-	A
7	BF, m, 69	T9	A	+	-	-	+	-	-	A
8	GD, f, 31	T4–T7	A	+	-	-	+	-	-	B
9	GA, f, 78	C5–C6	A	+	-	-	+	-	-	Deceased in ICU
10	BP, m, 74	T4	A	+	-	-	+	-	-	A
11	CA, m, 27	T10	A	+	-	-	+	-	-	B
12	BC, f, 19	T8	A	+	-	-	+	-	-	A
13	VQM, m, 73	C6–C7	A	+	-	-	+	-	-	Deceased in ICU
14	VME, m, 77	C5–C6	A	+	-	-	+	-	-	A
15	BJ, m, 20	C6–C7	A	+	-	-	+	-	-	A
16	PIM, f, 43	T4–T5	A	+	-	-	+	-	-	A
17	MS, f, 41	C5–C6	A	+	-	-	+	-	-	A
18	TC, m, 48	C7–T1	A	+	-	-	+	-	-	A
19	VN, m, 71	T5	A	+	-	-	+	-	-	A

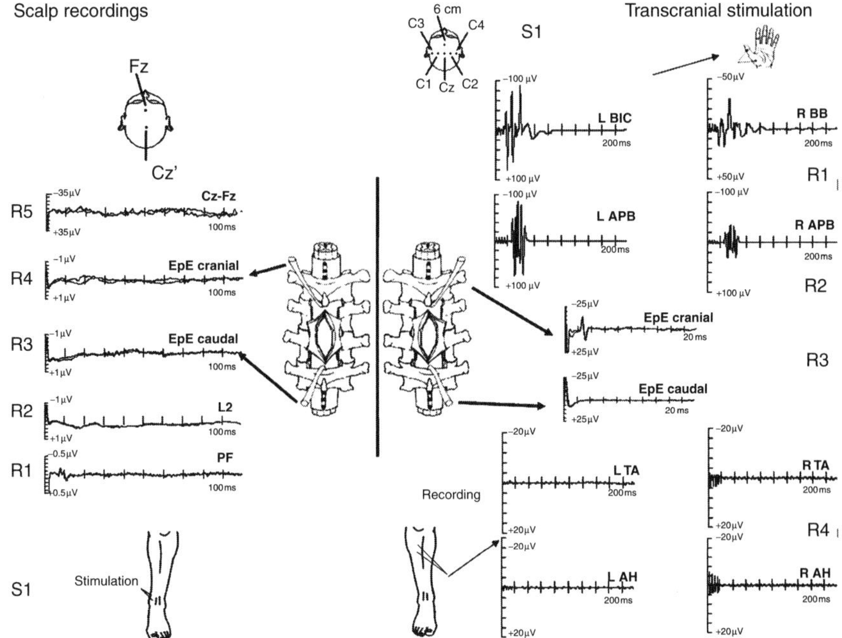

Figure 9–5 Patient with spinal cord injury at C5 and ASIA-A score with a presens of mMEPs from upper extremities (R1 and R 2), correctly predicting recovery of hand but not a leg function, due to the absence of mMEPs from low extremities and absence of D wave caudal to the lesion site.

In fact, many animal models of experimental spinal cord injury have demonstrated that epidural and muscle MEPs and epidural and cortical SEPs are sensitive measures of post-injury motor and sensory performance (Sudo, 1980a; Levy, 1983; Levy et al., 1984; 1987; Baskin & Simpson, 1987; Fehlings et al., 1987; Shiau et al., 1992; Jou, 2000; Arunkumar et al., 2001; Fukaya et al., 2003).

SEPs and MEPs have become a well-established method for intraoperatively testing spinal cord functional integrity in complex spine and spinal cord surgeries. Actually, two methodologies have been developed to intraoperatively elicit MEPs by transcranial electrical stimulation:

a) Recording the D wave directly from the epidural space (eMEPs) using single pulse stimulating technique (Boyd et al., 1986; Hicks et al.,1991);
b) Recording of MEPs in limb muscles (mMEPs) elicited by a multipulse stimulating technique (Pechstein et al., 1996).

The information provided by these two techniques is complementary, being the D wave generated by the direct activation of axons of fast-conducting fibers of the corticospinal tract (Patton & Amassian, 1954), while elicitability of mMEPs depend of facilitatory influence of cortical motor neurons, to the alfa motoneuronal pools of the spinal cord (Deletis & Kothbauer, 1998; Deletis et al., 2001a; 2001b; Deletis, 2002; Deletis & Sala, 2008).

Table 9–2 Results in Clinically Incomplete SCI at Time of Diagnosis

				SEPs			MEPs			
N.	**Pt.**	**Level**	**Pre-op ASIA**	**Caudal epidural**	**Cranial epidural**	**Scalp**	**Cranial D Wave**	**Caudal D Wave**	**Caudal mMEPs**	**ASIA at discharge or FU**
1	AG, m,70	Cervical	D (central cord)	+	-	-	+	+	+	D
2	GA, m 69	Cervical	C (central cord)	+	+	+	+	+	-	D
3	LP, m, 44	Cervical	D (central cord)	+	+	+	+	+	+	E
4	DM, m, 70	Thoracic	D (central cord)	+	+	+	+	+	+	D
5	PE, m, 27	Cervical	D	+	+	+	+	+	+	E
6	LSG, m 67	Thoracic	D	+	+	+	+	+	+	D
7	ZC, m, 34	Cervical	D (central cord)	+	+	+	+	+	+	D
8	RG, f, 39	Cervical	D	+	+	+	+	+	+	E
9	BF, f, 53	Cervical	D	+	+	+	+	+	+	E
10	MP, m, 36	Cervical	C (Central cord + Brown Sequard)	+	NP	+/-	NP	+	+/-	E

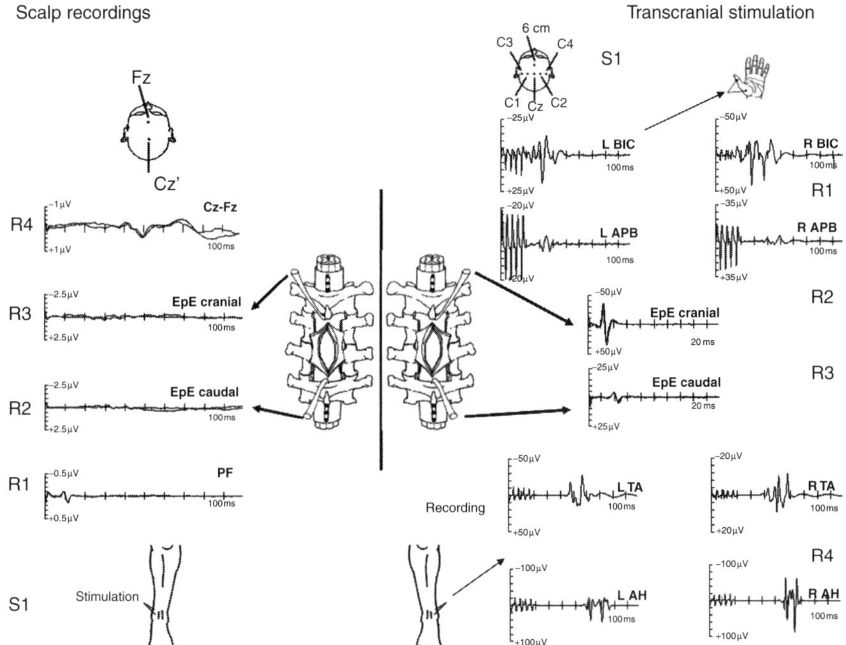

Figure 9–6 Patient with central cord syndrome at cervical level (nr. 7 of tab. 2), having low amplitude mMEPs from hand muscles (R2) with preserved mMEPs from lower limb muscles. The caudal D wave is clearly recordable, even with an amplitude lower than expected.

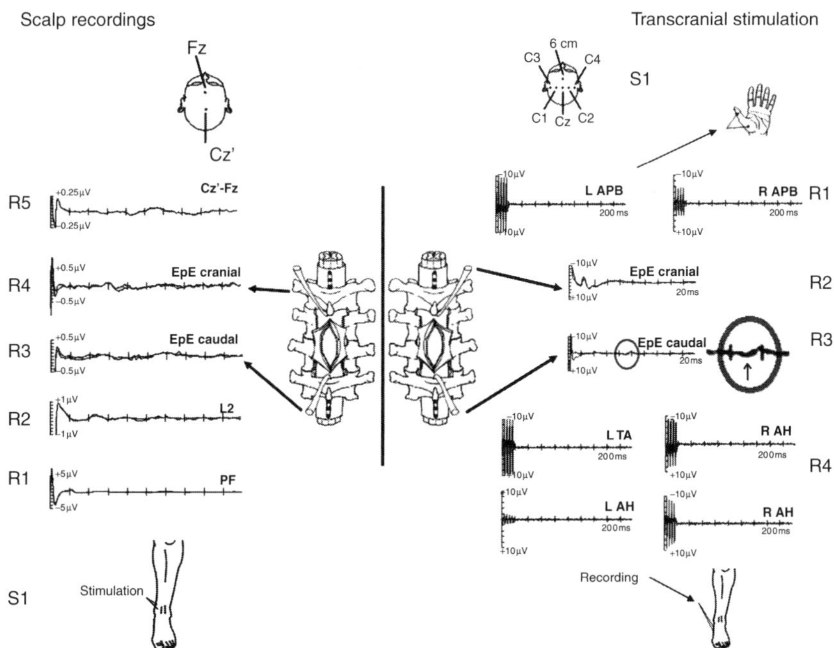

Figure 9–7 Neurologically incomplete spinal cord injured patient, having small amplitude and delayed latency of the D wave distally to the injured site, predicting good neurological recovery (R3, enlarged, marked within a circle).

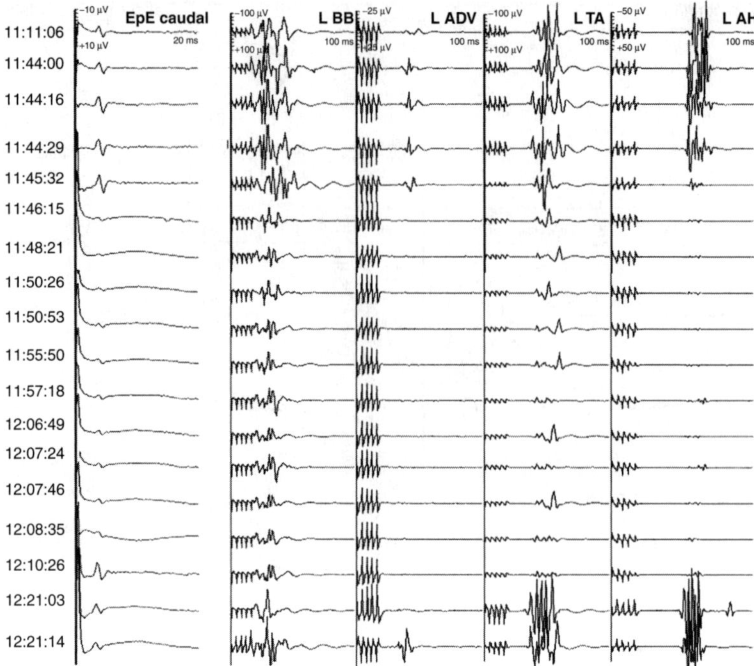

Figure 9–8 Neurologically incomplete spinal cord injured patient (Table 9–2, patient no. 7). During surgical maneuver for decompression-traction for spine alignment (starting at 11:45:32), deterioration of mMEPs with reduction of amplitude of the D wave occurred. Muscle MEPs and D wave started to return to the baseline after stopping maneuver (12:07:46) and completely recovered at the end of the surgery (12:21:14).

To the best of our knowledge, the combined intraoperative recording of mMEPs and eMEPs along with cSEPs and eSEPs in the patients with spinal and spinal cord trauma has not been previously reported. However, the intraoperative recording of mMEPs and eMEPs along with cSEPs and eSEPs allow for a separate assessment of motor and sensory functional integrity. Indeed, in a complete transverse section, one would expect to find the absence of both mMEPs and eMEPs caudally a lesion site, associated with the lack of SEPs cranially to the lesion. In incomplete SCI subjects, the presence of the D wave recorded caudal to the lesion site should be a reliable prognostic sign for the motor recovery. Finally, in neurologically uncompromised patients, the intraoperative monitoring of both motor and sensory functional integrity may reduce the risk of postoperative neurological deficit.

This study provides evidence, as expected, that the absence of both mMEPs and eMEPs caudal to the lesion site was associated with a lack of epidural and cortical SEPs cranially to the lesion site in complete spinal cord injury and the none affected recordings in uncompromised patients. Furthermore, the presence of D wave caudal to lesion site correctly predicts a good motor outcome.

Although the absence of muscle-MEPs and cortical SEPs in our patients with a complete clinical SCI correlates with a loss of motor and sensory function, there are several reasons why epidural recordings should be made. We shall give a brief outline why we recommend a combined use of these techniques.

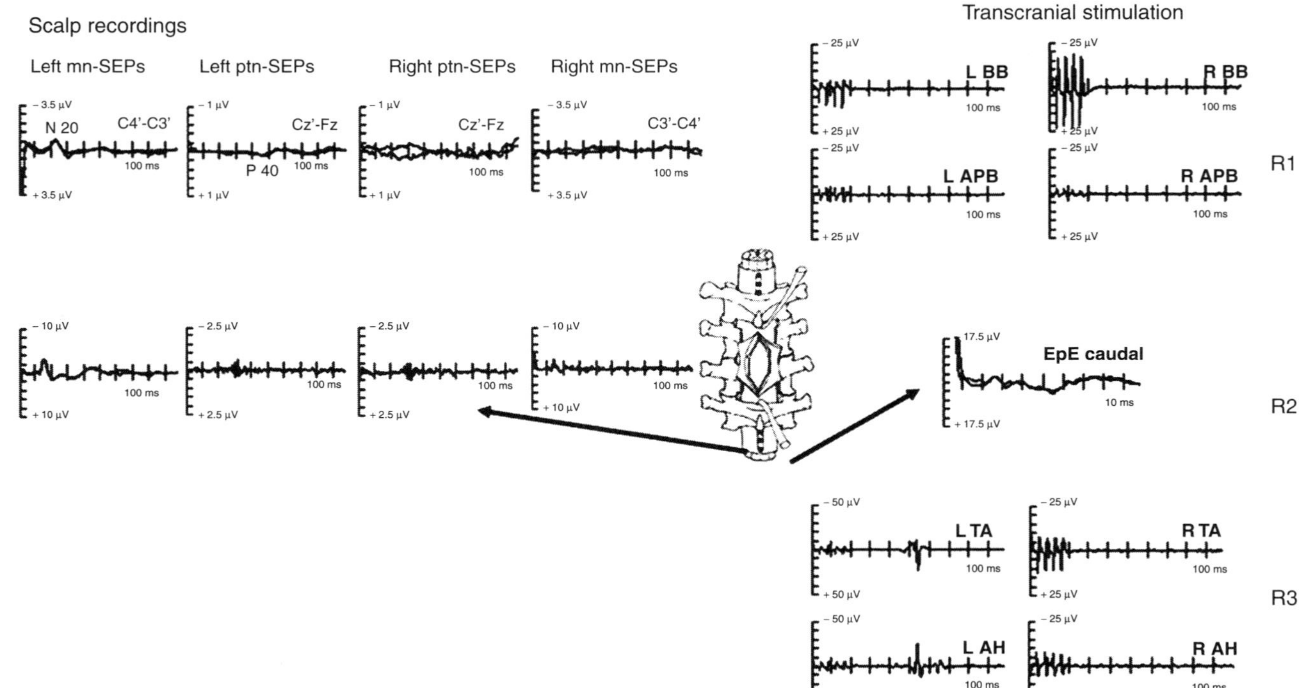

Figure 9–9 Spinal cord injured patient neurologically incomplete, having small amplitude caudal D wave, predicting good neurological recovery.

Epidural motor evoked potentials

A single electrical pulse produces a corticospinal "D wave" from direct cortical neuron axonal depolarization that can be recorded in the spinal epidural space: the D wave amplitude is a direct measure of the number of functioning fast-conducting fibers in the corticospinal tracts (Patton & Amassian, 1954). Since no synapses are involved between the stimulating and the recording site (the proximal axon of the cortical motoneuron is stimulated and the recording site is located caudal to the lesion site but cranially to the synapses at the alfa-motoneuron), the D wave has been considered the gold standard in the assessment of the integrity of the corticospinal tract (Deletis, 2002). There are numerous reports that demonstrate that if the D wave is lost during the removal of an intramedullary spinal cord tumor, the patient will suffer from profound, persistent motor deficit (Kothbauer et al., 1997; 1998; Morota et al., 1997; Cioni, 1999; Deletis, 2002; Deletis & Kothbauer, 1998). Although the absence of the D wave caudal to the lesion site strongly correlates with persistent motor deficits in our series, it has to be combined with mMEPs recording for a correct diagnosis.

In fact, in patients with intramedullary spinal cord tumor and patients who had previous irradiation of the spinal cord, the D wave may be absent, while mMEPs are still recordable (Kothbauer et al.,1997; 1998; Morota et al., 1997; Deletis 2002; Deletis & Kothbauer, 1998). It has been postulated that this phenomenon is due to a desynchronization of fast conducting fibers of the CT tract, induced by the pathological agent, with low-amplitude D waves caudal to the lesion site, up to the absence of the response (Deletis, 2002). Theoretically a similar phenomenon could be present in SCI and, therefore, the intraoperative recording of the D wave could be a potential predictive index of recovery. Indeed, an experimental study reported that as few as 10% of the corticospinal fibers were sufficient to support locomotion (Blight, 1983).

Muscle motor evoked potentials

There are relatively few reports of the use of mMEPs in SCI (Clarke et al., 1994; MacDonell & Donnan, 1995; Bondurant & Haghighi, 1997; McKay et al., 1997; Curt et al., 1998), and most of those describe the use of a transcranial magnetic stimulation. Transcranial magnetic stimulation has some advantages, the main one being that it is not painful. However, the magnetic stimulus indirectly activates corticospinal motoneurons transynaptically and therefore it is not a suitable technique for intraoperative use. Conversely, the motor cortex can be stimulated in the anesthetized subject by short duration, high frequency trains of electrical stimuli applied transcranially, producing several corticospinal volleys that combine to depolarize spinal motor neurons (Patton & Amassian, 1954; Taniguchi et al., 1993; Pechstein et al., 1996). The responses can be easily recorded from the muscles without averaging: mMEPs allow the evaluation of motor system from the cortex down to the neuromuscular junction, for an individual limb, and can be present even when SEPs are either lost or poorly defined (Taniguchi et al., 1993; Pechstein et al., 1996; Rodi et al., 1996; Cioni et al., 1999; Deletis et al., 2001a; 2001b).

Our study showed that the absence of muscle MEPs caudal to the lesion site correlates with persistent loss of ambulatory capacity: unfortunately, mMEPs alone may not be sufficient for a prognostic evaluation. Indeed, mMEPs are, at times, completely lost during surgery for intramedullary spinal cord tumors, but if the D wave amplitude is either stable or decreased by less than 50%, the patient will present additional transient motor deficit postoperatively but motor strength will be recovered hours or days after surgery (Deletis, 2002). This phenomenon ("transient paraplegia") is probably due to the surgically induced temporary inactivation of non-corticospinal descending tracts and the propriospinal system, while fast-conducting corticospinal fibers are mostly preserved (Deletis, 2002). The speculative mechanism of transient paraplegia has at least some similarity to the current hypothesis of proposed spinal shock (Ditunno et al., 2004).

Epidural somatosensory evoked potentials

After the introduction of epidural recording of SEPs by stimulation of peripheral nerves (Shimoji et al., 1971) various studies reported promising results in predicting and preventing surgically induced spinal cord injuries (Shimoji et al., 1971; Jones et al., 1985; Komatu et al., 1985; Forbes et al., 1991; Burke et al., 1992; Noordeen et al., 1997). Although many animal models of experimental spinal cord injury evidenced the role of epidural SEPs in testing the dorsal columns function (Sudo, 1980a; Baskin & Simpson, 1987; Jou, 2000; Arunkumar et al., 2001), there are only a few reports that propose its application in humans (Sudo, 1980b; Halter et al., 1989; Stetkarova et al.,1993; Tsirikos et al., 2004).

Sudo (1980b) recorded eSEPs on seven patients with cervical cord injury, suggesting that the eSEPs may be helpful in the assessment of how severely the spinal cord is involved. Although one case with complete SCI had responses cranial to the lesion level that yielded a positive deflection, according to a killed end potential at the level of cord lesion, this was not always the case for other subjects with complete SCI. In two studies conducted by the same group in the acute (Halter et al., 1989) and chronic phase (Stetkarova et al., 1993) of spinal cord injury, the eSEPs provided more information than did the surface recordings. In Tsirikos' large series (Tsirikos et al., 2004), 82 patients (40 with incomplete injury, 42 without preoperative neurological deficit) were studied intraoperatively with cortical and eSEPs to monitor the spinal cord function throughout surgery. They found that a persistent intraoperative decrement in SEP amplitude and poor restitution at completion of surgery is an indicator of there being a risk of postoperative neurological compromise.

Cortical SEPs

SEPs have been extensively studied in patients with spinal cord injury with absent cortical responses evoked by stimulation of peripheral nerves caudal to the lesion site associated with a complete injury (Perot & Vera, 1982; Rowed et al., 1978; York et al., 1983). Even if it is generally agreed that SEPs are no more effective in predicting outcome than is a proper examination (Kirshblum & O'Connor, 1998), clinical examination may be of limited value in subjects who are unresponsive and/or uncooperative, or in the presence of other trauma. SEPs can easily be recorded in the operating theatre without contamination of myogenic artifact activity, and it is possible to average a great number of responses so that the signal-to-noise ratio can be reduced. Intraoperative cortical SEPs can be used as a baseline to which further recordings can be compared: in fact, a return of the SEPs components in the initial stage of the SCI can lead to clinically detectable improvements in both motor and sensory function (Rowed et al., 1978; Spielholz et al., 1979; Dorfman et al., 1980; Young, 1982; Dimitrijevic et al., 1983; Gruninger & Ricker, 1991; Curt & Dietz, 1996; 1997). The main information SEPs carry relates to dorsal column activity, and the absence of cortical SEPs strongly correlates with an alteration of proprioception: these data are of paramount importance for the rehabilitation program. The fact that SEPs are inadequate to make a reliable assessment of the integrity of motor systems in the spinal cord may explain the contradictory results obtained when they are used as the sole technique to predict motor outcome (Kirshblum & O'Connor, 1998).

Safety

Intraoperative techniques, in particular transcranial electrical stimulation and spinal epidural recording electrodes, are generally considered safe in expert hands. None of our patients experienced any of the iatrogenic complications that have been described (Vandermeulen et al., 1994; MacDonald, 2002): no injury or infection due to electrode placement, no spinal epidural hematomas following insertion of epidural electrodes, no neurological complications associated with transcranial motor cortex stimulation, and no seizures occurred.

4. NEUROPHYSIOLOGICAL DETERMINATION OF THE SPINAL CORD INJURY SITE: THE KILLED-END POTENTIAL

Previous studies in experimental spinal cord injury have described the "so-called" killed-end potential (KEEP), also known as "final potential" or spinal cord evoked injury potential. Deecke and coworkers (1973) described a primate model, injured using controlled spinal cord compression, in which they measured afferent conduction of impulses initiated by sciatic nerve stimulation before and after injury. Before injury, a triphasic potential—with an initial positive component—was recorded from the dorsal surface of the cord. After injury, this response was abolished, and a huge positive monophasic potential appeared. This large monophasic positivity was explained as an impulse that approaches but does not reach the recording electrode because the fibers are interrupted. Interestingly, in some monkeys, it was still possible to record a slight positive deflection up to several millimeters rostral to the injury site. However, there was a steady decay in amplitude of this deflection cranially from the lesion up to an isoelectric line. Moreover, the latency of this response did not change, in spite of the fact that the recording electrode was moved rostrally. These two observations suggested that the positive deflection across the injury site was not an action potential but rather an electrotonic propagation. These potentials are conducted faster than true action potentials, but attenuate very rapidly and cannot sustain long-distance signalling.

Later, Schramm and colleagues (1983) examined spinal somatosensory evoked potentials in a slow graded compression model in cats. In the final stage of compression, they invariably recorded a small monophasic positive wave immediately rostral to the area of compression. They also attributed this response to electrotonic volume conduction from the activity of the dorsal white matter caudal to the compression site, as a neurophysiological landmark of complete conduction block. Further elucidation of the KEEP was provided by Schramm and coworkers in 1983 when they observed that with a gradual impairment of spinal cord conduction, the KEEP also developed gradually. Finally, in a serial recording along the spinal axis, they showed that the transition from the normal triphasic potential to the KEEP allowed for a precise localization of the lesion. The localizing value of the KEEP has been tested also in the clinical setting, although the report of KEEP recorded intraoperatively is anecdotal (Whittle, 1988, Katayama, 1988; Morioka, 1990).

Katayama and colleagues (1988) reported the preoperative determination of the level of spinal cord lesion in five patients with cervical injury. Electrodes were placed percutaneously under fluoroscopy at the cervical and thoracic epidural space. Spino-spinal evoked potentials were recorded in a monopolar fashion from the rostral electrode after stimulation from the electrode caudal to the injury site. In four patients they recorded a clear KEEP (large monophasic positivity) near the presumed level of injury. As the recording electrode was withdrawn stepwise to the proximity of the presumed level of cord injury, a small potential became apparent and its amplitude significantly increased near the center of the lesion. Yet the positive potential did not change in latency (electrotonic propagation). The presumed levels of lesion were confirmed at surgery, when the tip of the recording electrode appeared to be located at or a few millimeters caudal to the center of the lesion. In this study, Katayama emphasized that although a KEEP indicates a conduction block, it may not necessarily indicate complete and irreversible cord injury.

Morioka and coworkers (1990) described the KEEP in a patient with a cervicomedullary glioma. Interestingly, they used KEEP from SEPs after median nerve stimulation as a localizing landmark to decide the optimal level for myelotomy when the cord was swollen by the tumor and ultrasound failed to visualize the tumor clearly.

More recently, the KEEP has been investigated as a potential outcome measure for testing therapeutic agents in experimental spinal cord injury. Fukaya and colleagues (2003) tested the hypothesis that damage spreading after SCI can be evaluated by a progressive shift of the KEEP along the spinal cord. Furthermore, they assessed the effect of high doses of methylprednisolone on the spread of tissue damage. In the first six hours post-injury, they observed a clear shifting of the largest KEEP up to 2.5 mm rostral to the injury site, while at the site of lesion the KEEP decreased in amplitude. However, this spreading was less marked when methylprednisolone was administered to the cats within 30 minutes post-injury.

Overall, the KEEP appears to be a well documented neurophysiological marker of conduction block within the spinal cord. Yet it has been investigated primarily in the experimental setting, and mainly with regards to somatosensory evoked potentials or spino-spinal evoked potentials. There are no clinical studies on D wave KEEP.

Over the past few years, we have used intraoperative monitoring (IOM) techniques in 13 patients (11 males, two females) operated on within 72 hours after acute spinal cord injury. Posterior decompressive laminectomy and fixation were performed in 12 patients; an anterior decompression was done in one patient. The methodology was essentially the same as described earlier in this chapter, except for the additional recording of the D wave KEEP and the spinal SEPs KEEP. At the baseline, normal D wave and spinal SEP were recorded rostral and caudal to the injury site, respectively, using an epidural electrode placed after decompressive laminectomy. Once normal D wave cranial to the injury site and normal spinal SEPs caudal to the injury site were recorded, the electrode was moved stepwise either from rostral to caudal or vice versa at 1 cm steps, across the lesion site. This allowed us to identify the site were the potential was reversed, indicating the KEEP. Across the site of phase reversal, an isoelectric line was usually recorded. An example is given in Figure 9–10. All patients received methylprednisolone prior to surgery according to the National Acute Spinal Cord Injury Study protocol (Bracken et al. 1997).

Table 9–3 Correlation Between Intraoperative Neurophysiological Data and ASIA Scores

Pt.	Tc-MEP from limb muscles caudal to the level of injury	D wave caudal to the level of injury	Spinal SEPs rostral to the level of injury	D wave KEEP	Spinal SEPs KEEP	ASIA on admission	ASIA at discharge	ASIA at follow-up
GF	Absent	Questionable (absent)	Absent	Questionable (no)	Questionable (no)	A	B	D
TM	Unmonitorable (anesthesia)	Unmonitorable (anesthesia)	Unmonitorable (cortical SEPs only)	Unmonitorable (L1)	Unmonitorable (L1)	C	D	D
SS	Absent	Absent	Absent	Yes	Yes	A	A	A
TC	Absent	Present	Present	No	No	C	D	E
SG	Absent	Absent	Absent	No	No	D	D	D
PMK	Absent	Unmonitorable (anterior approach)	Unmonitorable (anterior approach)	Unmonitorable (anterior approach)	Unmonitorable (anterior approach)	A	A	A
CG	Absent	Absent	Absent	Yes	Yes	A	A	A
AM	Present	Unmonitorable (L1)	Present	Unmonitorable (L1)	Unmonitorable (L1)	D	D	D
DRG	Absent	Absent	Absent	Yes	Yes	A	A	A
SB	Absent	Present	Present	No	No	D	D	D
KA	Absent	Absent	Absent	Questionable (no)	Questionable (no)	A	A	B
TG	Present	Unmonitorable	Present	No	No	D	D	D
ZC	Absent	Absent	Absent	Yes	Yes	A	A	A

On admission, seven patients were ASIA-A, two patients were ASIA-C, and four patients were ASIA-D. Time between SCI and surgery was 7.5 hours (median); the range was 3.5 to 24 hours. After surgery, these patients were followed with a mean follow-up time of 11.3 months (range, 4–22). At surgery, caudal to the level of the lesion, mMEPs were absent in all but two ASIA-D patients, and unmonitorable in one because of myorelaxation. D wave caudal to the level of injury was absent in six patients (five ASIA-A, one ASIA-D), present in two (one ASIA-C, one ASIA-D), unmonitorable in four patients (three because of low spinal cord level, one because of anterior surgical approach), and questionable in one (ASIA-A). Spinal SEPs cranial to the level of the lesion were absent in seven, present in four (one ASIA-C, three ASIA-D) and unmonitorable in two patients. A D wave and spinal SEP KEEP was recorded in four patients: these four patients were ASIA-A on admission and remained ASIA-A at the follow-up (Figure 9–10).

In the other two patients with no D wave caudal to the lesion (one ASIA-A, one—with extradural hematoma—ASIA-D), neurological status were unchanged at

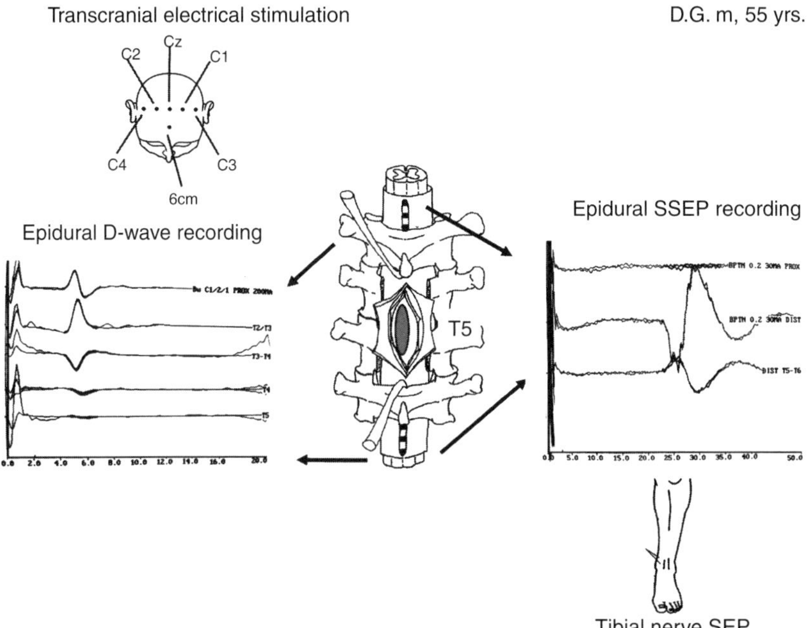

Figure 9–10 Intraoperative recordings of a 55-year-old male who arrived in surgery eight hours after a motor vehicle accident. He presented with a T5 vertebral fracture and spinal cord injury (SCI). On neurological examination he was ASIA-A on admission. *Left panel*: D wave recordings after transcranial electrical stimulation (TES). D wave is present cranial to the level of SCI (T3). A killed-end potential occurs at the T3–T4 spinal cord level, with an inverted polarity followed by a flat line. *Middle panel*: schematic illustration of an exposed spinal cord with D wave recording electrodes rostral and caudal to the lesion site. *Right panel*: Spinal somatosensory evoked potentials—recorded by the same epidural electrodes as those used to record the D wave after tibial nerve stimulation. An inversion polarity followed by a flat line is clearly visible when moving the recording electrodes upwards across the injury site.

discharge from hospital, but one recovered to ASIA-B at the follow-up. The patient with questionable D waves on admission (ASIA-A) recovered to ASIA-B at discharge and ASIA-D at the follow-up. In conclusion, this preliminary study provides evidence that the presence of a KEEP can be a clinical neurophysiological marker indicating irreversible and complete SCI.

5. CONCLUSIONS

This study demonstrates the feasibility, reliability, and safety of an intraoperative assessment of spinal cord function in spine and spinal cord trauma. As one would expect, the absence of both mMEPs and eMEPs caudal to the lesion site associated with the lack of cortical and epidural SEPs cranial to the lesion site strongly correlates with a poor outcome in complete SCI. Conversely, the presence of a D wave caudal to the lesion provides information on positive motor outcome, even if muscle MEPs are not present.

In neurologically uncompromised SCI patients or in incomplete patients, the continuous intraoperative monitoring of motor and sensory tract functional integrity can be beneficial and may help the surgeon detect and reduce an adjunctive intraoperative injury to the spinal cord that can be devastating for patients and influence their quality of life. The intraoperative electrophysiological testing allows the definition of an individual "neurophysiological profile," which is of utmost importance in order to provide prognosis and, therefore, to objectively test the efficacy of therapeutic measures.

References

Arunkumar, M. J., Srinivasa Babu, K., Chandy, M. J. "Motor and somatosensory evoked potentials in a primate model of experimental spinal cord injury." *Neurology India* 49 (2001): 219–224.

Baskin, D. S., Simpson, R. K., Jr. "Corticomotor and somatosensory evoked potential evaluation of acute spinal cord injury in the rat." *Neurosurgery* 20 (1987): 871–877.

Blight, A. R. "Cellular morphology of chronic spinal cord injury in the cat: Analysis of myelinated axons by line sampling." *Neuroscience* 10 (1983): 521–543.

Bondurant, C. P., Haghighi, S. S. "Experience with transcranial magnetic stimulation in evaluation of spinal cord injury." *Neurological Research* 19 (1997): 497–500.

Boyd, S. G., Rothwell, J. C., Cowan, J. M., et al. "A method of monitoring function in corticospinal pathways during scoliosis surgery with a note on motor conduction velocities." *Journal of Neurology, Neurosurgery, and Psychiatry* 49 (1986): 251–257.

Bracken, M. B., Shepard, M. J., Holford, T. R., et al. "Administration of methylprednisolone for 24 or 48 hours or tirilazad mesylate for 48 hours in the treatment of acute spinal cord injury. Results of the Third National Acute Spinal Cord Injury Randomized Controlled Trial. National Acute Spinal Cord Injury Study." *Journal of the American Medical Association* 277 (1997): 1597–1604.

Bridwell, K. H., Anderson, P. A., Boden, S. D., Vaccaro, A. R., Zigler, J. E. "What's new in spine surgery." *The Journal of Bone & Joint Surgery* 86 (2004): 1587–1596.

Burke, D., Hicks, R., Stephen, J., Woodforth, I., Crawford, M. "Assessment of corticospinal and somatosensory conduction simultaneously during scoliosis surgery." *Electroencephalography & Clinical Neurophysiology* 85 (1992): 388–396.

Burns, A. S., Ditunno, J. F. "Establishing prognosis and maximizing functional outcomes after spinal cord injury: A review of current and future directions in rehabilitation management." *Spine* 26 (2001): S137–S145.

Cioni, B., Meglio, M., Rossi, G. F. "Intraoperative motor evoked potentials monitoring in spinal neurosurgery." *Archives Italiennes de Biologie* 137 (1999): 115–126.

Clarke, C. E., Modarres-Sadeghi, H., Twomey, J. A., Burt, A. A. "Prognostic value of cortical magnetic stimulation in spinal cord injury." *Paraplegia* 32, 8 (1994): 554–560.

Costa, P., Bruno, A., Bonzanino, M., et al. "Somatosensory- and motor evoked potential monitoring during spine and spinal cord surgery." *Spinal Cord* 45 (2007): 86–91.

Curt, A., Dietz, V. "Traumatic cervical spinal cord injury: Relation between somatosensory evoked potentials, neurological deficit, and hand function." *Archives of Physical Medicine and Rehabilitation* 77 (1996): 48–53.

Curt, A., Dietz, V. "Ambulatory capacity in spinal cord injury: Significance of somatosensory evoked potentials and ASIA protocol in predicting outcome." *Archives of Physical Medicine & Rehabilitation* 78 (1997): 39–43.

Curt, A., Keck, M. E., Dietz, V. "Functional outcome following spinal cord injury: significance of motor evoked potentials and ASIA scores." *Archives of Physical Medicine & Rehabilitation* 79 (1998): 81–86.

Deecke, L., Tator, C. H. "Neurophysiological assessment of afferent and efferent conduction in the injured spinal cord of monkeys." *Journal of Neurosurgery* 39, 1 (1973): 65–74.

Deletis, V., Kothbauer, K. "Intraoperative neurophysiology of the corticospinal tract." In *Spinal Cord Monitoring*, edited by E. Stalberg, H. S. Sharma, Y. Olsson, 421–444. Vienna, Austria: Springer, 1998.

Deletis, V., Isgum, V., Amassian, V. E. "Neurophysiological mechanisms underlying motor evoked potentials in anesthetized humans: Part 1. Recovery time of corticospinal tract direct waves elicited by pairs of transcranial electrical stimuli." *Clinical Neurophysiology* 112 (2001a): 438–444.

Deletis, V., Rodi, Z., Amassian, V. E. "Neurophysiological mechanisms underlying motor evoked potentials in anesthetized humans: Part 2. Relationship between epidurally and muscle recorded MEPs in man." *Clinical Neurophysiology* 112 (2001b): 445–452.

Deletis, V. "Intraoperative neurophysiology and methodologies used to monitor the functional integrity of the motor system." In *Neurophysiology in Neurosurgery*, edited by V. Deletis, J. L. Shils, 25–51. New York: Academic Press, 2002.

Deletis, V., Sala, F. "Corticospinal tract monitoring with D- and I-waves from the spinal cord and muscle MEPs from limb muscles." In *Handbook of Clinical Neurophysiology*. Vol. 8: *Intraoperative Monitoring of NeuralFunction e* functiondited by M. R. Nuwer, 235–251. Amsterdam, Netherlands: Elsevier, 2008.

DiCindio, S., Theroux, M., Shah, S., et al. "Multimodality monitoring of transcranial electric motor and somatosensory evoked potentials during surgical correction of spinal deformity in patients with cerebral palsy and other neuromuscular disorders." *Spine* 28 (2003): 1851–1856.

Dimitrijevic, M. R., Prevec, T. S., Sherwood, A. M. "Somatosensory perception and cortical evoked potentials in established paraplegia." *Journal of Neurological Sciences* 60 (1983): 253–265.

Ditunno, J. F., Little, J. W., Tessler, A., Burns, A. S. "Spinal shock revisited: a four-phase model." *Spinal Cord* 42 (2004): 383–395.

Dorfman, L. J., Perkash, I., Bosley, T. M., Cummins, K. L. "Use of cerebral evoked potentials to evaluate spinal somatosensory function in patients with traumatic and surgical myelopathies." *Journal of Neurosurgery* 52 (1980): 654–660.

Fehlings, M. G., Tator, C. H., Linden, R. D., Piper, I. R. "Motor evoked potentials recorded from normal and spinal cord-injured rats." *Neurosurgery* 20 (1987): 125–130.

Forbes, H. J., Allen, P. W., Waller, C. S., et al. "Spinal cord monitoring in scoliosis surgery. Experience with 1,168 cases." *Journal of Bone & Joint Surgery* 73 (1991): 487–491.

Fukaya, C., Katayama, Y., Kasai, M., Kurihara, J., Maejima, S., Yamamoto, T. "Evaluation of time-dependent spread of tissue damage in experimental spinal cord injury by killed-end evoked potential: effect of high-dose methylprednisolone." *Journal of Neurosurgery* 98 Suppl 1 (2003): 56–62.

Gruninger, W., Ricker, K. "Somatosensory cerebral evoked potentials in spinal cord diseases." *Paraplegia* 9 (1991): 206–215.

Halter, J. A., Haftek, I., Sarzynska, M., Dimitrijevic, M. R. "Spinal cord evoked injury potentials in patients with acute spinal cord injury." *Journal of Neurotrauma* 6 (1989): 231–245.

Hawryluk, G. W. J., Rowland, J., Kwon, B. K., Fehlings, M. G. "Protection and repair of the injured spinal cord: a review of completed, ongoing, and planned clinical trials for acute spinal cord injury. A review." *Neurosurgical Focus* 25 (2008): E14.

Hicks, R. G., Burke, D. J., Stephen, J. P. "Monitoring spinal cord function during scoliosis surgery with Cotrel-Dubousset instrumentation." *Medical Journal of Australia* 154 (1991): 82–86.

Hilibrand, A. S., Schwartz, D. M., Sethuraman, V., Vaccaro, A. R., Albert, T. J. "Comparison of transcranial electric motor and somatosensory evoked potential monitoring during cervical spine surgery." *Journal of Bone & Joint Surgery* 228 (2003): 1851–1856.

Jones, S. J., Carter, L., Edgar, M. A., et al. "Experience of epidural spinal cord monitoring in 410 cases." In *Spinal Cord Monitoring,* edited by J. Schramm, S. J. Jones, 215–220. Berlin: Springer-Verlag, 1985.

Jones, S. J., Harrison, R., Koh, K. F., Mendoza, N., Crockard, H. A. "Motor evoked potential monitoring during spinal surgery: responses of distal limb muscles to transcranial cortical stimulation with pulse trains." *Electroencephalography & Clinical Neurophysiology* 100 (1996): 375–383.

Jou, I. M. "Effects of core body temperature on changes in spinal somatosensory evoked potential in acute spinal cord compression injury. An experimental study in the rat." *Spine* 25 (2000): 1878–1885.

Kirshblum, S. C., O'Connor, K. C. "Predicting neurological recovery in traumatic cervical spinal cord injury." *Archives of Physical Medicine & Rehabilitation* 79 (1998): 1456–1466.

Katayama, Y., Tsubokawa, T., Yamamoto, T., Hirayama, T., Maejima, S. "Preoperative determination of the level of spinal cord lesions from the killed end potential." *Surgical Neurology* 29 (1998): 91–94.

Katayama, Y., Tsubokawa, T., Sugitani, S. et al. "Assessment of spinal cord injury with multimodality evoked spinal cord potentials: Part I. Localization of lesions in experimental spinal cord injury." *Neuro-Orthopedics* 1 (1986): 130–141.

Komatu, S., Kikuchi, S., Sasaki, T., et al. "Detection of spinal cord ischemia in surgery of the thoracoabdominal aorta using spinal cord potentials." *Surgical Treatment* 153 (1985): 214–215.

Kothbauer, K., Deletis, V., Epstein, F. J. "Intraoperative spinal cord monitoring for intramedullary surgery: an essential adjunct." *Paediatric Neurosurgery* 26 (1997): 247–254.

Kothbauer, K., Deletis, V., Epstein, F. J. "Motor evoked potential monitoring for intramedullary spinal cord tumor surgery: correlation of clinical and neurophysiological data in a series of 100 consecutive procedures." *Neurosurgical Focus* 4 (1998): Article 1 available at http://www.aans.org/journals/online_j/may98/4.

Kraus, J. F., Silberman, T. A., McArthur, D. L. "Epidemiology of spinal cord injury." In *Principles of Spine Surgery*, edited by E. C. Benzel, D. W. Cahill, P. McCormack, 41–58. New York: McGraw-Hill, 1996.

Levy, W. J. "Spinal evoked potentials from the motor tracts." *Journal of Neurosurgery* 58 (1983): 38–44.

Levy, W. J., McCaffrey, M., York, D. H., Tanzer, F. "Motor evoked potentials from transcranial stimulation of the motor cortex in cats." *Neurosurgery* 15 (1984): 214–227.

Levy, W. J., McCaffrey, M., Hagichi, S. "Motor evoked potential as a predictor of recovery in chronic spinal cord injury." *Neurosurgery* 20 (1987): 138–142.

MacDonald, D. B., Al Zayed, Z., Khoudeir, I., Stigsby, B. "Monitoring scoliosis surgery with combined multiple pulse transcranial electric motor and cortical somatosensory evoked potentials from the lower and upper extremities." *Spine* 28 (2003): 194–203.

MacDonald, D. B. "Safety of intraoperative transcranial electrical stimulation motor evoked potential monitoring." *Journal of Clinical Neurophysiology* 19 (2002): 416–429.

MacDonell, R. A. L., Donnan, G. A. "Magnetic cortical stimulation in acute spinal cord injury." *Neurology* 45 (1995): 303–306.

McKay, W. B., Stokic, D. S., Dimitrijevic, M. R. "Assessment of corticospinal function in spinal cord injury. Using transcranial motor cortex stimulation: a review." *Journal of Neurotrauma* 14 (1997): 539–348.

Morioka, T., Fujii, K., Mitani, M., Fukui, M. "Intraoperative localization of a cervicomedullary glioma from the killed end potential: illustrative case." *Neurosurgery* 26 (1990): 1038–1041.

Morota, N., Deletis, V., Constantini, S., Kofler, M., Cohrn, H., Epstein, F. J. "The role of motor evoked potentials during surgery for intramedullary spinal cord tumors." *Neurosurgery* 41 (1997): 1327–1336.

National Cord Injury Database in the United States: Available at www.spinalcord.uab.edu.

Noordeen, M. H. H., Lee, J., Gibbons, C. E. R., et al. "Spinal cord monitoring in operations for neuromuscular scoliosis." *The Journal of Bone & Joint Surgery* 79 (1997): 53–57.

Nuwer, M. R., Dawson, E. G., Carlson, L. G., Kanim, L. E., Sherman, J. E. "Somatosensory evoked potential spinal cord monitoring reduces neurological deficits after scoliosis surgery: results of a large multicenter survey." *Electroencephalography & Clinical Neurophysiology* 96 (1995): 6–11.

Patton, H. D., Amassian, V. E. "Single and multiple unit analysis of cortical stage of pyramidal tract activation." *Journal of Neurophysiology* 17 (1954): 345–363.

Pechstein, U., Cedzich, C., Nadstawek, J., Schramm, J. "Transcranial high-frequency repetitive electrical stimulation of recording myogenic motor evoked potential with the patient under general anesthesia." *Neurosurgery* 39 (1996): 335–344.

Pelosi, L., Lamb, J., Grevitt, M., Mehdian, S. M. H., Webb, J. K., Blumhardt, L. D. "Combined monitoring of motor and somatosensory evoked potentials in orthopedic spinal surgery." *Clinical Neurophysiology* 113 (2002): 1082–1091.

Perot, P. L., Vera, C. L. "Scalp-recorded somatosensory evoked potentials to stimulation of nerves in the lower extremities and evaluation of patients with spinal cord trauma." *Annals of the New York Academy of Sciences* 388 (1982): 359–368.

Quiñones-Hinojosa, A., Lyon, R., Zada, G., et al. "Changes in transcranial motor evoked potentials during intramedullary spinal cord tumor resection correlate with postoperative motor function." *Neurosurgery* 56 (2005): 982–993.

Rodi, Z., Deletis, V., Morota, N., et al. "Motor evoked potentials during brain surgery." *Pflügers Archives* 431 Suppl 2 (1996): R291–R292.

Rowed, D. W., McLean, J. A. G., Tator, C. H. "Somatosensory evoked potentials in acute spinal cord injury: prognostic value." *Surgical Neurology* 9 (1978): 203–210.

Schramm, J., Krause, R., Shigeno, T., Brock, M. "Experimental investigation on the spinal cord evoked injury potential." *Journal of Neurosurgery* 59 (1983): 485–492.

Sekhon, L. H. S., Fehlings, M. G. "Epidemiology, Demographics, and pathophysiology of acute spinal cord injury." *Spine* 26 (2001): S2–S12.

Shiau, J. S., Zappulla, R. A., Nieves, J. "The effect of graded spinal cord injury on the extrapyramidal and pyramidal motor evoked potentials of the rat." *Neurosurgery* 30 (1992): 76–84.

Shimoji, K., Higashi, H., Kano, T. "Epidural recording of spinal electrogram." *Electroencephalography & Clinical Neurophysiology* 30 (1971): 236–239.

Spielholz, N. I., Benjamin, M. V., Engler, G., Ransohoff, J. "Somatosensory evoked potentials and clinical outcome in spinal cord injury." In *Neural Trauma*, edited by A. J. Popp, R. S. Bourke, L. R. Nelson, H. K. Kimelberg, 217–222. New York: Raven Press, 1979.

Stetkarova, I., Halter, J. A., Dimitrijevic, M. R. "Surface and epidural lumbosacral spinal cord evoked potentials in chronic spinal cord injury." *Journal of Neurotrauma* 10 (1993): 315–326.

Stripling, T. E. "The cost of economic consequences of traumatic spinal cord injury." *Paraplegia News* 8 (1990): 50–54.

Sudo, N. "Clinical application of the evoked spinal cord potentials. Part 1. Neurophysiological assessment of the evoked spinal cord potentials in experimental cord trauma—with reference to cord compression and ischemia." *Nippon Seikeigeka Gakkai Zasshi* 54 (1980a): 1631–1647.

Sudo, N. "Clinical application of the evoked spinal cord potentials. Part 2: Neurophysiological assessment of the evoked spinal cord potentials in cervical lesion." *Nippon Seikeigeka Gakkai Zasshi* 54 (1980b): 1649–1659.

Taniguchi, M., Cedzich, C., Schramm, J. "Modification of cortical stimulation under general anesthesia; technical description." *Neurosurgery* 32 (1993): 219–226.

Tsirikos, A. I., Aderinto, J., Tucker, S. K., Noordeen, H. H. "Spinal cord monitoring using intraoperative somatosensory evoked potentials for spinal trauma." *Journal of Spinal Disorders & Techniques* 17 (2004): 385–394.

Vandermeulen, E. P., van Aken, H., Vermylen, J. "Anticoagulants and spinal–epidural anesthesia." *Anesthesia & Analgesia* 79 (1994): 1165–1177.

Whittle, I. R. "Intraoperative recording of the killed-end potential." *Surgical Neurology* 30 (1988): 162.

York, D. H., Watts, C., Raffensberger, M., Spagnolia, T., Joyce, C. "Utilization of somatosensory evoked cortical potentials in spinal cord injury-prognostic limitations." *Spine* 8 (1983): 832–839.

Young, W. "Correlation of somatosensory evoked potentials and neurological findings in spinal cord injury." In *Early Management of Acute Spinal Cord Injury*, edited by C. H. Tator, 153–165. New York: Raven Press, 1982.

10

Transcutaneous Lumbar Posterior Root Stimulation for Motor Control Studies and Modification of Motor Activity after Spinal Cord Injury

KAREN MINASSIAN, URSULA HOFSTOETTER, AND FRANK RATTAY

CONTENTS

1. Introduction
2. Background
3. Methodology of Transcutaneous Spinal Cord Stimulation
4. Biophysics of Transcutaneous Spinal Cord Stimulation
5. Electromyographic Features of PRM Reflexes Elicited by Transcutaneous Stimulation of the Lumbosacral Spinal Cord
6. Electrophysiological Characteristics of PRM Reflexes
    6.1. Double Stimulation
    6.2. Tendon Vibration
7. Transcutaneous Stimulation Applied Over the Lumbosacral Spinal Cord and Cauda Equina
8. The PRM Reflex and the H Reflex
9. PRM Reflexes Applied to Extend H Reflex Studies to Multiple Muscles Simultaneously
10. Continuous Transcutaneous Spinal Cord Stimulation to Modify the Activity of Neural Circuits
    10.1. Control of Spasticity
    10.2. Augmentation of Neural Control of Locomotion
11. Conclusions
References

1. INTRODUCTION

Clinical assessment of the severity of spinal cord injury includes the evaluation of the patient's ability to perform voluntary movements. As part of this assessment, detecting reflex and automatic contributions of infra-injury spinal neural circuits to these movements is essential. Electrophysiological studies of human spinal cord reflex circuitry can be traced back for a century (Hoffmann, 1910; 1918; Magladery et al., 1951; Pierrot-Deseilligny & Burke, 2005a). Noninvasive methods for recording spinal reflexes were developed and helped assess the function of the spinal cord below a lesion (Magladery et al., 1952; Paillard, 1955). Experimental studies in spinalized animals on the capacity of the spinal cord to control movement advanced the understanding of the nature of spinal reflexes (Sherrington, 1910; Creed et al., 1932; Renshaw, 1940; Lloyd, 1943) and of higher level circuits in the organization of spinal locomotion, such as central pattern generators (Brown, 1911; Grillner & Zangger, 1979). Locomotor central pattern generators residing within the mammalian lumbar spinal cord can produce rhythmic, alternating activities of flexor and extensor motoneurons in the absence of input from higher centers and proprioceptive feedback (Grillner, 1985). The view that humans possess a spinal locomotor pattern generator similar to the circuits described in animal species after complete spinal lesions has been supported by several independent observations (Bussel et al., 1988; Calancie et al., 1994; Dimitrijevic et al., 1998; Calancie, 2006; Nadeau et al., 2010). Harnessing the potential of such neural circuits and augmenting their activity to supplement altered descending control are principal strategies for restoring motor function after spinal cord injury. In order to achieve this goal, the evaluation of the condition and operation of these functional circuits in spinal cord injured individuals is essential. We have recently developed a method for transcutaneous spinal cord stimulation that can be used for noninvasive investigations of lumbar neural circuits' function in human subjects. The same technique can be applied as a neuroaugmentative method for the control of spinal spasticity and the enhancement of neural control of locomotion after spinal cord injury. In this chapter we shall describe this novel method for the stimulation of the lumbosacral spinal cord in humans. By elaborating the underlying biophysical principles, we will identify sensory fibers within the posterior roots as the directly stimulated neural structures. The electrophysiology of muscle responses to the electrical stimuli, referred to as "posterior root-muscle reflexes", will be addressed, and their similarity to the soleus Hoffmann reflex (H reflex) will be discussed. The potential of transcutaneous spinal cord stimulation to modulate the central state of excitability of lumbar cord circuits, when the stimulation mode is changed from the application of single pulses to trains of stimuli, will be illustrated on the basis of two cases.

2. BACKGROUND

Epidural spinal cord stimulation used for modifications of impaired motor activity has provided a unique approach for electrophysiological studies of the spinal cord in humans. Epidural electrodes placed over the lumbar spinal cord in spinal cord injured individuals stimulate afferent fibers of multiple posterior roots. The stimulated afferents activate spinal neuronal circuitries and can thus provide access to the spinal cord physiology caudal to the site of a spinal cord lesion. Low-rate epidural stimulation (2 Hz) applied to the lumbar spinal cord of motor complete spinal cord injured subjects evokes brief contractions in several lower limb muscles bilaterally in response to each pulse. It was already recognized in earlier neurophysiological studies that these "muscle twitches" were due to reflexes initiated by large-diameter afferents within the posterior roots (Dimitrijevic, 1983; Dimitrijevic et al., 1983; Murg et al., 2000). The responses were evoked in muscles associated with the posterior roots close to the stimulating cathode. They were recorded electromyographically as compound muscle action potentials in the lower limb muscles, with short latencies and characteristic recovery cycles when tested by double stimuli (Minassian et al., 2004). The responses were identified as posterior root-muscle reflexes (PRM reflexes), named according to their initiation and recording sites (Jilge et al., 2004a; Minassian et al., 2004; 2007a) and following the nomenclature of "dorsal root-ventral root reflexes" in the classical electrophysiological studies in cats of Renshaw (1940) and Lloyd (1943). Evoked at low repetition rates, PRM reflexes have rather simple electrophysiological characteristics, with constant latencies, consistent waveforms of compound muscle action potentials, and rather invariant peak-to-peak amplitudes during constant stimulation conditions (Minassian et al., 2004; Hofstoetter, 2009). Under such conditions, PRM reflexes are monosynaptic responses (Murg et al., 2000; Minassian et al., 2004; 2007a) similar to the Hoffman reflex (H reflex) classically recorded from the soleus muscle in response to stimulation of the posterior tibial nerve (Hoffmann, 1910; 1918; Schieppati, 1987). Posterior root afferents are equally directly activated when epidural stimulation is applied at a frequency of 25 Hz–50 Hz. At such frequencies, however, the lumbar spinal cord, isolated from supraspinal structures by traumatic injury, was shown to generate rhythmic, locomotor-like flexion and extension activity in the paralyzed lower limbs (Rosenfeld et al., 1995; Dimitrijevic et al., 1998). The rhythmic activities consisted of a series of stimulus-triggered PRM reflexes (Minassian et al., 2004; 2007a). The rhythmicity consisted of alternation between two phases. A phase of successively elicited and modulated PRM reflexes was followed by a phase of PRM reflex suppression. The data suggested that the tonic drive to the lumbar spinal cord via afferents of multiple posterior roots was producing parallel effects. Along with the repetitive elicitation of PRM reflexes, the stimulated afferents transsynaptically activated lumbar locomotor circuits due to temporal summation processes (Minassian et al., 2004; Jilge et al., 2004b). The locomotor networks were in turn modifying and coordinating the PRM reflex activity at multiple segmental levels. It should be noted that, while the neural signals generated by the electrical stimulation were delivered via segmental afferent input pathways, their non-patterned repetitive nature is rather characteristic for tonic descending signals from supraspinal structures (Pearson & Gordon, 2000).

In this chapter, it will be reported how the capacity of spinal cord stimulation to activate spinal neuronal circuitries via segmental afferent projections can be utilized by a recently developed transcutaneous stimulation method (Dimitrijevic et al., 2004; Minassian et al., 2007b). Having all advantages of a noninvasive technique, transcutaneous spinal cord stimulation can be widely applied in motor control studies as well as for modification of movement after spinal cord injury or other neurological disorders. The technique uses rather large stimulating electrodes placed over the lower back and abdomen that consistently stimulate posterior roots of L2 to S2 spinal cord segments at moderate stimulus intensities. The specific, localized depolarizations of posterior root fibers in spite of the distant stimulation are made feasible by the tissue heterogeneity of the volume conductor in-between the electrodes and by the neuroanatomy of the terminal spinal cord (Ladenbauer et al., 2010). The vertebral bones have a low electrical conductivity (Geddes & Baker, 1967), but the vertebral column is not a continuous bony structure in its inferior to superior course. Its transversal electrical resistance is reduced by the ligaments between the spinous processes and laminae, and by the intervertebral discs between the vertebral bodies (Gu et al., 2002). Particularly at the lowest thoracic and lumbar vertebrae, containing the lumbosacral spinal cord and the cauda equina, the posterior aspect of the vertebral canal is only partially shielded by bony structures. Within the vertebral canal, the excitation threshold of the posterior root fibers is considerably reduced by their bends and the non-uniformities along the axons at their entries into the spinal cord. The influence of axon-bending on excitation thresholds, as well as of passing anatomical structures with different electrical conductivities, has been repetitively described in modeling studies of epidural spinal cord stimulation (Coburn, 1985; Struijk et al., 1993; Rattay et al., 2000; Minassian et al., 2007a). Computer simulations of transcutaneous spinal cord stimulation recently confirmed that these anatomical factors are also essentially contributing to the low thresholds for posterior root stimulation (Ladenbauer et al., 2010; Danner et al., 2011). The effect of fiber bending on excitation thresholds is in fact well known from transcranial stimulation. Sharp changes of the fiber direction of pyramidal cells in the motor cortex result in action potential initiation at these bends when electrical (Iles, 2005; Wongsarnpigoon & Grill, 2008) or magnetic stimulation is applied (Maccabee et al., 1993; Amassian & Maccabee, 2006).

Figure 10–1 compares the electromyographic activity of brief contractions (twitches) of lower limb muscles evoked by transcutaneous and epidural stimulation in an incomplete spinal cord injured person. The responses evoked by the transcutaneous technique have compound muscle action potential morphology similar to the PRM reflexes elicited by epidural stimulation, and the same onset latencies. Responses elicited by the transcutaneous stimulation applied over the terminal spinal cord are PRM reflexes (Minassian et al., 2007b) initiated at the same sites as by epidural stimulation (Ladenbauer et al., 2010). The similarities of PRM reflexes elicited by either technique imply that transcutaneous stimulation depolarizes at least a subset of the neural structures activated by implanted epidural leads.

3. METHODOLOGY OF TRANSCUTANEOUS SPINAL CORD STIMULATION

Different set-ups of surface electrodes can elicit PRM reflexes in lower limb muscles. Here, we will focus on a method with the skin electrodes placed over the lower back and abdomen that consistently activated quadriceps, hamstrings, tibialis anterior, and triceps surae bilaterally in people with an intact nervous system (Minassian et al., 2007b; Hofstoetter et al., 2008) and in individuals with motor complete or incomplete spinal cord injury (Minassian et al., 2010). The electrical phenomena produced by this configuration of skin electrodes were also studied in detail by computer modeling (Ladenbauer et al., 2010; Danner et al., 2011). Stimulation is performed using commercially available self-adhesive transcutaneous electrical

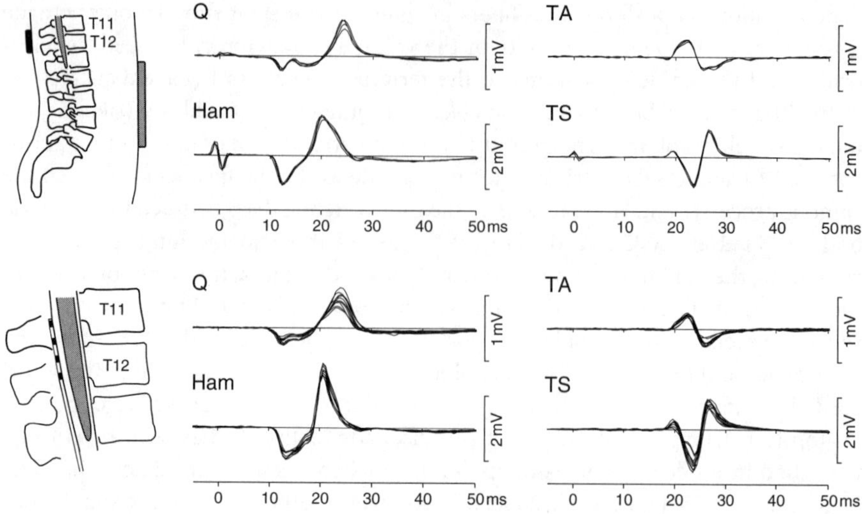

Figure 10–1 Posterior root-muscle reflexes of quadriceps (Q), hamstrings (Ham), tibialis anterior (TA), and triceps surae (TS) evoked by transcutaneous and epidural spinal cord stimulation. All recordings were derived during a single session from an incomplete spinal cord injured individual classified as AIS C. Epidural spinal cord stimulation-data were collected during the trial phase prior to full implantation, with the epidural lead being connected to an external stimulator (Model 3625 Test Stimulator, Medtronic, Inc., Minneapolis, MN). Epidural stimulation was applied at 5 Hz, the lowest frequency provided by the test stimulator. The frequency of transcutaneous stimulation was 0.2 Hz. Onset latencies of PRM reflexes evoked by epidural stimulation were Q: 10.30 ± 0.27 ms; Ham: 11.48 ± 0.20 ms; TA: 19.81 ± 0.29 ms; TS: 19.24 ± 0.48 ms; and for the transcutaneous stimulation technique, they amounted to Q: 10.05 ± 0.25 ms; Ham: 10.68 ± 0.22 ms; TA: 18.93 ± 0.94 ms; TS: 18.60 ± 0.20 ms. Time "0" of the *x*-axis corresponds to the onset of epidural stimulus application, and in case of transcutaneous stimulation, to the edge between first and second phase of a biphasic stimulus (see Section 3, Methodology, below). Peak-like biphasic deflections occurring at onset of transcutaneous stimulation are artifacts due to volume conduction of the generated electrical field.

neural stimulation (TENS) electrodes. Stimulation electrodes are a pair of round electrodes with diameters of 5 cm. They are placed over the paravertebral skin on each side of the spine (Figure 10–2). This paravertebral electrode pair is positioned between the T11 and T12 spinous processes to stimulate the lumbosacral spinal cord (Lang, 1984) or more caudally for cauda equina stimulation (Cohen et al., 1991). Reference electrodes are a pair of large rectangular electrodes covering the lower abdomen. The two electrodes of each pair are connected to function as a single electrode. In fact, the exact dimensions and shapes of the electrodes are not essential. Yet, the large reference electrodes ensure low current density and correspondingly less voltage drop near the abdomen. Hence a larger portion of the total stimulation voltage is available under the paravertebral electrodes, with a stronger stimulating effect near the spine.

Symmetrical, biphasic rectangular pulses (1 ms + 1 ms width) delivered by a constant-voltage stimulator were empirically found to require rather low stimulus intensities to elicit PRM reflexes in the lower limbs (28.6 V–34.3 V, impedance

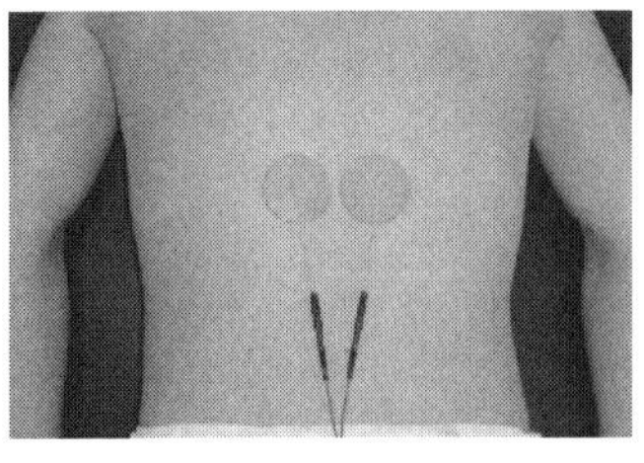

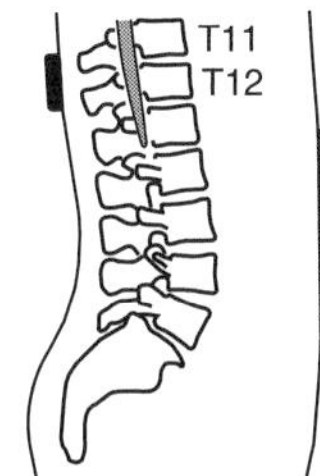

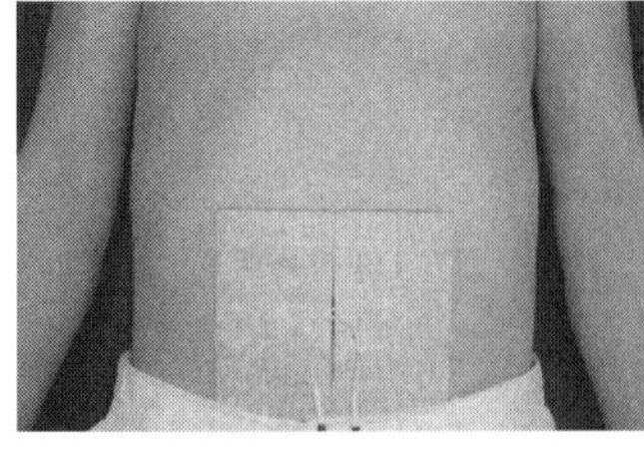

Figure 10–2 Electrode placement for transcutaneous elicitation of posterior root-muscle reflexes in the lower limbs.

700 Ω–900 Ω; Minassian et al., 2007b; Hofstoetter et al., 2008; Ladenbauer et al., 2010). The electrodes were connected to the stimulator such that the paravertebral electrodes were the cathode and the abdominal electrodes the anode when the polarity of stimulation was changed at the edge between the first and second phases of the biphasic stimulus. With such stimulation, neural elements are stimulated, that is, action potentials are elicited, at this abrupt change of polarity.

4. BIOPHYSICS OF TRANSCUTANEOUS SPINAL CORD STIMULATION

The immediate effects of electrical stimulation upon neural structures can be described by the theory of electricity and volume conduction. Therefore, computer modeling is an appropriate approach for obtaining theoretical knowledge on generated current flow and neural activation. The analysis of different substructures of a neuron has shown that the part most excitable by externally applied electrical stimulation is the myelinated axon. As a consequence of the high value of the membrane capacitance of the soma compared to that of the area of a node of Ranvier, the probability of exciting a nerve at the soma region is low (Porter, 1963; Nowak & Bullier, 1998; Rattay, 1998; 1999). Myelinated fibers are more excitable than unmyelinated ones, and large-diameter fibers have lower thresholds than thinner ones (Ranck, 1975; Rattay, 1987; 1990; Roth, 1994). The relationship between the excitation threshold and the fiber diameter is not linear, and thresholds for small-diameter fibers dramatically increase (Veltink et al., 1988; Struijk et al., 1993).

Low excitation thresholds of an axon require sudden changes of the external potential generated during a stimulus pulse and acting along the fibers. This follows from the activating-function concept, which predicts low threshold sites for external stimulation at the maxima of the second derivative of the external potential along the fiber path (Rattay, 1998; 1999). Such sudden changes can result from a focal electrical stimulation applied close to a long axon. The electrical field produced by transcutaneous spinal cord stimulation, however, is rather diffuse within the vertebral canal (Figure 10–3).

In the widespread electrical field, abrupt changes in the voltage profile along axons are caused by non-uniformities of the anatomy along the fiber path. Such anatomical influences cause localized, low threshold sites of posterior root fibers at their entries

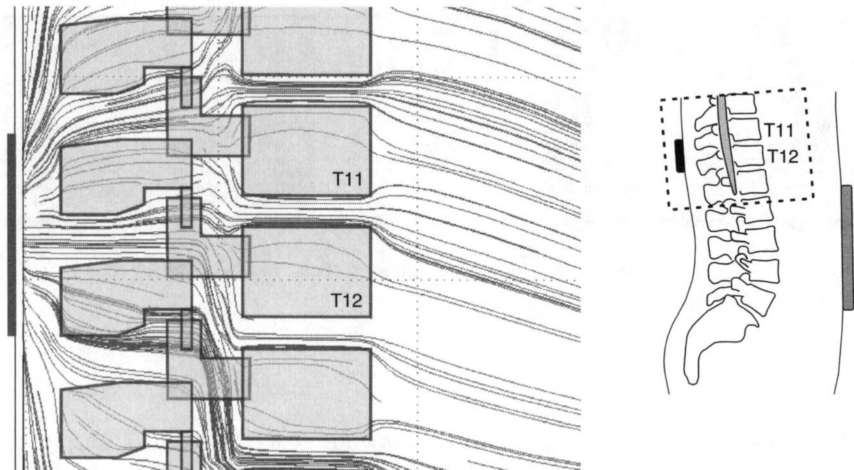

Figure 10–3 Computer-simulated current flow within a 2 mm layer at the mid-sagittal plane and at the rostrocaudal level of the stimulating electrode placed over the T11–T12 vertebrae. Of the various anatomical structures included in the volume conductor model, only the vertebral bones are shown. The density of the displayed lines of current flow is proportional to the current density. Current penetrates the vertebral canal predominantly through the better-conducting anatomical structures between the bony structures of the spine. For details of the computer model, see Ladenbauer et al. (2010).

into the spinal cord (Ladenbauer et al., 2010). The higher thresholds of anterior root fibers at the level of the terminal spinal cord are a consequence of their trajectories. When exiting the spinal cord, they have a different orientation with respect to the generated electrical field than the trajectories of the posterior roots, which is unfavorable for the external cathodic stimulation and increases their thresholds. Modeling studies suggest low thresholds of anterior root fibers at their exits from the spinal canal (Ladenbauer et al., 2010; Danner et al., 2011).

The electrical potential field generated by transcutaneous spinal cord stimulation and evaluated along straight longitudinal fibers within the posterior white matter lacks substantial changes (Danner et al., 2011). Consequently, thresholds of straight posterior column fibers are high. Even when considering axonal branches (Struijk et al., 1992), computer simulations suggest that the thresholds of posterior column fibers are three times higher than the thresholds of posterior root fibers (Danner et al., 2011). Yet, of all intraspinal neural structures, posterior column fibers superficially located within the white matter, with rather large diameters and multiple collaterals, can be assumed to have lowest thresholds (Holsheimer, 2002). Thus, the electrical activation of other tracts would require even higher stimulus intensities, and direct electrical stimulation of gray matter structures can be excluded with stimulus intensities applied in human neurophysiological studies. It should be noted that even intraspinal microelectrodes inserted into the spinal cord gray matter in animal studies excite nearby fibers in passage, like axonal branches of afferents, at lower intensities than other co-localized neuronal structures (Renshaw, 1940; Gaunt et al., 2006).

To summarize the biophysical background, transcutaneous spinal cord stimulation can produce localized depolarizations and controlled recruitment of specific neural structures in spite of the non-focused electrical field. There is a considerable discontinuity of the threshold spectrum of the various neuronal structures within the generated field, and large-diameter posterior root fibers have the lowest thresholds and can be selectively recruited. It can be further concluded that neural structures within the spinal cord are not directly electrically stimulated but transsynaptically activated by posterior root stimulation.

5. ELECTROMYOGRAPHIC FEATURES OF PRM REFLEXES ELICITED BY TRANSCUTANEOUS STIMULATION OF THE LUMBOSACRAL SPINAL CORD

A single pulse applied through surface electrodes placed over the T11–T12 spinous processes evokes PRM reflexes bilaterally in the L2–S2 innervated lower limb muscles. Figure 10–4 displays electromyographic recordings of PRM reflexes produced in a

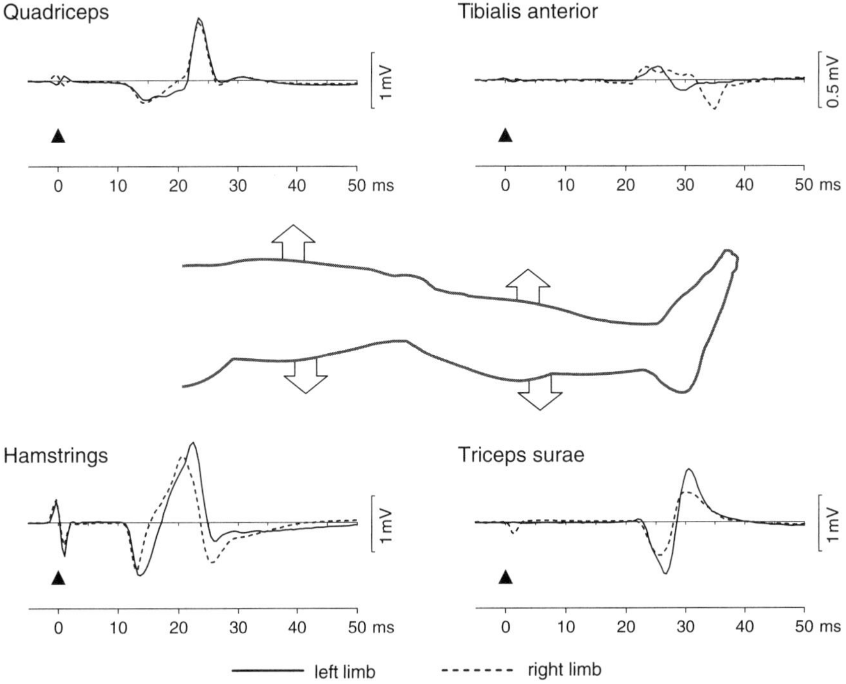

Figure 10–4 Electromyographic characteristics of posterior root-muscle reflexes evoked by a single pulse applied over the T11–T12 interspinous space and recorded from the surface of left and right lower limb muscles. Stimulus intensity was 28 V, and the common threshold for recruiting all studied muscles was 25 V. Time "0" of the *x*-axis corresponds to the onset of the second, effectively activating, phase of the biphasic stimulus pulse of 1 ms + 1 ms duration. Black arrowheads mark the time of action potential initiation within the posterior root afferents. Open arrows indicate the standardized recording sites. Data derived from a subject with intact nervous system in supine position.

Table 10–1 Electrophysiological Parameters of Posterior Root-muscle Reflexes Evoked in Lower Limbs.

Muscle	Onset latency [ms]	Peak-to-peak amplitude [μV]
Quadriceps	10.3 ± 1.1	848.0 ± 735.9
Hamstrings	11.2 ± 0.4	1683.4 ± 986.7
Tibialis anterior	19.1 ± 0.9	449.4 ± 356.9
Triceps surae	19.7 ± 1.1	2686.0 ± 2060.2

Transcutaneous spinal cord stimulation with paravertebral electrodes over the T11–T12 spinous processes was applied at the lowest intensity (common threshold) that elicited responses in all muscles bilaterally (28.6 ± 6.3 V group average, 1 ms + 1 ms-biphasic pulses). Values are given as mean ± standard deviation and were derived from eight subjects with intact nervous system and mean height of 181 cm (Minassian et al., 2007b). Recording sites as indicated in Figure 10–4.

subject with intact nervous system at 1.1 times the common threshold value; that is, the lowest stimulus intensity evoking PRM reflexes in all studied muscles. The example illustrates characteristic electromyographic features of PRM reflexes recorded from the different muscles.

The electromyographic signal evoked by a PRM reflex can be distinguished from other signals detected, and the muscle, from which the PRM reflex is recorded, can be identified by inspecting the compound muscle action potential shape and its time parameters. The PRM reflex of quadriceps has the most invariant compound muscle action potential waveform, with a triphasic configuration observed in humans with spinal cord injury as well as with intact nervous system in response to spinal cord stimulation. Hamstrings show the most inter-individual variability of compound muscle action potential waveforms, with three to five phases and an initial positive (i.e., downward) deflection. PRM reflexes of tibialis anterior and triceps surae have bi- or triphasic compound muscle action potentials . Table 10–1 gives average values of onset latencies and peak-to-peak amplitudes of PRM reflexes. Onset latencies of PRM reflexes are longer in the distal muscles due to the longer efferent limb of the respective reflex arcs. In people with an intact nervous system, PRM reflex amplitudes are generally larger in hamstrings than in quadriceps, and they are larger in triceps surae than in tibialis anterior.

The recordings displayed in Figure 10–4 show some asymmetries between PRM reflexes evoked in the muscles of the left and right lower limbs. Asymmetries of response amplitudes at the common threshold intensity generally amount to 20% of the mean amplitudes of both sides (Minassian et al., 2007b). Such asymmetries cannot be completely compensated for in all muscles by adjusting the positions of the paravertebral stimulating electrodes. The asymmetries are most probably due to the electrical field generated and anatomical asymmetries like of the mediolateral spinal cord position in the thecal sac (Holsheimer et al., 1995), as well as physiological left-right differences.

6. ELECTROPHYSIOLOGICAL CHARACTERISTICS OF PRM REFLEXES

6.1. Double Stimulation

There is a prolonged period of excitability changes of PRM reflexes of up to 10 seconds following a prior stimulus applied to the lumbosacral spinal cord (Minassian et al., 2009). The posterior root volley generated by the first pulse of a double stimulation alters the excitability of the spinal neuronal circuitries. The altered excitability in turn affects the response to the afferent volley produced by the second pulse when applied in close succession. Potential mechanisms involved in these modifications are presynaptic inhibition of Ia terminals, recurrent inhibition of motoneurons, and secondary contributions like from Golgi tendon organs activated by the first muscle twitch (Pierrot-Deseilligny & Burke, 2005a; 2005b). Taking into account that transcutaneous spinal cord stimulation recruits afferents of multiple posterior roots, facilitation from close synergists or disynaptic inhibition from antagonists might also influence successively elicited PRM reflexes (Delwaide et al., 1976).

Figure 10–5 depicts PRM reflexes induced by pairs of stimuli delivered at different inter-stimulus intervals. A stimulus applied 40 ms after a conditioning one did not evoke PRM reflexes in any of the studied muscles. PRM reflexes of the thigh muscles could be elicited 60 ms after the preceding stimulus and attained large amplitudes when evoked after an interval of 120 ms. Recovery of PRM reflexes in the lower leg muscles required longer periods. Low-amplitude responses were elicited by the second pulse of a pair at intervals of 120 ms, and PRM reflexes were still of low amplitudes at an interval of 300 ms in tibialis anterior and triceps surae. In general, the excitability curve investigating the time course of amplitude changes of a test PRM reflex elicited at progressively increasing intervals after a conditioning PRM reflex is different in the thigh than in the leg muscles. PRM reflexes in the thigh muscles demonstrate an early recovery, attaining an initial peak at inter-stimulus intervals of 120 ms–200 ms, followed by a phase of reduced excitability and a later,

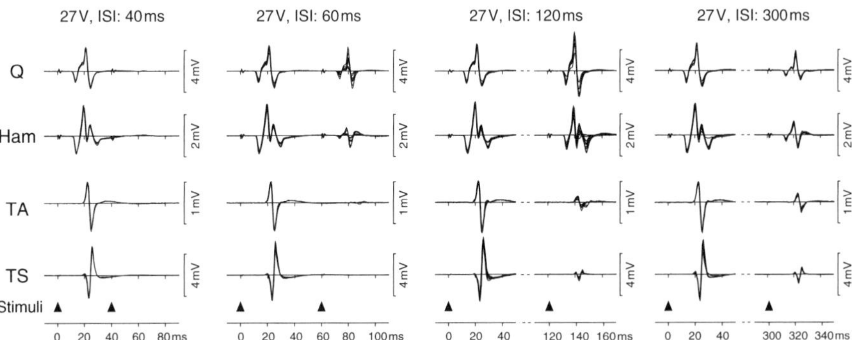

Figure 10–5 Posterior root-muscle reflexes of quadriceps (Q), hamstrings (Ham), tibialis anterior (TA), and triceps surae (TS) elicited by paired stimuli of same intensity delivered at different inter-stimulus intervals (ISI). Five stimulus-triggered traces are shown superimposed for each muscle and condition. Recordings derived from a subject with intact nervous system while supine.

gradual recovery. The initial recovery of PRM reflexes in the lower leg muscles peaks at 250 ms–300 ms, but the peak is less expressed. When evoked five seconds later than the first stimulus, PRM reflexes recovered to within 91% to 96% of their control amplitudes. Applying pairs of stimuli is a simple and time-effective method to distinguish PRM reflexes from M waves that would be elicited in response to direct anterior root stimulation (Courtine et al., 2007; Minassian et al., 2007b; Hofstoetter et al., 2008; Dy et al., 2010). Inter-stimulus intervals of 50 ms or less should be used for that purpose, while keeping in mind that the amount of recovery varies with the size of the conditioning and test reflexes (Minassian et al., 2004).

6.2. Tendon Vibration

Another characteristic of the PRM reflex is its attenuation when vibration is applied to the patellar tendon, the tendons of the hamstrings at the back of the knee, or the Achilles tendon. Figure 10–6 shows PRM reflexes evoked once every five seconds prior, during, and after vibration is applied to the Achilles tendon. The afferent input to the spinal cord produced by the unilateral Achilles tendon vibration considerably suppressed the PRM reflexes in all of the studied muscles ipsilateral to vibration. The widespread effect of vibration, while less expressed, could be also detected in the contralateral side (Minassian et al., 2007b). Note that the effect of vibration upon PRM reflexes is also depending on the initial response magnitudes; large-amplitude PRM reflexes are reduced in size, and small-amplitude PRM reflexes can be completely suppressed. The vibration-induced suppression is due to various mechanisms, probably including presynaptic inhibition and a partial occlusion of input to the spinal cord carried via large afferents, and is a further indication of the reflex origin of the responses evoked by transcutaneous spinal cord stimulation (Mao et al., 1984). As an alternative to the double-stimulus paradigm, vibration can be applied to identify PRM reflexes.

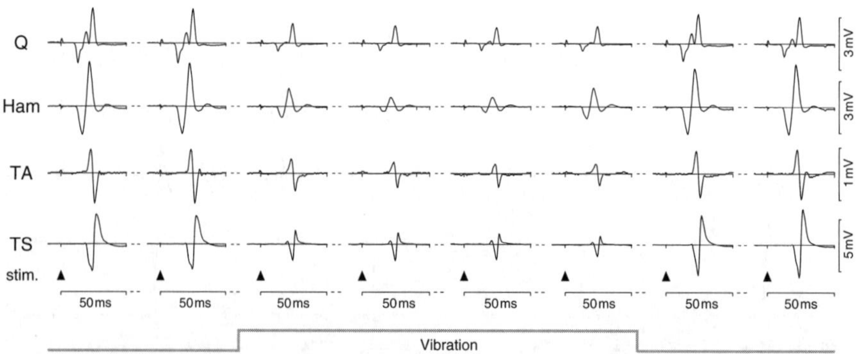

Figure 10–6 Effect of Achilles tendon vibration on posterior root-muscle reflexes of ipsilateral quadriceps (Q), hamstrings (Ham), tibialis anterior (TA), and triceps surae (TS). Transcutaneous stimulation was applied over the T11–T12 interspinous space at a rate of 0.2 Hz and with constant stimulus intensity of 20 V. Recordings derived from a subject with intact nervous system in supine position. The examined lower limb was positioned with the Achilles tendon resting on the vibrator.

7. TRANSCUTANEOUS STIMULATION APPLIED OVER THE LUMBOSACRAL SPINAL CORD AND CAUDA EQUINA

PRM reflexes can be evoked in lower limb muscles by stimulation applied over the lowest thoracic vertebrae, corresponding to the level of the lumbar spinal cord, as well as over the whole extent of lumbar vertebrae that contains the cauda equina. The arrangement of the spinal roots characteristically changes from the lumbosacral spinal cord in inferior direction (Wall et al., 1990; Cohen et al., 1991). At the terminal spinal cord, the posterior root fibers are separated from the anteriorly located motor fibers. At the cauda equina, the posterior and anterior roots progressively approach each other and reach anterolateral sites at their respective intervertebral exits. At these exits, posterior and anterior roots of the same segment are located close to each other and assume similar trajectories. These facts result in a spatial pattern of spinal roots anatomy (as illustrated in Figure 10–7), and the evoked muscle responses reflect that anatomy (Minassian et al., 2007b).

PRM reflexes to graded transcutaneous lumbosacral spinal cord stimulation are characterized by increasing amplitudes without changes in the onset latency or compound muscle action potential shape (Figure 10–8A). Small-amplitude M waves or

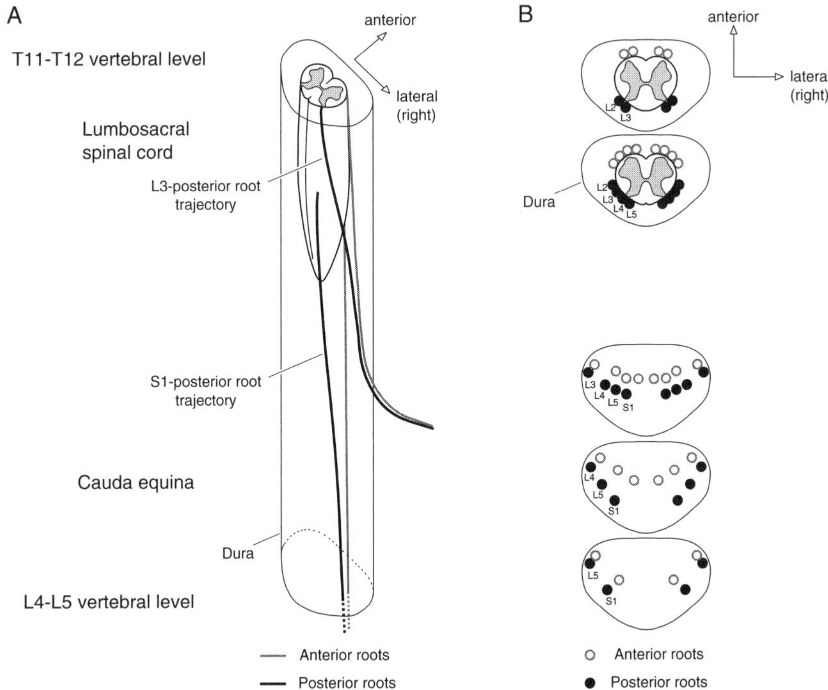

Figure 10–7 Spinal root anatomy at the terminal spinal cord and cauda equina. *A.* Drawing of trajectories of L3- and S1-posterior and anterior root fibers. *B.* Schematic diagrams of the positions of intrathecal posterior and anterior roots at different cross sections (Wall et al., 1990; Cohen et al., 1991); superior to inferior positions of cross sections are in accordance to A. Note that the motor and (multifascicular) sensory bundles are larger than indicated by the circles, and the intrathecal anatomy is more crowded by the roots than shown in the simplified sketches.

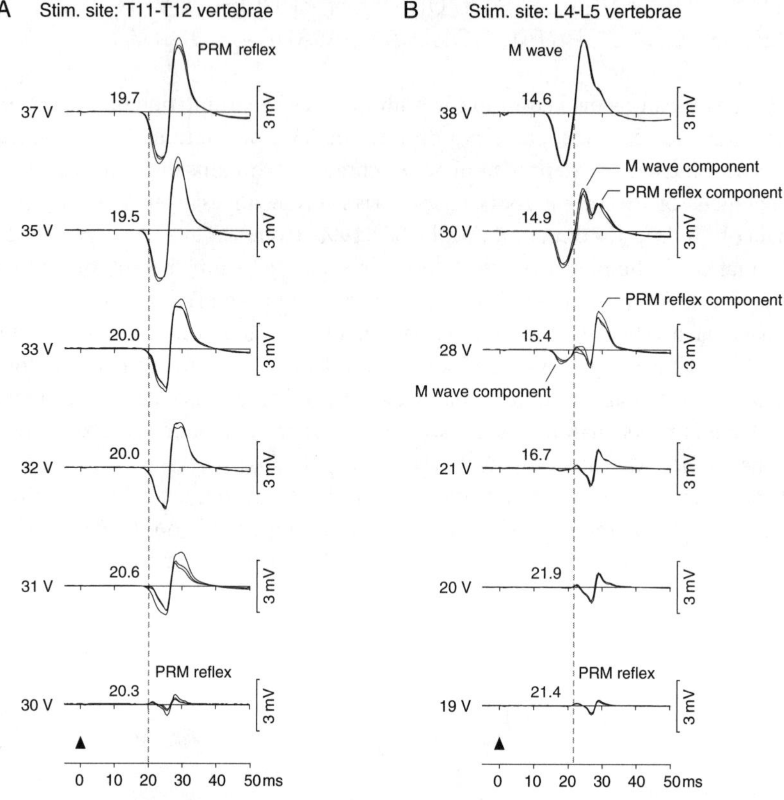

Figure 10–8 Triceps surae responses evoked by graded stimulation applied transcutaneously over the lumbosacral spinal cord (*A*) and cauda equina (*B*). Onset latencies [ms] of responses are given by inserted values. Vertical dashed lines are indicating latencies of the threshold responses, marking the characteristic onset of a monosynaptic response elicited at the respective stimulation site. Three stimulus-triggered responses are shown superimposed for every muscle and given stimulus intensity. All recordings were collected during the same session in a subject with intact nervous system while supine.

M wave contamination of the PRM reflex can occur in quadriceps, yet the elicitation of M waves is an uncommon finding (Minassian et al., 2007b). Stimulation of the cauda equina at incremental intensities, on the other hand, results in a characteristic sequence of PRM reflex and direct M wave elicitation. The example presented in Figure 10–8B shows that the recruitment of afferents and efferents at the cauda equina is similar to mixed peripheral nerve stimulation. As expected, PRM reflexes are evoked at threshold intensity, and they have the same waveform as PRM reflexes evoked in the same muscle from the more superior stimulation site, but with slightly longer latency. When increasing the stimulus intensity above threshold, there is initially a progressive increase in the response amplitudes, without changes of latencies or compound muscle action potential shapes. Stronger stimulation produces additional, earlier electromyographic components and an abrupt shortening of the response latencies. The short-latency components increase in size with yet stronger stimulation along with a progressive decrease of the PRM reflex components. These early potentials are in fact M wave components. The detected electromyographic signals are composite compound muscle action potentials with the M wave superimposed onto the PRM reflex activity due to the short difference between the reflex and direct pathway lengths.

Characteristic responses evoked by cauda equina stimulation via L4–L5 placed paravertebral electrodes are shown in Figure 10–9. At low intensity, PRM reflexes are evoked in hamstrings, tibialis anterior, and triceps surae, with average latencies of 13.3 ± 1.0 ms, 21.1 ± 1.0 ms, and 21.3 ± 1.1 ms (Minassian et al., 2007b). These latencies are longer by 2.1 ms, 2.0 ms, and 1.6 ms, respectively, than the latencies of PRM reflexes produced by stimulation over the T11–T12 vertebrae, due to the more distant sites of posterior root afferent depolarization. With increased intensity, M waves are produced in the lower leg muscles that are fused with the PRM reflex, as well as small-amplitude M wave components in the hamstrings. Concomitantly, a short-latency response is evoked in quadriceps that is a pure M wave. The elicitation of only M waves in quadriceps is a characteristic finding when stimulation is applied to the lower cauda equina. The spinal roots associated with quadriceps have already exited the thecal sac at this inferior stimulation site, and the M waves are most probably elicited in the corresponding anterior roots at the intervertebral foramina. In the other muscles, the latency difference between PRM reflexes at threshold stimulation and M waves at increased intensity suggests that the direct responses are due to depolarization of anterior root motor axons, also at rather distal sites, most probably at their exists from the vertebral canal (Maccabee et al., 1996; Ladenbauer et al., 2010; Danner et al., 2011).

8. THE PRM REFLEX AND THE H REFLEX

The Hoffman reflex or H reflex results from the stimulation of large-diameter group Ia muscle spindle afferents in a mixed peripheral nerve and the monosynaptic excitation of homonymous alpha-motoneurons by the evoked afferent volley. PRM reflexes as described above have some similarities to the H reflex, such as (1) constant latencies, waveforms, and amplitudes of the surface-recorded compound muscle action

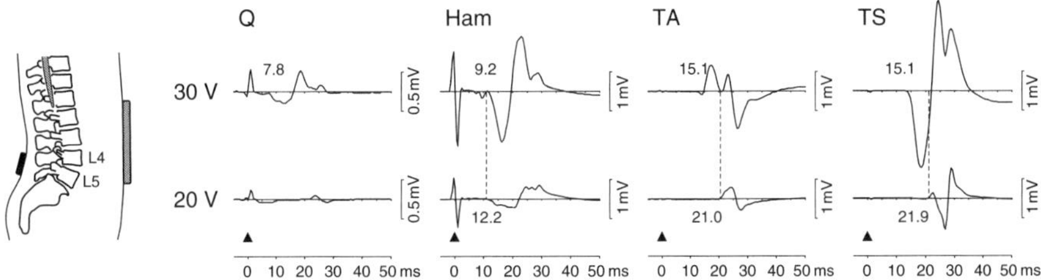

Figure 10–9 Responses evoked by cauda equina stimulation via stimulating electrodes placed over the L4–L5 spinous processes in quadriceps (Q), hamstrings (Ham), tibialis anterior (TA), and triceps surae (TS). Inserted values are onset latencies; vertical dashed lines mark the latencies of PRM reflexes elicited at threshold intensity. M waves only were evoked in Q. Each trace is the average of three responses that were derived from the same series of recordings as used for Figure 10–8B.

potentials during constant conditions; (2) excitability changes for several seconds when a prior stimulus is given; and (3) attenuation of response amplitudes during Achilles tendon vibration (Mao et al., 1984; Pierrot-Deseilligny & Burke, 2005a; Minassian et al., 2007b). The PRM reflex and the H reflex are both evoked by stimulation of the same type of sensory axons, with the PRM reflex initiated at proximal sites close to the spinal cord (Figure 10–10).

There are nevertheless some differences between the PRM reflex and the H reflex. As a result of the short afferent limb of the PRM reflex arc (Figure 10–10B), the latency of the triceps surae PRM reflex corresponds to 63.2 ± 1.2% of the H reflex delay (Minassian et al., 2007b). Other dissimilarities can arise from the distinct neural activities produced at the different stimulation sites. The stimulation of a mixed peripheral nerve at increased stimulus intensities activates motor axons in addition to the sensory fibers. The former produces the M wave that precedes the H reflex in the electromyographic recording (Figure 10–10A), as well as antidromic action potentials in the efferents that cancel the reflexively generated signals in the same motor axon (Schieppati, 1987). On the other hand, transcutaneous stimulation applied over the spinal cord and cauda equina can be controlled to selectively recruit sensory fibers within the posterior roots that are anatomically separated from the motor fibers located in the anterior roots (Minassian et al., 2007b; Kitano & Koceja, 2009; Ladenbauer et al., 2010). Peripheral stimulation can evoke a monosynaptic reflex in a single muscle or muscle group. Stimulation of multiple posterior roots, on the other hand, usually activates afferents involved in the myotatic reflex arcs of agonists and antagonists simultaneously. Thus, PRM reflexes of different muscles evoked

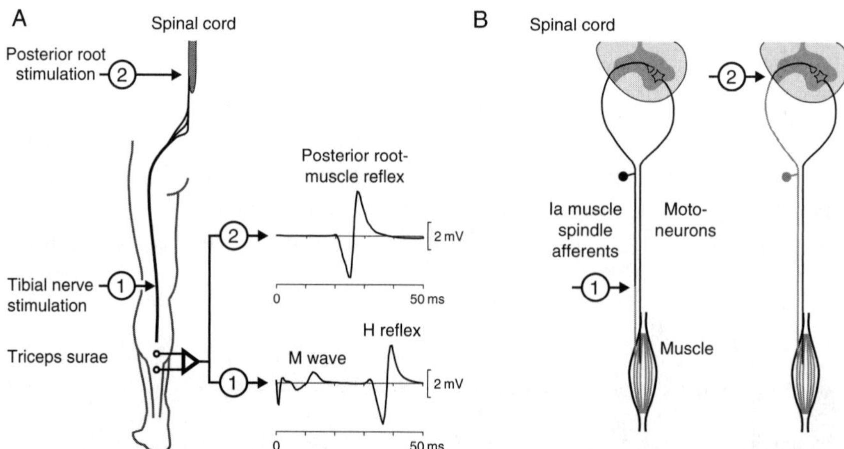

Figure 10–10 Comparison of elicitation and recording of the H reflex and posterior root-muscle reflex of triceps surae and illustration of the involved neural pathways. *A*. The H reflex is classically evoked by transcutaneous electrical stimulation of the posterior tibial nerve in the popliteal fossa. The posterior root-muscle reflex of the same muscle is elicited in the same group of sensory fibers, but close to the spinal cord. Both reflexes are recorded electromyographically as compound muscle action potential from the surface of the muscle with similar morphology. *B*. The volleys initiated in the group Ia muscle spindle afferents evoked at different distances from the spinal cord provide direct excitatory input to motoneurons in the ventral horn of the spinal cord gray matter.

in series and in close succession can potentially affect each other (Delwaide et al., 1976). Note that monosynaptic reflexes in many muscles can be evoked by posterior root stimulation that are not commonly evoked by stimulation of the corresponding peripheral nerve.

9. PRM REFLEXES APPLIED TO EXTEND H REFLEX STUDIES TO MULTIPLE MUSCLES SIMULTANEOUSLY

Due to the direct connections of Ia afferents to motoneurons, the monosynaptic reflex was recognized as a means for investigating excitability changes of the motoneuron pool supplied by the stimulated nerve (Renshaw, 1940). After pioneering investigations in the 1950s (Magladery & McDougal, 1950; Magladery et al., 1951; Paillard, 1955), the H reflex became a major noninvasive tool in human motor control studies.

The H reflex is characteristically modulated by voluntary movements at the ankle. Voluntary ankle dorsiflexion depresses the soleus H reflex. Several mechanisms contribute to this depression, one being reciprocal Ia inhibition (Pierrot-Deseilligny & Burke, 2005c). On the other hand, slight voluntary activation of soleus increases the excitability of the H reflex in the same muscle. Figure 10–11 shows that these motor tasks have very similar effects on the PRM reflex in triceps surae (Minassian et al., 2007b). The electrophysiological similarities of the PRM reflex with the H reflex suggest its applicability in neurophysiological studies.

PRM reflexes can extend H reflex studies of a single muscle to the simultaneous assessment of synaptic transmission of two-neuron reflex arcs at multiple segmental levels (Hofstoetter et al., 2008). This is relevant because motor control involves many muscles with state- and dynamic phase-dependent changes of their functional roles, independently as well as within different synergies. Hofstoetter and colleagues (2008) reported on the effect of postural maneuvers incorporating the whole body on the regulation of multiple lower-limb PRM reflexes in upright standing humans with an intact nervous system. One observation was the reproducible and characteristic modification of PRM reflexes of all studied muscles during leaning forward and

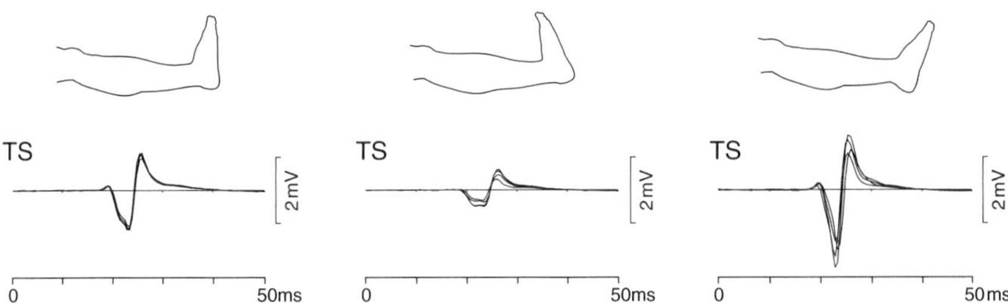

Figure 10–11 Effect of ipsilateral voluntary ankle dorsiflexion and plantar flexion upon posterior root-muscle reflexes of triceps surae (TS) during unchanged stimulation conditions. Posterior root-muscle reflexes were evoked by transcutaneous stimulation applied over the T11–T12 spinous processes in a subject with intact nervous system while supine. Responses shown on the left side were evoked during relaxation and serve as controls.

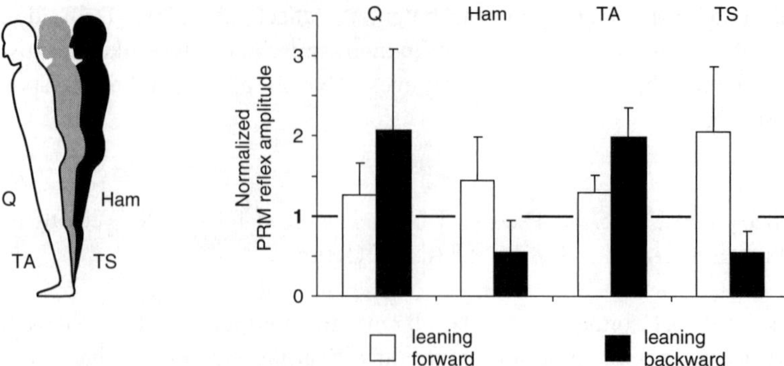

Figure 10–12 Posterior root-muscle reflexes elicited in quadriceps (Q), hamstrings (Ham), tibialis anterior (TA), and triceps surae (TS) while leaning forward and backward at the ankle from neutral standing. Bars represent peak-to-peak amplitudes of conditioned posterior root-muscle reflexes normalized to controls evoked during upright standing position; group results were derived from three subjects with intact nervous system.

backward of the body from a neutral upright standing position (Figure 10–12). PRM reflexes were facilitated while leaning forward in hamstrings and in triceps surae as well as tibialis anterior (Figure 10–12, white bars). Facilitation of both lower leg muscles was most probably due to the necessity to stiffen the ankle joint during the task. Leaning backward resulted in facilitation of PRM reflexes in the anterior compartments of thigh and lower leg (quadriceps and tibialis anterior) and a suppression of the responses of the posterior compartments (Figure 10–12, black bars). No background electromyographic activity was produced in hamstrings and triceps surae while leaning backward. The suppression of the PRM reflexes in these muscle groups demonstrated that there was not only an absence of motor drive to the posterior compartments but also an active suppression. The methodological advancement to simultaneously record the level of activity of multiple spinal motor nuclei during combinations of postural-automatic and volitional-skilful movements can be a promising new approach to learning how postural and volitional motor control is contributing to functional movements from standing to locomotion.

10. CONTINUOUS TRANSCUTANEOUS SPINAL CORD STIMULATION TO MODIFY THE ACTIVITY OF NEURAL CIRCUITS

Epidural spinal cord stimulation as a neuromodulation therapy has been introduced in the late 1960s in the treatment of chronic, intractable pain (Shealy et al., 1967) based on the "gate theory" of pain proposed by Melzack and Wall (1965). The control of painful neuropathies is still the major application. The role of epidural spinal cord stimulation was expanded by the observation of improved motor function in a multiple sclerosis patient being treated for pain (Cook & Weinstein, 1973). Various applications other than pain control were reported shortly thereafter. The effect in suppressing spasticity in people with chronic complete spinal cord injury was described by Richardson and McLone (1978) and later studies (e.g., Dimitrijevic et al., 1986a; 1986b).

Based on these findings, epidural stimulation in the control of severe lower limb spasticity following chronic spinal cord injury was revisited, with the electrodes specifically placed over the lumbar enlargement of the spinal cord (Pinter et al., 2000). A remarkable antispastic effect across multiple lower limb muscles was demonstrated when targeting the upper lumbar posterior roots with a stimulation frequency within a range of 50 Hz–100 Hz. The stimulation most probably enhanced the activity of inhibitory spinal cord circuits and increased the level of presynaptic inhibition. The lumbar spinal cord segments targeted in the control of lower limb spasticity correspond to the respective levels in the mammalian spinal cord that contain neural circuits involved in hind limb locomotion control (Barthélemy et al., 2007; Gerasimenko et al., 2008). In patients with chronic complete spinal cord injuries being treated for spasticity, Dimitrijevic and colleagues found that continuous epidural stimulation could generate rhythmic, locomotor-like flexion and extension movements in the paralyzed lower limbs (Rosenfeld et al., 1995; Dimitrijevic et al., 1998). Locomotor-like activities were most readily produced by continuous stimulation of the upper lumbar spinal cord at a frequency within a range of 25 Hz–60 Hz. It was thus demonstrated that the human lumbar spinal cord contains neural circuitries involved in the control of muscle tone and in the coordination of oscillating motor outputs. These circuitries can be activated by tonic neural signals delivered via segmental afferent input pathways.

Early work has begun to investigate the clinical relevance of epidural spinal cord stimulation to enhance locomotor activity in motor complete or incomplete spinal cord injured people. Specifically, the interaction of tonic epidural lumbar spinal cord stimulation and phasic proprioceptive feedback input generated by assisted treadmill stepping has been addressed. In two chronic, motor complete spinal cord injured individuals the rhythmic electromyographic activity produced by partial body weight-supported, assisted treadmill stepping was immediately augmented when epidural stimulation was supplied at a frequency of 20 Hz–50 Hz (Minassian et al., 2005; 2007a). Rhythmic activity was produced in muscles that did not respond to passive treadmill stepping alone, and the timing of the activity could be shifted relative to the stepping cycle. Independent functional stepping, however, was not achieved. Following a period of extensive locomotor training over 26 months, rhythmic activity generated by assisted treadmill stepping was enhanced by additionally applying epidural stimulation in a spinal cord injured individual with no clinically detectable voluntary motor function below the lesion (Harkema et al., 2011). In two persons with chronic motor-incomplete spinal cord injury, who were no functional ambulators, continuous epidural spinal cord stimulation at a frequency of 40 Hz–60 Hz could facilitate recovery of functional walking, when applied during partial weight-bearing therapy (Herman et al., 2002; Huang et al., 2006).

Transcutaneous lumbar spinal cord stimulation, just like epidural stimulation, predominantly activates large-diameter afferent fibers bilaterally in several posterior roots and rootlets. This similarity of the immediate effects upon neural input structures to the spinal cord implies that tonic transcutaneous stimulation can be used to modify altered activity of neural circuits after spinal cord injury. In the following section, two cases will be presented, reporting on the application of the noninvasive stimulation technique in the modification of spasticity and in the augmentation of neural control of locomotion. The two cases are based on multiple recordings derived from two different incomplete spinal cord injured subjects.

10.1. Control of Spasticity

The effect of tonic transcutaneous spinal cord simulation in modifying different manifestations of lower limb spasticity was tested by the assessment of the subject's residual voluntary and reflex functions before and after continuous stimulation for 30 minutes.

The evaluation was derived from segments of the brain motor control assessment (BMCA; see Chapter 8). BMCA is based on principles of the neurological evaluation of upper motoneuron dysfunctions. The aim is the assessment of the subject's spasticity and altered motor control following spinal cord injury. The protocol conducted here included BMCA-segments to detect muscle responses to passive stretch, clonus, exaggerated responses to plantar stimulation, as well as changes in the control of volitional motor tasks (Sherwood et al., 1996; 2000). Motor outputs were detected by multichannel electromyography with surface electrodes placed over quadriceps, hamstrings, tibialis anterior, triceps surae, and lower back and abdomen. The key information of the BMCA is contained in the overall temporal pattern of activity across the multiple lower limb muscles (Lee et al., 2004).

The subject was a male, age 32, with traumatic spinal cord injury in a stable condition (12 years post-injury), a motor level at C4-C5, classified as D according to the American Spinal Injury Association (ASIA) impairment scale (AIS). The subject had preserved stretch and cutaneo-muscular reflexes below the level of the lesion. Motor scores ranged from 3–5 in the right and 1–4 in the left lower limb muscles. The subject's ambulation ability was 16 according to the WISCI II scale; that is, 10 meters over ground walking with two crutches, without braces or physical assistance (Morganti et al., 2005). Clonogenic activities strongly interfered with the subject's ability to ambulate.

For transcutaneous lumbar spinal cord stimulation, the paravertebral skin electrodes were at first placed over the T11–T12 spinous processes. The stimulation site was monitored by applying single stimuli and recording PRM reflexes from quadriceps, hamstrings, tibialis anterior, and triceps surae in a supine position. The placement of the paravertebral skin electrodes was subsequently adjusted to result in lower thresholds of the PRM reflexes evoked in quadriceps than in triceps surae, a criterion similar to that of the application of epidural spinal cord stimulation in the control of spasticity (Murg et al., 2000; Pinter et al., 2000). The stimulation of posterior root afferents was verified by testing the reflex nature of the elicited responses with double stimuli with interstimulus intervals of 50 ms and 30 ms.

With the designated electrode placement, the stimulation mode was then changed to continuous stimulation at 50 Hz. The stimulus intensity was slowly increased starting from 0 V to allow the subject to adapt to the stimulation-induced effects. The sequence of these effects was, first, sensory perception of the stimulation below the paravertebral and subsequently the abdominal electrodes, followed by contractions of these muscles. With further increase of stimulus intensity, the subject reported paraesthesiae that started in the feet and then spread to the posterior and anterior lower legs, and eventually to the posterior and anterior thighs. At a stimulus intensity producing paraesthesiae covering most of the lower limb dermatomes, yet below threshold for eliciting PRM reflexes, the stimulation was continuously applied for another 30 minutes. The subject remained lying supine on the examination bed for this period. After termination of the stimulation, temporary carryover effects were examined by performing the same assessment protocol as prior to the stimulation session. Exemplary results of this evaluation are illustrated in Figures 10–13 and 10–14.

Passive unilateral hip and knee flexion and extension movements performed by the examiner initially evoked passive stretch responses with a spread of activity to all studied ipsilateral muscles (Figure 10–13A, *left*). Activities were reduced to a large degree after stimulation (Figure 10–13A, *right*). A rapid manual stretch of the Achilles tendon with the leg extended elicited a clonogenic activity in triceps surae, with spread of activity to hamstrings and tibialis anterior (Figure 10–13B, *left*). Except for a brief reflex response to the tendon stretch in the calf, there was an absence of activity following the same maneuver after stimulation (Figure 10–13B, *right*). During the control assessment, plantar stimulation with a blunt rod, similar to the test for the Babinski reflex, resulted in a withdrawal-like response involving all ipsilateral muscles (Figure 10–13C, *left*). The pattern of response to plantar stimulation was altered and the overall activities reduced during the post–spinal cord stimulation assessment (Figure 10–13C, *right*). Continuous transcutaneous spinal cord

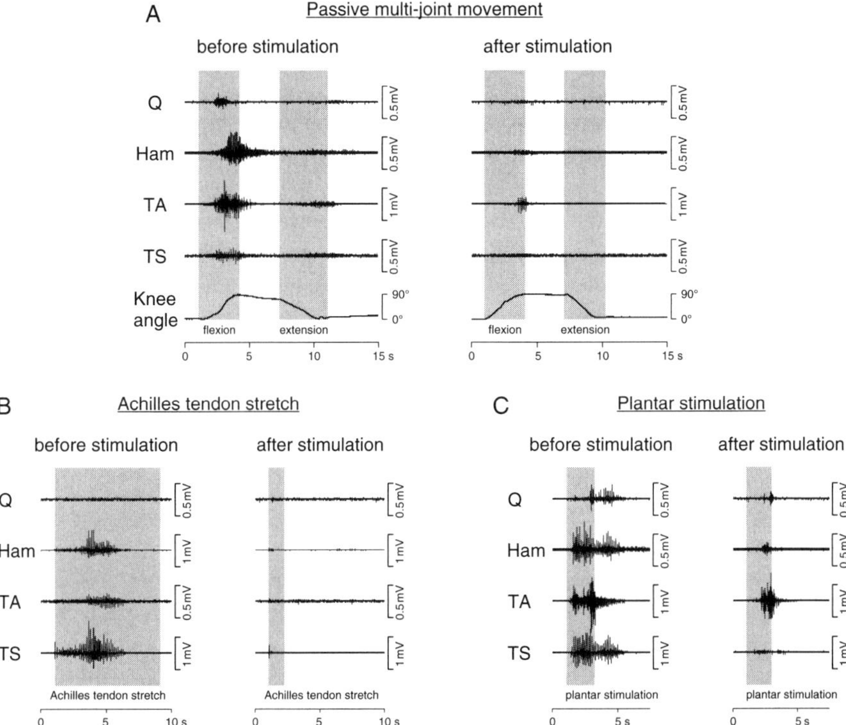

Figure 10–13 Electrophysiological assessment of manifestations of spasticity before and after tonic transcutaneous spinal cord stimulation. *A*. Passive hip and knee flexion-extension movements imposed by an examiner. *B*. Attempt to elicit a clonus by a brisk stretch of the Achilles tendon. *C*. Plantar surface stimulation with a blunt rod. Electromyographic activities of right quadriceps (Q), hamstrings (Ham), tibialis anterior (TA), and triceps surae (TS) and goniometer recordings of knee movements. Stimulation was applied for 30 minutes at 50 Hz and 22 V, corresponding to 85% threshold of eliciting PRM reflexes in Q. Incomplete spinal cord injured subject classified as AIS D.

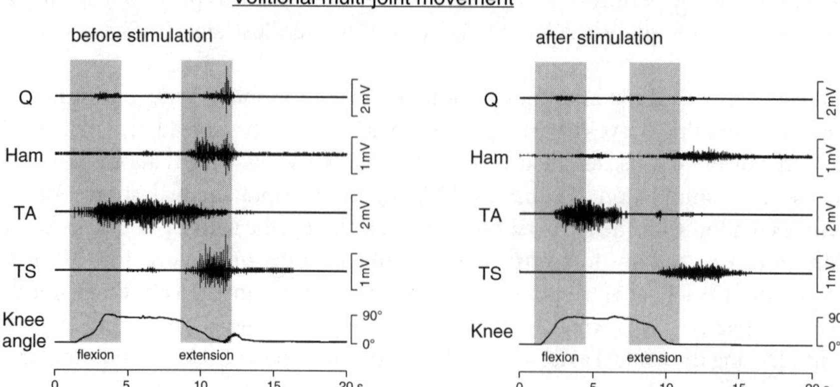

Figure 10–14 Electromyographic activity recorded from quadriceps (Q), hamstrings (Ham), tibialis anterior (TA), and triceps surae (TS) during volitional hip and knee flexion and extension movements before and after continuous transcutaneous spinal cord stimulation applied for 30 minutes. Shaded bars marking the times during which the subject was asked by the examiner to perform each maneuver. Recordings are from the same subject and the same evaluation session as in Figure 10–13.

stimulation also temporarily modified motor unit activation patterns during a volitional motor task (Figure 10–14). The subject in supine position was instructed to pull his knee up with the foot off the bed, and after five seconds to extend the leg before relaxing it back down the examination bed. Before stimulation, the subject was able to lift the foot from the supporting surface with some delay after the command cue. When asked to extend the leg again, the activity in the ankle flexor could not be immediately terminated, and the movement of the limb was achieved by nonselective activation of thigh and leg muscles. Assessment after stimulation demonstrated changes of the pattern of activity across the lower limb muscles during the volitional multi-joint movement, including selectivity and task-appropriate timing of muscle activation. The post-stimulus modification of the volitional motor task was also reflected by changes in the performance of the movement as documented by the electrogoniometric recording at the knee joint. The subject reported that the perceived beneficial effects lasted for two to several hours after the assessment time of the different stimulation sessions.

Stimulation-related changes of the subject's ambulation ability were assessed by the 10-meter walk test on two different days. The times the subject needed to walk 10 meters with two crutches at a secure gait speed were 49 seconds and 54 seconds before stimulation. After continuous transcutaneous spinal cord stimulation at 50 Hz was applied for 30 minutes in a supine position, the measured times were 32 seconds and 35 seconds. One obvious effect following stimulation was a definitive reduction of the clonogenic activities that normally interfered with the subject's volitional stepping movements.

Spasticity is recognized as one of the most common disabling and bothersome complications affecting spinal cord injured individuals, with about 70% being spastic one year after injury (Biering-Sørensen et al., 2006). Severe spasticity interferes with the patient's residual ability to perform voluntary movements, can hinder effective rehabilitation, and leads to a reduction of independence and quality of life.

Despite its high prevalence, effective suppression of spasticity, while maintaining or even enhancing volitional movement capabilities, has remained difficult. Tonic transcutaneous stimulation of the lumbar spinal cord could be a promising noninvasive neuromodulative approach to reduce spasticity and augment residual motor function. Therapeutic benefit would be based on the carryover effects of stimulation after single treatments. This duration might be prolonged with repetitive application of the intervention method. Temporary carryover effects are known from functional electrical stimulation (FES) of peripheral nerves (Stein et al., 1999), and it is well accepted that activity-dependent plasticity results from repetitive activation of the CNS via sensory pathways (Liberson et al., 1961; Dietz & Harkema, 2004; Lynskey et al., 2008).

10.2. Augmentation of Neural Control of Locomotion

The potential of transcutaneous stimulation of the lumbar spinal cord to facilitate stepping will be illustrated in an incomplete spinal cord injured person. The subject was a female, age 28, with a motor level at T8-T9 following a vascular event, classified as AIS D. She was in a chronic, stable condition (10 years post-injury). The subject had preserved stretch and cutaneo-muscular reflexes below the level of the lesion, and motor scores ranged from 3–5 in the right and 2–4 in the left lower limb muscles. She could walk over ground with two crutches, without braces and physical assistance (WISCI II scale of 16) and required 23 seconds to walk 10 meters. She was not a community or homebound functional ambulator.

The subject was assessed with respect to electromyographic activity and hip and knee joint movements during active stepping on a moving treadmill belt without assistance from therapists and without body-weight support (Figure 10–15A and B, *left side*). In a standing position, transcutaneous stimulation was then applied to the lumbar spinal cord at a frequency of 30 Hz. Stimulus intensity was slowly increased to a sensory level producing paraesthesiae in the lower limb dermatomes but without generating responses in the thigh and leg muscles. With the stimulation being continuously applied at that intensity, the treadmill was again activated. During active stepping, stimulation consistently augmented electromyographic activity in all muscles in a gait-phase–appropriate manner and modified the execution of the movement (Figure 10–15A, *right side*). The stick-figures calculated from the electrogoniometric data illustrate the changes of kinematics of the joints (Figure 10–15B, *right side*). An obvious immediate effect of stimulation was the augmentation of a fluid multi-joint flexion movement with improved foot clearance. An increased stride length could be deduced from the lower number of gait cycles at the same stepping speed. Changes in produced muscle forces could be inferred from these alterations of movement. The subject reported an effortless, near-automatic initiation of the flexion movement and improved stability during stance. All muscle activities were volitionally controlled, and when the treadmill belt movement was stopped, they could be terminated by the subject in spite of the stimulation being continuously applied. Thus, in motor incomplete spinal cord injured individuals, transcutaneous spinal cord stimulation can combine with residual descending supraspinal commands (and step-related proprioceptive feedback) to augment locomotor output and modify gait kinematics.

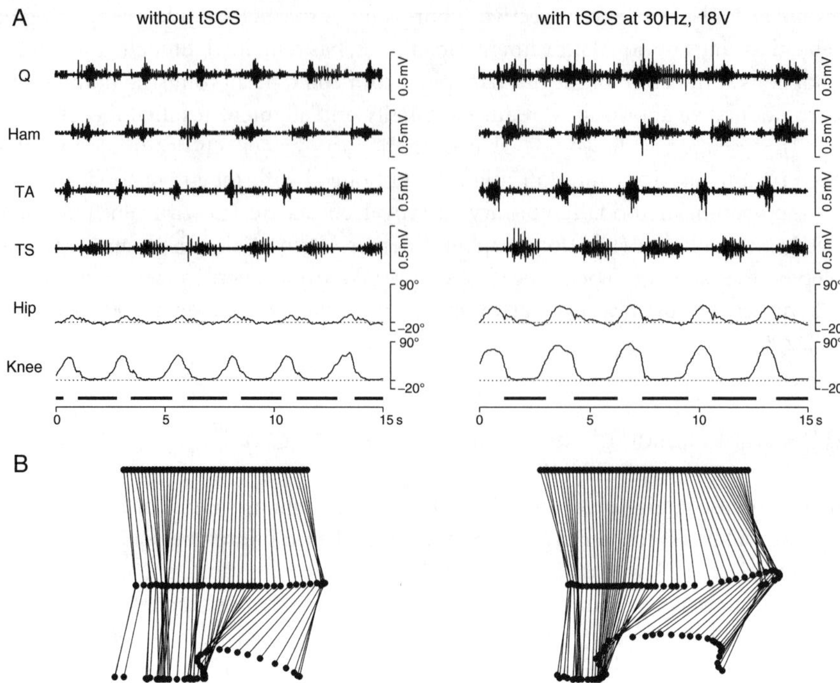

Figure 10–15 Active stepping on a treadmill at 1.6 km/h of an incomplete spinal cord injured person (AIS D) without (*left column*) and during (*right column*) the application of continuous transcutaneous spinal cord stimulation. *A*. Electromyographic activities of right quadriceps (Q), hamstrings (Ham), tibialis anterior (TA), and triceps surae (TS), and goniometer recordings of hip and knee angles. Horizontal bars mark stance phases. *B*. Stick figures calculated from the hip and knee angle recordings as shown in *A*, averaged from 10 consecutive gait cycles. Manual assistance and body weight support were not required. Stimulation was applied over the T11–T12 spinous processes at 30 Hz and an intensity generating paraesthesiae in the lower limb dermatomes during continuous stimulation without eliciting PRM reflexes in the lower limbs during standing.

11. CONCLUSIONS

We presented a noninvasive method for the stimulation of posterior root afferent fibers of the L2 to S2 spinal cord segments in humans. The selective stimulation of posterior root fibers by skin electrodes was discussed in the context of the electrical phenomena produced by transcutaneous spinal cord stimulation. Locally enhanced electrical field gradients leading to the depolarization of posterior root fibers resulted from the curved paths of the axons and sudden changes in tissue conductivity along the axons at their entries into the spinal cord. The electrically stimulated afferents make synaptic contacts onto spinal motoneurons and interneurons processing information from the periphery and integrating supraspinal information to generate motor outputs (Jankowska, 1992). Transsynaptically, the stimulation exerted effects through specific reflex pathways or through higher-level circuits in the organization of spinal locomotion.

Methodologically, the induced effects partially depend on the repetition rate of stimulation. Single stimuli applied over the lumbar spinal cord elicit PRM reflexes simultaneously in many lower limb muscles. Due to its similarity to the H reflex, the PRM reflex can become an important measure in studies of sensorimotor integration and plasticity of the central nervous system in humans (Hofstoetter et al., 2008; Knikou, 2008). Double-stimulus paradigms to explore excitability (recovery) curves of PRM reflexes (Minassian et al., 2009) may be useful to assess the integrated influence of various factors that alter the test PRM reflex gain. The H reflex recovery curve tested via double stimulation has been previously used in evaluating spinal motoneuron pool excitability in various motor disorders of central origin (Magladery et al., 1952). Paired PRM reflexes test the excitability states of myotatic reflex arcs of several muscles, as well as the functional relationships between them (Delwaide et al., 1976), and may provide several parameters for the characterization of specific factors that alter the test reflex. In individuals with spinal cord injury, "tonic external drives" can be applied transcutaneously to the spinal cord below the lesion to activate intrinsic, structurally preserved neural circuits. The generated neural activity contributes to the central state of activity of neural circuits that are (partially) deprived of descending supraspinal input. The activation of circuits involved in the control of muscle tone and movement can lead to suppression of spasticity and augmentation of residual volitional movement. Repetitive stimulation of posterior roots can increase our understanding of the spinal cord physiology caudal to the site of a spinal cord lesion. This method will be of particular value when the subjects under evaluation are paralyzed, and can be complementary to methods assessing lumbar circuitries via fast- and slow-conducting descending pathways.

Transcutaneous posterior root stimulation can become an important assessment and intervention procedure meeting the principles of restorative neurology: (1) for the assessment of mechanisms responsible for neurological deficits and (2) for the improvement of impaired nervous system function through modification of altered neural control.

References

Amassian, V. E., Maccabee, P. J. "Transcranial magnetic stimulation." *Conference Proceedings of the IEEE Engineering in Medicine and Biology Society* 1 (2006): 1620–1623.

Barthélemy, D., Leblond, H., Rossignol, S. "Characteristics and mechanisms of locomotion induced by intraspinal microstimulation and dorsal root stimulation in spinal cats." *Journal of Neurophysiology* 97 (2007): 1986–2000.

Biering-Sørensen, F., Nielsen, J. B., Klinge, K. "Spasticity-assessment: a review." *Spinal Cord* 44 (2006): 708–722.

Brown, T. G. "The intrinsic factors in the act of progression in the mammal." *Proceedings of the Royal Society London B* 84 (1911): 309–319.

Bussel, B., Roby-Brami, A., Azouvi, P., Biraben, A., Yakovleff, A., Held, J. P. "Myoclonus in a patient with spinal cord transection. Possible involvement of the spinal stepping generator." *Brain* 111 (1988): 1235–1245.

Calancie, B., Needham-Shropshire, B., Jacobs, P., Willer, K., Zych, G., Green, B. A. "Involuntary stepping after chronic spinal cord injury. Evidence for a central rhythm generator for locomotion in man." *Brain* 117 (1994): 1143–1159.

Calancie, B. "Spinal myoclonus after spinal cord injury." *Journal of Spinal Cord Medicine* 29 (2006): 413–424.

Coburn, B. "A theoretical study of epidural electrical stimulation of the spinal cord. Part II: Effects on long myelinated fibers." *IEEE Transactions in Biomedical Engineering* 32 (1985): 978–986.

Cohen, M. S., Wall, E. J., Kerber, C. W., Abitbol, J. J., Garfin, S. R. "The anatomy of the cauda equina on CT scans and MRI." *Journal of Bone and Joint Surgery* (British) 73 (1991): 381–384.

Cook, A. W., Weinstein, S. P. "Chronic dorsal column stimulation in multiple sclerosis. Preliminary report." *New York State Journal of Medicine* 73 (1973): 2868–2872.

Courtine, G., Harkema, S. J., Dy, C. J., Gerasimenko, Y. P., Dyhre-Poulsen, P. "Modulation of multisegmental monosynaptic responses in a variety of leg muscles during walking and running in humans." *Journal of Physiology* 582 (2007): 1125–1139.

Creed, R. S., Denny-Brown, D. E., Eccles, J. C., Liddell, E. G. T., Sherrington, C. S. *Reflex Activity of the Spinal Cord*. London: Oxford University Press, 1932.

Danner, S. M., Hofstoetter, U. S., Ladenbauer, J., Rattay, F., Minassian, K. "Can the human lumbar posterior columns be stimulated by transcutaneous spinal cord stimulation? A modeling study." *Artificial Organs* 35 (2011): 257–262.

Delwaide, P. J., Cordonnier, M., Charlier, M. "Functional relationships between myotatic reflex arcs of the lower limb in man: investigation by excitability curves." *Journal of Neurology, Neurosurgery and Psychiatry* 39 (1976): 545–554.

Dietz, V., Harkema, S. J. "Locomotor activity in spinal cord–injured persons." *Journal of Applied Physiology* 96 (2004): 1954–1960.

Dimitrijevic, M. M., Dimitrijevic, M. R., Illis, L. S., Nakajima, K., Sharkey, P. C., Sherwood, A. M. "Spinal cord stimulation for the control of spasticity in patients with chronic spinal cord injury: I. Clinical observations." *Central Nervous System Trauma* 3 (1986a): 129–144.

Dimitrijevic, M. R. "Neurophysiological evaluation and epidural stimulation in chronic spinal cord injury patients." In *Spinal Cord Reconstruction*, edited by C. C. Kao, R. P. Bunge, P. J. Reier, 465–474. New York: Raven Press, 1983.

Dimitrijevic, M. R., Dimitrijevic, M. M., Kern, H., Minassian, K., Rattay, F. "Electrophysiological characteristics of H-reflexes elicited by percutaneous stimulation of the cauda equina." In *Program No. 417.11. Abstract Viewer/Itinerary Planner*. Washington, D.C.: Society for Neuroscience, 2004.

Dimitrijevic, M. R., Faganel, J., Sherwood, A. M. "Spinal cord stimulation as a tool for physiological research." *Applied Neurophysiology* 46 (1983): 245–253.

Dimitrijevic, M. R., Gerasimenko, Y., Pinter, M. M. "Evidence for a spinal central pattern generator in humans." *Annals of the New York Academy of Science* 860 (1998): 360–376.

Dimitrijevic, M. R., Illis, L. S., Nakajima, K., Sharkey, P. C., Sherwood, A. M. "Spinal cord stimulation for the control of spasticity in patients with chronic spinal cord injury: II. Neurophysiological observations." *Central Nervous System Trauma* 3 (1986b): 145–152.

Dy, C. J., Gerasimenko, Y. P., Edgerton, V. R., Dyhre-Poulsen, P., Courtine, G., Harkema, S. J. "Phase-dependent modulation of percutaneously elicited multisegmental muscle responses after spinal cord injury." *Journal of Neurophysiology* 103 (2010): 2808–2820.

Gaunt, R. A., Prochazka, A., Mushahwar, V. K., Guevremont, L., Ellaway, P. H. "Intraspinal microstimulation excites multisegmental sensory afferents at lower stimulus levels than local alpha-motoneuron responses." *Journal of Neurophysiology* 96 (2006): 2995–3005.

Geddes, L. A., Baker, L. E. "The specific resistance of biological material—a compendium of data for the biomedical engineer and physiologist." *Journal of Medical and Biological Engineering* 5 (1967): 271–293.

Gerasimenko, Y., Roy, R. R., Edgerton, V. R. "Epidural stimulation: Comparison of the spinal circuits that generate and control locomotion in rats, cats and humans." *Experimental Neurology* 209 (2008): 417–425.

Grillner, S. "Neurobiological bases of rhythmic motor acts in vertebrates." *Science* 228 (1985): 143–149.

Grillner, S., Zangger, P. "On the central generation of locomotion in the low spinal cat." *Experimental Brain Research* 34 (1979): 241–261.

Gu, W. Y., Justiz, M. A., Yao, H. "Electrical conductivity of lumbar anulus fibrosis: effects of porosity and fixed charge density." *Spine* 27 (2002): 2390–2395.

Harkema, S., Gerasimenko, Y., Hodes, J., et al. "Effect of epidural stimulation of the lumbosacral spinal cord on voluntary movement, standing, and assisted stepping after motor complete paraplegia: a case study." *Lancet* 377 (2011): 1938–1947.

Herman, R., He, J., D'Luzansky, S., Willis, W., Dilli, S. "Spinal cord stimulation facilitates functional walking in a chronic, incomplete spinal cord injured." *Spinal Cord* 40 (2002): 65–68.

Hoffmann, P. "Beitrag zur Kenntnis der menschlichen Reflexe mit besonderer Berücksichtigung der elektrischen Erscheinungen." *Archives of Anatomy and Physiology* 1 (1910): 223–246.

Hoffmann, P. "Über die Beziehungen der Sehnenreflexe zur willkürlichen Bewegung und zum Tonus." *Zeitschrift für Biologie* 68 (1918): 351–370.

Hofstoetter, U. S. "Model of spinal cord reflex circuits in humans: Stimulation frequency-dependence of segmental activities and their interactions." Ph.D. dissertation, Vienna University of Technology, 2009. Accessible at http://www.ub.tuwien.ac.at/diss/AC07806007.pdf.

Hofstoetter, U. S., Minassian, K., Hofer, C., Mayr, W., Rattay, F., Dimitrijevic, M. R. "Modification of reflex responses to lumbar posterior root stimulation by motor tasks in healthy subjects." *Artificial Organs* 32 (2008): 644–648.

Holsheimer, J. "Which neuronal elements are activated directly by spinal cord stimulation?" *Neuromodulation* 5 (2002): 25–31.

Holsheimer, J., Barolat, G., Struijk, J. J., He, J. "Significance of the spinal cord position in spinal cord stimulation." *Acta Neurochirurgica* Suppl 64 (1995): 119–124.

Huang, H., He, J., Herman, R., Carhart, M.R. "Modulation effects of epidural spinal cord stimulation on muscle activities during walking." *IEEE Transactions on Neural Systems and Rehabilitation Engineering* 14 (2006): 14–23.

Iles, J. F. "Simple models of stimulation of neurones in the brain by electric fields." *Progress in Biophysics and Molecular Biology* 87 (2005): 17–31.

Jankowska, E. "Interneuronal relay in spinal pathways from proprioceptors." *Progress in Neurobiology* 38 (1992): 335–378.

Jilge, B., Minassian, K., Rattay, F., et al. "Initiating extension of the lower limbs in subjects with complete spinal cord injury by epidural lumbar cord stimulation." *Experimental Brain Research* 154 (2004a): 308–326.

Jilge, B., Minassian, K., Rattay, F., Dimitrijevic, M. R. "Frequency-dependent selection of alternative spinal pathways with common periodic sensory input." *Biological Cybernetics* 91 (2004b): 359–376.

Kitano, K., Koceja, D. M. "Spinal reflex in human lower leg muscles evoked by transcutaneous spinal cord stimulation." *Journal of Neuroscience Methods* 180 (2009): 111–115.

Knikou, M. "The H-reflex as a probe: pathways and pitfalls." *Journal of Neuroscience Methods* 171 (2008): 1–12.

Ladenbauer, J., Minassian, K., Hofstoetter, U. S., Dimitrijevic, M. R., Rattay, F. "Stimulation of the human lumbar spinal cord with implanted and surface electrodes: a computer simulation study." *IEEE Transactions in Neural Systems Rehabilitation Engineering* 18 (2010): 637–645.

Lang, J. "Morphologie und funktionelle Anatomie der Lendenwirbelsäule und des benachbarten Nervensystems—1. Rückenmark." In *Neuroorthopädie 2—Lendenwirbelsäulenerkrankungen mit Beteiligung des Nervensystems*, edited by D. Hohmann, B. Kügelgen, K. Liebig, M. Schirmer, 3–9. Berlin: Springer, 1984.

Lee, D. C., Lim, H. K., McKay, W. B., Priebe, M. M., Holmes, S. A., Sherwood, A. M. "Toward an objective interpretation of surface EMG patterns: a voluntary response index (VRI)." *Journal of Electromyography and Kinesiology* 14 (2004): 379–388.

Liberson, W. T., Holmquest, H. J., Scott, D., Dow, M. "Functional electrotherapy: stimulation of the peroneal nerve synchronized with the swing phase of the gait of hemiplegic patients." *Archives of Physical Medicine and Rehabilitation* 42 (1961): 101–105.

Lloyd, D. C. P. "Reflex action in relation to pattern and peripheral source of afferent stimulation." *Journal of Neurophysiology* 6 (1943): 111–120.

Lynskey, J. V., Belanger, A., Jung, R. "Activity-dependent plasticity in spinal cord injury." *Journal of Rehabilitation Research and Development* 45 (2008): 229–240.

Maccabee, P. J., Amassian, V. E., Eberle, L. P., Cracco, R. Q. "Magnetic coil stimulation of straight and bent amphibian and mammalian peripheral nerve in vitro: locus of excitation." *Journal of Physiology* 460 (1993): 201–219.

Maccabee, P. J., Lipitz, M. E., Desudchit, T., et al. "A new method using neuromagnetic stimulation to measure conduction time within the cauda equina." *Electroencephalography and Clinical Neurophysiology* 101 (1996): 153–166.

Magladery, J. W., McDougal, D. B. Jr. "Electrophysiological studies of nerve and reflex activity in normal man. I. Identification of certain reflexes in the electromyogram and the conduction velocity of peripheral nerve fibers." *Bulletin of the Johns Hopkins Hospital* 86 (1950): 265–290.

Magladery, J. W., Porter, W. E., Park, A. M., Teasdall, R. D. "Electrophysiological studies of nerve and reflex activity in normal man. IV. The two-neurone reflex and identification of certain action potentials from spinal roots and cord." *Bulletin of the Johns Hopkins Hospital* 88 (1951): 499–519.

Magladery, J. W., Teasdall, R. D., Park, A. M., Languth, H. W. "Electrophysiological studies of reflex activity in patients with lesions of the nervous system. I. A comparison of spinal motoneurone excitability following afferent nerve volleys in normal persons and patients with upper motor neurone lesions." *Bulletin of the Johns Hopkins Hospital* 91 (1952): 219–244.

Mao, C. C., Ashby, P., Wang, M., McCrea, D. "Synaptic connections from large muscle afferents to the motoneurons of various leg muscles in man." *Experimental Brain Research* 56 (1984): 341–350.

Melzack, R., Wall, P. D. "Pain mechanisms: a new theory." *Science* 150 (1965): 971–979.

Minassian, K., Hofstoetter, U. S., Tansey, K., Rattay, F., Mayr, W., Dimitrijevic, M. R. "Transcutaneous stimulation of the human lumbar spinal cord: Facilitating locomotor output in spinal cord injury." *Society for Neuroscience Abstracts* 286 (2010).

Minassian, K., Hofstoetter, U. S., Rattay, F., Mayr, W., Dimitrijevic, M. R. "Posterior root-muscle reflexes and the H reflex in humans: Electrophysiological comparison." In *Program No. 658.12. 2009 Neuroscience Meeting Planner.* Chicago: Society for Neuroscience, 2009.

Minassian, K., Jilge, B., Rattay, F., et al. "Stepping-like movements in humans with complete spinal cord injury induced by epidural stimulation of the lumbar cord: electromyographic study of compound muscle action potentials." *Spinal Cord* 42 (2004): 401–416.

Minassian, K., Persy, I., Rattay, F., Dimitrijevic, M. R. "Peripheral and central afferent input to the lumbar cord." *Biocybernetics and Biomedical Engineering* 25 (2005): 11–29.

Minassian, K., Persy, I., Rattay, F., Pinter, M. M., Kern, H., Dimitrijevic, M. R. "Human lumbar cord circuitries can be activated by extrinsic tonic input to generate locomotor-like activity." *Human Movement Science* 26 (2007a): 275–295.

Minassian, K., Persy, I., Rattay, F., Dimitrijevic, M. R., Hofer, C., Kern, H. "Posterior root-muscle reflexes elicited by transcutaneous stimulation of the human lumbosacral cord." *Muscle and Nerve* 35 (2007b): 327–336.

Morganti, B., Scivoletto, G., Ditunno, P., Ditunno, J. F., Molinari, M. "Walking index for spinal cord injury (WISCI): criterion validation." *Spinal Cord* 43 (2005): 27–33.

Murg, M., Binder, H., Dimitrijevic, M. R. "Epidural electric stimulation of posterior structures of the human lumbar spinal cord: 1. Muscle twitches—a functional method to define the site of stimulation." *Spinal Cord* 38 (2000): 394–402.

Nadeau, S., Jacquemin, G., Fournier, C., Lamarre, Y., Rossignol, S. "Spontaneous motor rhythms of the back and legs in a patient with a complete spinal cord transection." *Neurorehabilitation and Neural Repair* 24 (2010): 377–383.

Nowak, L. G., Bullier, J. "Axons, but not cell bodies, are activated by electrical stimulation in cortical gray matter. II. Evidence from selective inactivation of cell bodies and axon initial segments." *Experimental Brain Research* 118 (1998): 489–500.

Paillard, J. *Réflexes et régulations d'origine proprioceptive chez l'homme*. Paris: Arnette, 1955.

Pearson, K., Gordon, J. "Locomotion." In *Principles of Neural Science,* 4th edition, edited by E. R. Kandel, J. H. Schwartz, T. M. Jessell, 737–755. New York: McGraw-Hill, 2000.

Pierrot-Deseilligny, E., Burke, D. "General methodology." In *The Circuitry of the Human Spinal Cord: Its Role in Motor Control and Movement Disorders,* 1–62. Cambridge, U.K.: Cambridge University Press, 2005a.

Pierrot-Deseilligny E, Burke D. "Monosynaptic Ia excitation and post-activation depression." In *The Circuitry of the Human Spinal Cord: Its Role in Motor Control and Movement Disorders,* 63–112. Cambridge, U.K.: Cambridge University Press, 2005b.

Pierrot-Deseilligny E, Burke D. "Reciprocal Ia inhibition." In *The Circuitry of the Human Spinal Cord: Its Role in Motor Control and Movement Disorders, 195–243.* Cambridge, U.K.: Cambridge University Press, 2005c.

Pinter, M. M., Gerstenbrand, F., Dimitrijevic, M. R. "Epidural electrical stimulation of posterior structures of the human lumbosacral cord: 3. Control of spasticity." *Spinal Cord* 38 (2000): 524–531.

Porter, R. "Focal stimulation of hypoglossal neurons in the cat." *Journal of Physiology* 169 (1963): 630–640.

Ranck, J. B. "Which elements are excited in electrical stimulation of mammalian central nervous system: A review." *Brain Research* 98 (1975): 417–440.

Rattay, F. "Ways to approximate current-distance relations for electrically stimulated fibers." *Journal of Theoretical Biology* 125 (1987): 339–349.

Rattay, F. *Electrical Nerve Stimulation*. Vienna: Springer, 1990.

Rattay, F. "Analysis of the electric excitation of CNS neurons." *IEEE Trans Biomedical Engineering* 45 (1998): 766–772.

Rattay, F. "The basic mechanism for the electrical stimulation of the nervous system." *Neuroscience* 89 (1999): 335–346.

Rattay, F., Minassian, K., Dimitrijevic, M. R. "Epidural electrical stimulation of posterior structures of the human lumbosacral cord: 2. Quantitative analysis by computer modeling." *Spinal Cord* 38 (2000): 473–489.

Renshaw, B. "Activity in the simplest spinal reflex pathways." *Journal of Neurophysiology* 3 (1940): 373–387.

Richardson, R. R., McLone, D. G. "Percutaneous epidural neurostimulation for paraplegic spasticity." *Surgical Neurology* 9 (1978): 153–155.

Rosenfeld, J. E., Sherwood, A. M., Halter, J. A., Dimitrijevic, M. R. "Evidence of a pattern generator in paralyzed subject with spinal cord stimulation." *Society for Neuroscience Abstracts* 21 (1995): 688.

Roth, B. J. "Mechanisms for electrical stimulation of excitable tissue." *Critical Reviews in Biomedical Engineering* 22 (1994): 253–305.

Schieppati, M. "The Hoffmann reflex: a means of assessing spinal reflex excitability and its descending control in man." *Progress in Neurobiology* 28 (1987): 345–376.

Shealy, C. N., Mortimer, J. T., Reswick, J. B. "Electrical inhibition of pain by stimulation of the dorsal columns: preliminary clinical report." *Anesthesia and Analgesia* 46 (1967): 489–491.

Sherrington, C. S. "Flexion-reflex of the limb, crossed extension reflex and the stepping reflex and standing." *Journal of Physiology* 40 (1910): 28–121.

Sherwood, A. M., Graves, D. E., Priebe, M. M. "Altered motor control and spasticity after spinal cord injury: subjective and objective assessment." *Journal of Rehabilitation Research and Development* 37 (2000): 41–52.

Sherwood, A. M., McKay, W. B., Dimitrijevic, M. R. "Motor control after spinal cord injury: assessment using surface EMG." *Muscle and Nerve* 19 (1996): 966–979.

Stein, R. B. "Functional electrical stimulation after spinal cord injury." *Journal of Neurotrauma* 16 (1999): 713–717.

Struijk, J. J., Holsheimer, J., van der Heide, G. G., Boom, H. B. "Recruitment of dorsal column fibers in spinal cord stimulation: influence of collateral branching." *IEEE Transactions in Biomedical Engineering* 39 (1992): 903–912.

Struijk, J. J., Holsheimer, J., Boom, H. B. "Excitation of dorsal root fibers in spinal cord stimulation: a theoretical study." *IEEE Transactions in Biomedical Engineering* 40 (1993): 632–639.

Veltink, P. H., van Alsté, J. A., Boom, H. B. "Simulation of intrafascicular and extraneural nerve stimulation." *IEEE Transactions in Biomedical Engineering* 35 (1988): 69–75.

Wongsarnpigoon, A., Grill, W. M. "Computational modeling of epidural cortical stimulation." *Journal of Neural Engineering* 5 (2008): 443–454.

Wall, E. J., Cohen, M. S., Abitbol, J. J., Garfin, S. R. "Organization of intrathecal nerve roots at the level of the conus medullaris." *Journal of Bone and Joint Surgery* (U.S.) 72 (1990): 1495–1499.

Epilogue

NILS G. ANDRESEN, BYRON A. KAKULAS, GERTA VRBOVA, AND MILAN R. DIMITRIJEVIC

This monograph brings together the "state of the art" regarding the injured spinal cord, and in particular of the restorative neurology of motor control after spinal cord injury. Each chapter is written by an expert drawing on their vast personal experience in the field. Until recently, knowledge of human spinal cord neurophysiology was crude and largely dependent on clinico-pathological correlations. Several decades ago this all changed, when poly-EMG for assessment of motor function and evoked potentials for sensory modalities were first applied in human spinal cord injury (SCI).

Beginning with basic observations, knowledge of spinal cord neurophysiology has accumulated over the years and evolved to the point of providing major insights into the disordered function that results from human SCI. Such information, gathered from a patient by using the most sophisticated assessment techniques, allows us to know what has gone awry and how to treat it. Thus, a number of interventions, physical and pharmacological, including electrical stimulation of the spinal cord, FES, reconstructive neurosurgery, and robotics, have been developed to improve residual spinal cord functions and thus upgrade the rehabilitative status of the SCI patient. It is important to point out that even a small gain may make a significant difference in the ability of a person with SCI to participate in the activities that make up and provide a good quality of life.

Included within this body of work is an account of the neuropathology of SCI. The benefit of such knowledge is to allow clinico-pathological correlation so that the treating physician or therapist has in his or her "mind's eye" an idea of the underlying condition of the spinal cord. In addition, it provides essential information for the neuroscientists who seek to "cure" SCI, by describing the disorganized anatomy of the injured spinal cord that they are trying to regenerate, whether it be with stem cells, tissue transplants, or bridges with or without trophic factors, or by other methods. Among the many insights provided by the neuropathological findings is the remarkable fact that, in the majority of human SCI, there is usually some white matter traversing the lesion. This preserved white matter offers a substrate for the restorative neurologist to exploit. For those whose injury is severe enough to cause complete paralysis, the term *discomplete* was introduced to describe lesions that spare enough white matter to allow translesional modulation of motor excitability. Initially greeted with some skepticism, this neuropathological observation from human material supports this concept of discomplete SCI. The contents of this monograph rest upon this foundation provided by the neuropathology. Each chapter has addressed a particular aspect of neurophysiology and restorative neurology, be it basic neuroscience or applied neurophysiology, biological interventions, neurosurgery, or robotics. However, one essential requirement that must be met prior to any of the described treatment methods being applied to the SCI patient is the detailed assessment of the patient's status by brain motor control assessment (BMCA; see Chapter 8).

The spinal cord is part of the central nervous system (CNS), and its neuronal circuitry is essential for motor control. It contains sophisticated mechanisms that in normal individuals carry out complex functions when called upon by other parts of the CNS. When the connections between these neuronal circuits in the spinal cord and the rest of the CNS are damaged by injury, there are essentially only two ways that recovery of function can be achieved: (1) by restoring the precise connections between the severed segments of the spinal cord; (2) by using the existing neuronal circuitry of the spinal cord below the lesion together with the few surviving connections with the brain. This book attempts to provide material to support the novel approach that restorative neurology takes toward spinal cord injury. It proposes and substantiates the idea that, rather than focusing on the deficits and loss of function caused by spinal cord injury, it is more advantageous to elucidate, in each injured individual, the specific functions available, and then to build upon them by designing a protocol that combines intervention and continual assessment in order to optimize its effectiveness and thus improve recovery.

During the second half of the twentieth century and the beginning of this century, progress was made by experimental scientists who explored the possibility of restoring the connections between the disconnected parts of the spinal cord. However, this hard-earned progress was not sufficient to have a serious impact on the treatment of spinal cord injury in humans (Chap. 5). There are serious biological reasons for these difficulties. The connections between different neurons in the adult mammalian CNS are highly specific and ordered, and to remain so, the system has developed mechanisms that protect them from any arbitrary, new, and possibly disorderly connections. It will therefore be difficult to overcome these natural protective mechanisms and to induce regenerative processes. We are left with the second approach—to augment surviving capabilities—and this monograph provides a wealth of information regarding current assessment and restoration methods used in this process. This restorative approach was boosted by the discovery that, in mammals (including humans), the spinal cord contains neuronal circuits referred to as *pattern generators* that can execute complex, repetitive motor tasks. These can be used to generate movement either by activating them by the remaining connections with the brain, or by externally applied stimuli (Chapter 10).

The damage caused by spinal cord injury is unique for each individual. Thus, the first step in designing a protocol for how best to use the preserved functions for restoring coordinated movement has to be an accurate inventory of what is available in that patient. Methods for accurate assessment and evaluation of these remaining functions are therefore key elements in determining the appropriate treatment of each individual. The most up-to-date and imaginative methods to reveal residual motor control that is not seen using conventional neurological examination are presented here in a form that can be used by any therapist with access to modern facilities. Having established the availability of residual motor control within the injured individual, clinical interventions designed to utilize these functions are described and illustrated through examples to show for whom they would be suitable and how they should be applied. Through this process, the "new anatomy" of the injured spinal cord where some connections with the brain are left can often be utilized to promote the recovery of function. These interventions are based on our understanding of motor control, and much of the book has explained the basic principles that guide us in the choice and application of treatment. Moreover, knowledge of the motor control generated by healthy, non-injured individuals and the changes that occur with spinal cord injury, described in this book, allow us not only to use this information to refine the diagnosis, but also to guide the restoration of movement in injured individuals. This, together with advances in the availability of sophisticated electronic devices, will make us able to externally affect the excitability of structures within the CNS, including those in the spinal cord, thus opening new avenues for reestablishing function.

This book illustrates the feasibility of this approach, which uses both invasive and noninvasive methods. Biomedical engineers are making great advances in designing new equipment, complex electrical stimulating devices that, together with feedback mechanisms, can be applied to help reestablish coordinated control of structures such as nerves and muscles below the site of the injury. It is therefore important that these structures be kept in as good condition as possible by preventing changes that follow inactivity and denervation. Procedures that can be successfully applied to this end are part of this monograph, a useful guide to all who are trying to look after individuals with spinal cord injury.

Reconstructive surgery—where the ability of peripheral nerves to support regeneration could provide a useful tool with which to bypass the damaged portion of the spinal cord and connect paralyzed sections of the body directly to the brain—could provide a way to alleviate the loss of function. However, this is still a developing field, and, with time, we will gain a better understanding of the mechanisms that allow the establishment of connections between different parts of the nervous system. Nevertheless, reconstructive surgery, particularly in combination with the imaginative use of electronic devices, is ready to be of use in restorative neurology of spinal cord injury. This does not apply to the advances made in enhancing and utilizing the regenerative capacity of the damaged pathways and loss of cells in the injured spinal cord. Here, the better understanding of the mechanisms that control regeneration, survival of various implanted neurons, and other cells obtained in recent years shows promise, but its application to treatment of the damaged human spinal cord is disappointing. There is a good account of the present state of knowledge on the subject in this monograph, and we hope that it will be useful in the future.

The spinal cord as a part of the CNS that is strongly involved in motor control has capabilities to control body motor function and outside interactions until it is injured and separated, partially or (seldom) even completely, from the brain. This new condition wherein spinal cord motor control is not fully integrated with the rest of the CNS plays a dual role. (1) The spinal cord below the injury is contributing to the clinical picture of spinal cord with altered function and recognized as a clinical syndrome with impaired motor functions. (2) If we look to the injured spinal cord, not as a source of disability, but as a spinal cord with potential motor functions, then clinically and neurophysiologically assessed residual spinal function can be seen as a resource for restoration of movement.

In this book we described principles of *restorative neurology* of the injured spinal cord, and we illustrated through clinical examples how and for whom such practice can be conducted, and outlined assessment and intervention procedures that can help clinicians add the practice of restorative neurology to their approach to chronic spinal cord injury.

In some way, it is paradoxical to capitalize on the injured spinal cord for recovery of neurocontrol of movement if we are under the impression that the person is suffering from injury. However, if we approach spinal cord injuries by assessing functional conditions of spinal cord motor control, then, with additional intervention, we are able to restore functional connections between previously linked hierarchical systems, with partially preserved function. We can then expect to restore motor control with functional outcome, but based on newly established anatomical conductivity and functional outcome.

This clinical practice and ongoing human research in the restorative neurology of spinal cord injury is not a phenomenon of the last few years: actually, such programs have been working for the last 50 years in quite a few different medical centers around the world. The question we should ask is why this approach is not yet more popular when available. A probable explanation is that the knowledge of human neurosciences, and particularly the science of motor control of the injured spinal cord, is not yet widespread, since even widely available human neurophysiology has been more used as a part of diagnostic protocols than for therapeutic interventions.

What can we expect today and tomorrow from the restorative neurology of spinal cord injury? Existing, contemporary equipment for assessment and neurophysiological intervention will definitely help us see that interest in such assessment and treatment become more widespread and be based on the application of human neurosciences in the clinical programs for treatment of spinal cord injury. Moreover, we can expect that development of the neurobiology of the repair of spinal cord injury will become part of restorative neurology, and, as such, be involved in the repair of neurocontrol for movement recovery by closely monitoring the pathophysiology of the spinal cord after injury.

Even with ever-advancing technology, we will always have a significant number of spinal cord injury people. Ultimately, the most successful future will come from prevention of the pathological effects of spinal cord injury. At the same time, we should not neglect the fact that, with neurophysiological monitoring during the acute phase of spinal cord injury, it will be possible to guide treatment using the direct evidence of preserved but impaired complex spinal cord functions. There are numerous practical and biological reasons for preventing the effects of disuse and relieving temporary blocks in conduction and processing within and across the injury zone. Thus, this book on chronic spinal cord injury discusses only motor control and not other problems such as altered sensation and pain. We do expect that neuromonitoring of spinal cord function will become a routine part of clinical programs in medical centers that specialize in the treatment of spinal cord injury.

The most important contribution of this book is that it offers a new perspective. It suggests that any person involved in the care or therapy of people suffering from spinal cord injuries should not focus on establishing observed deficits through the use of methods that ignore, replace, or subjugate surviving capabilities, but instead, concentrate on the most effective use of these residual structures and functions to restore and improve function still further.

Appendix I

A Manual for the Neurophysiological Assessment of Motor Control

The Brain Motor Control Assessment (BMCA) Protocol

W. BARRY McKAY, ARTHUR M. SHERWOOD, AND SIMON F. T. TANG

CONTENTS

1. Introduction
2. Standards for Recording fEMG BMCA Protocols
   2.1. Study Setup
3. Sequence of Motor Tasks (Table I–2)
4. Relaxation
5. Reinforcement Maneuvers
6. Voluntary Movement
7. Passive Stretch
8. Tendon Tap Reflexes
9. Manual Clonus Elicitation
10. Tonic Vibratory Response (TVR)
11. Withdrawal Suppression (Plantar Stimulation Response Suppression—PRS)
12. Optional Segment for All Protocols
13. Sitting and Standing

1. INTRODUCTION

The Brain Motor Control Assessment (BMCA) is a functional electromyography (fEMG) method that records electrical activity from several appropriately selected muscles through surface EMG (sEMG) electrodes during the performance or attempted performance of standard volitional and reflex motor tasks. The method is used to characterize impaired motor control and has a rich history of theoretical and technological development through contributions made by many researchers from laboratories located around the world. Initially designed to confirm paralysis and provide evidence of translesional conduction in severe spinal cord injury (SCI), the BMCA protocol and the analytical tools associated with it have evolved into an objective and quantitative measure of essential motor control components for use in assessing all neurological disorders known to impair motor function.

Protocols have been developed for the assessment of neck, shoulders, arms, hands, trunk, and lower limbs that contain the common components of relaxation, voluntary excitation via reinforcement maneuvers (Jendrassik, etc.) and specific movement tasks, reflex responsiveness, and volitional modification of reflex excitability. The validity and utility of data collected under any of these BMCA protocols depend on adherence to standards that control the technical quality of the recording instrumentation, condition of the skin–electrode interface, rigorous administration of the protocol of motor tasks, and the ability of the examiner to control the recording environment, recognize and control artifactual signals, and manage the understanding and cooperation of the person being tested.

2. STANDARDS FOR RECORDING fEMG BMCA PROTOCOLS

1. The recording instrument specifications must meet published standards for sEMG recording including a minimum bandpass of 10 Hz to 500 Hz with high common mode rejection ratio for differential amplification.
2. The condition of the recording instrument and its settings are confirmed by recording a short segment of calibration into the data file as the first data collected with filter and amplification settings used for the BMCA data collection.
3. The frequency bandpass for BMCA is at least 30 Hz to 500 Hz, and digitizing sample rate is at least 1000 Hz. The frequency composition of sEMG is 10 Hz to 450 Hz (ISEK). Electrode and wire artifacts are found in the lower end of that range and need to be reduced as much as is possible. Therefore, the 30 Hz high-pass setting may be used to stabilize the baseline and reduce such low-frequency artifacts without appreciably diminishing sEMG information content.
4. Display sensitivity is the same for all sEMG channels, 50 μV per display unit. This allows the examiner to perform continuous quality control and to recognize minimal motor unit activation. During recording, it is more important to monitor low-amplitude noise and motor unit activity than the large sEMG patterns.
5. The examination is carried out with the test subject in the supine position on a comfortable examination table or bed. Padding or mattress compliance and bedding must not impede performance of volitional tasks by weak individuals.
6. Electrodes are placed in pairs for differential recording, oriented parallel to the long axis of each muscle, centered on the muscle belly for a standard set

of muscles predetermined by protocol (Table I–1). The wider the spacing, the larger will be the volume of muscle recorded. Some electrodes on the market are manufactured as attached pairs providing consistent spacing. More recently, electrodes with preamplifier circuitry located directly on the electrodes have become available. Such electrodes provide improved performance and eliminate cable-movement artifacts.

7. Skin at the location of the electrodes is prepared to provide intraelectrode impedances of less than 5 KΩ. This preparation is performed by cleaning the skin with alcohol and gentle abrasion using commercially available conductive pastes commonly used in EEG laboratories. "Active" electrodes with built-in pre-amplification require only alcohol cleaning of the skin.
8. Electrodes, regardless of type, must be well-fixed to the skin to minimize movement of their recording surfaces relative to the skin. Such movement generates large high-energy artifacts and low-frequency instability that contaminate the desired signals significantly.
9. Electrodes are connected to the appropriate input channel of the device as specified by the standard protocol. (Polarity, distal electrode into the negative input, is observed when transcranial motor cortex, spinal cord, or peripheral nerve stimulation is to be applied as additional test items to expand beyond the standard volitional and reflex sections of the BMCA protocol.)
10. Connections of electrodes to appropriate channels are confirmed through recording into the data file a short "electrode test" segment in which artifacts are induced in each channel in sequence by mechanically disturbing the electrodes (Figure I–1). It may be necessary to reduce the high-pass filter setting to allow this relatively low-frequency artifact to be registered. The high-pass filter setting must be restored before continuing data collection.
11. Data signal quality is monitored throughout the recording, and artifacts such as those radiated by the power-line or that result from electrode failures must be addressed immediately whenever encountered (Figure I-2).
12. The data acquisition is continuous and stored in a single recorded file. It starts from testing the electrodes (item #9 above) and continues until the end of the protocol of tasks as determined by standard protocol (Table I–2).
13. Annotations are placed into the record throughout the recording to label protocol tasks and describe extra-protocol events.
14. An audible and/or visible (for use in hearing-impaired subjects) cue, operated by a button held by the examiner, is tested, and the subject's ability to hear or see the tone or light is confirmed before beginning the examination. This cue is also recorded as an event marker in the data file.
15. All protocols begin with quiet relaxation for five minutes in the supine position. For expanded protocols described later, when in the upright suspended position, five minutes are also recorded; but for sitting or standing-unsupported protocols, only one minute is required.
16. Subjects are carefully instructed using recommended scripts and encouraged to make their best effort. Instructions and tasks can be

repeated as necessary to acquire the minimum number of "best-effort" trials specified for the particular protocol segment being presented, usually three trials. The examiner must remain vigilant and confirm that the instructions are understood by the test subject and provide re-instruction when judged necessary.

17. A brief cue (tone or light) and event mark is given to begin and end the five-minute relaxation section for data reduction and analysis purposes.
18. *Reinforcement* tasks are cued with a three-second tone/light. *For this and subsequent sections of the recording, complete sEMG silence is obtained or 30 seconds is allowed to pass before tasks are repeated or a new task is begun (referred to as the "relaxation standard").* This section requires that three repetitions, separated by a minimum of five seconds each, be performed for each task.
19. *Voluntary* movement tasks are cued and marked with a five-second tone/light for each phase of the movement. The relaxation standard is observed, and three "best-effort" trials are recorded for each voluntary task.
20. *Passive* movements are individually denoted with a brief mark at the beginning and end of each phase but are not audibly or visually cued. The relaxation standard is observed, and three repetitions of each task are recorded. It may be necessary to repeat the relaxation instructions. Tasks should be repeated, with re-instruction, if the examiner perceives assistance during the movement.
21. *Tendon taps* are delivered manually at approximately one per second, 10 times, for each location examined. The relaxation standard applies.
22. Attempts to manually elicit *clonus* are repeated three times for each joint tested, and the relaxation standard is observed.
23. *Vibration* is delivered for 30 seconds to each site tested, and the relaxation standard applies.
24. *Plantar stimulation* is delivered using the handle of the tendon tap hammer to perform the J-shaped stroke used to elicit Babinski's sign. The handle tip is moved along the plantar surface, beginning on the heel, up toward the toes, and across the ball of the foot. Three trials are performed on each side. The series is then repeated after instructing the subject to suppress the response by enforced relaxation, not stiffening, of the limbs.
25. *Additional segments can be added to the end of this protocol to examine specific stimulus-related responses, control of sitting, standing, and walking, or other questions of interest to the clinician or clinical researcher.*
26. Following any additional protocol segments, the electrodes are removed and the skin is cleaned of conductive paste and examined for irritation. Irritated skin should be treated with antibiotic ointment.

Adherence to these principles and standards allows the calculated parameter values obtained to be reliably compared across repeated BMCA sessions in the same person, across populations of persons with similar diagnoses, across populations of different diagnoses, and across laboratories with different examiners in different geographic locations.

Appendix Table I–1 Example of 16-Channel sEMG Montages for Examining Motor Control in the Upper Limbs, Trunk, and Lower Limbs

Channels	SIDE	MUSCLES		
		Upper Limbs	**Trunk**	**Lower Limbs**
1	RIGHT	Upper Trapezius	Upper Trapezius	Quadriceps
2		Biceps Brachii	Pectoralis Major	Hip Adductor
3		Triceps Brachii	Latissimus Dorsi	Medial Hamstring
4		Wrist Flexors	Intercostal	Tibialis Anterior
5		Wrist Extensors	Rectus Abdominis (para-umbilical)	Triceps Surae
6		Adductor Pol Brevis	External Oblique	Extensor Digitorum Brevis
7		Adductor Dig Quinti	Paraspinal (T12)	Short Toe Flexors
8	LEFT	Upper Trapezius	Upper Trapezius	Quadriceps
9		Biceps Brachii	Pectoralis Major	Hip Adductor
10		Triceps Brachii	Latissimus Dorsi	Medial Hamstring
11		Wrist Flexors	Intercostal	Tibialis Anterior
12		Wrist Extensors	Rectus Abdominis (para-umbilical)	Triceps Surae
13		Adductor Pol Brevis	External Oblique	Extensor Digitorum Brevis
14		Adductor Dig Quinti	Paraspinal (T12)	Short Toe Flexors
15		Open/spare	Open/spare	Open/spare
16		Event Marker	Event Marker	Event Marker

2.1. Study Setup

The key to a good recording of surface EMG is the proper preparation of the skin during the placement of electrodes. When using passive electrodes, it is always necessary to clean with alcohol and slightly abrade the skin under the electrodes in order to reach an impedance of 5 KΩ or less between electrodes as is the standard for electroencephalographic (EEG) testing. Otherwise, recorded signals will be contaminated by electrical fields from power lines and electrical devices (Figure I–2). When using active electrodes with pre-amplifiers built into the electrode, simply cleaning with alcohol should be adequate.

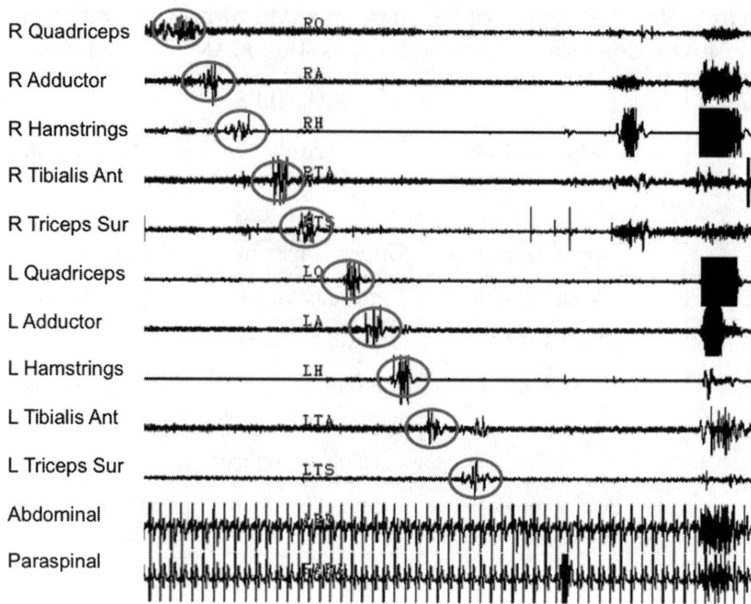

Appendix Figure I–1 Verification of sEMG channels and marking channels. Note that this "stripchart" display confirms that electrodes are properly connected to the instrument by recording the movement artifact sequentially induced in each channel by tapping the electrodes with amplifier low-pass filters set to allow such artifacts to pass.

Figure I–1 shows a typical lower-limb recording "stripchart" display of the brief setup segment for electrode testing, with filters set to allow lower-frequency, approximately 1 Hz, movement artifacts to pass. This stripchart display will be used throughout this manual to prepare the reader to recognize electrophysiological patterns in the form in which they will appear during a typical recording session. It is also important to test the manual event marker(s) used by the examiner to both cue the subject and mark points in the recording that will be needed for use by the computer data-reduction software. The examiner must also confirm that the subject can perceive the cuing tone. A visual cue such as a light placed in the visual field of the subject can be substituted for the auditory tone. Any movement-sensors or video recordings should also be verified during this setup section of the BMCA. Once all signals have been verified, the sEMG channel filter settings should be set to 30 Hz to 500 Hz and the subject instructed for the beginning of the examination section of the protocol. The 30 Hz high-pass setting will greatly reduce the movement artifacts recorded during the BMCA examination. If it does not, electrode fixation and wire movement must be examined and controlled. The minimum computer analog-to-digital conversion sampling rate should be 1 KHz to fully represent the 500 Hz band-pass setting on the amplifiers.

Artifact identification and annotation should be carefully performed throughout the recording session. Figure I–2 illustrates the second of the two most common artifacts encountered during the BMCA session. Since the BMCA is often expected to recognize very low sEMG signal levels, 5 μV minimum, such artifacts must be

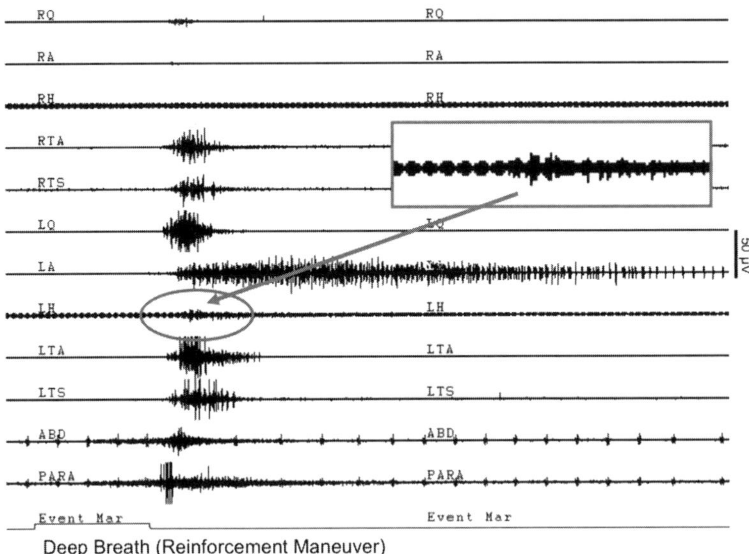

Appendix Figure I–2 High-impedance electrode pairs pick up radiated power-line interference that can make recognition and quantification of the signal difficult. The event mark denotes the three-second tone used to "cue" the subject. The left hamstring muscle shows such an artifact illustrating the effect on sEMG recognition in the enlarged inset. As with Figure I–1 and for subsequent figures, illustrations were taken from a "scrolling stripchart" display acquired as they appeared during recording, and channel abbreviations are: Right (R) and Left (L) Quadriceps (Q), Adductor (A), Hamstring (H), Tibialis Anterior (TA) and Triceps Surae (TS) along with para-umbilical Rectus Abdominis (ABD) and bilateral T12 Paraspinal (PARA).

controlled. They are usually caused by high-impedance electrode pairs that will pick up radiated power-line and other electrical interference. Other sources may be the location of sEMG signal-carrying cables being too close to power cables. Other sources include powered hospital beds or examination tables. Often, disconnecting such items and other unused electrical devices from power during the recording session is all that is needed to remove these artifacts. A final source can be fluorescent lighting, under some conditions. However, properly prepared electrode impedances should not pick up power-line artifacts from the room lighting unless there are electrical faults in its circuitry. The preceding technical standards for instrumentation setup and record-verification insure that, whatever instrumentation is used to record the BMCA, all inter- and intra-individual differences in motor control patterns recorded are of physiological and not technological origin.

For the core protocol, all maneuvers are attempted in the supine position and repeated three times each. Examiners should be trained to recognize and eliminate artifacts that can and do appear during the recording session. They should also learn to make proper annotations that label event marks and describe extra-protocol events that may occur. It is those annotations that allow anomalous data to be properly interpreted in post-study data reduction and analysis.

Appendix Table I–2 Motor Task Sequence Protocols for Upper Limb, Trunk and Lower Limb Motor Control Assessment

	Protocol		
	Upper Limb	**Trunk**	**Lower Limb**
	Supine position		
	Electrode test		
Relaxation	**5 minutes**		
Reinforcement	Deep breath		
	Neck flexion against resistance		
	Jendrassik		
	Bilateral shoulder shrug		
Voluntary	Unilateral elbow flexion and extension hand pronated	Voluntary cough	Bilateral hip and knee flexion and extension
	Unilateral wrist extension hand pronated	Maximum inspiration (blocked airway - pressure gauge)	Unilateral hip and knee flexion and extension
	Unilateral wrist flexion hand supinated	Maximum expiration (blocked airway—pressure gauge)	Bilateral ankle dorsi- and plantar flexion
	Unilateral grip and release	Unilateral shoulder abduction and adduction	Unilateral ankle dorsi- and plantar flexion
		Unilateral elbow flexion and extension	
		Bilateral hip and knee flexion and extension	
		Unilateral hip and knee flexion and extension	
Passive	Unilateral elbow flexion and extension	Unilateral shoulder abduction and adduction	Unilateral hip and knee flexion and extension
	Unilateral wrist extension hand pronated	Unilateral elbow flexion and extension	Unilateral ankle dorsi- and plantar flexion

Appendix Table I–2 (Continued)

	Protocol		
	Upper Limb	**Trunk**	**Lower Limb**
	Unilateral wrist flexion hand supinated	Unilateral hip and knee flexion and extension	
Tendon taps	Biceps brachii		Quadriceps (Patellar)
	Triceps brachii		Triceps surae (Achilles)
	Wrist extensors		
	Wrist flexors		
Vibration	Biceps brachii		Quadriceps (Patellar)
	Triceps brachii		Triceps surae (Achilles)
	Wrist extensors		
	Wrist flexors		
Clonus	Wrist extension		Quadriceps (Patellar)
			Triceps surae (Achilles)
			Unilateral plantar surface stimulation
			with volitional suppression
		Sitting position—unsupported	
		30 sec Quiet sitting	
		10 sec Lean forward	
		10 sec Lean right	
		10 sec Lean left	
		Standing position—unsupported or supported	
		(Optional)	
		Quiet standing—3 minutes	
		Lean forward—10 seconds	
		Lean right—10 seconds	
		Lean left—10 seconds	
		One step forward (lead right)	
		One step forward (lead left)	
		5 steps (in place, self-paced)	

3. SEQUENCE OF MOTOR TASKS (TABLE I–2)

For all recordings, the protocol sequence begins with five minutes of relaxation in the supine position followed by reinforcement maneuvers, which include deep breath, Jendrassik, and neck flexion against resistance. Next, subjects attempt a series of bilateral and unilateral, single- and multi-joint voluntary movements. Regardless of their ability to accomplish the requested motor task, they should be encouraged to do their best, as sEMG is very sensitive and can record even trace activity. These voluntary tasks were chosen because they are simple to instruct and perform and are common movements performed by everyone during normal activities of daily living. Passive movements are then performed, followed by tendon and vibration reflexes. Attempts are made to manually elicit clonus. This series completes the upper-limb protocol. For lower-limb studies, plantar surface stimulation to elicit cutaneomuscular reflexes is performed and repeated with instructions to relax and suppress the response. At this point, before the study is ended or the subject is brought to the sitting or standing position (trunk protocol), transcranial magnetic or electrical stimulation may be applied as an option to acquire threshold and conduction-time data from the corticospinal system. The standard trunk protocol continues with sitting and standing tasks. Standing tasks may be added to the lower-limb protocol as well. Descriptions of the lower-limb protocol tasks, instructions to test subjects, and examples of typically recorded events follow.

4. RELAXATION

Five minutes of relaxation in the supine position begins and ends with a silent event mark to trigger automated analysis. *The test subject is told: "Please place your arms on your chest and relax. Are you comfortable? Do you need a cover for warmth? Please try to relax to the best of your ability. Try not to fall asleep, but should you do so, it will not be a problem. It is important that you relax and keep any voluntary movement to a minimum until I tell you that the five minutes have elapsed. Do you have any questions? Please begin the relaxation period."* It is important to note that the instructions for the BMCA must be cognitively simple and easily reproduced. However, the instructions may be repeated and rephrased or translated as needed for the test subject to understand and respond to the best of their true ability.

Motor events recorded during the relaxation period are of two basic varieties: episodic and continuous. Episodic events include fasciculation potentials (Figure I–3) and withdrawal-like "spasms" (Figure I–4) that can continue into other segments of the BMCA recording (Figure I–5). The first of these patterns are suggestive of denervation as seen in peripheral nerve injury. This form of background activity is distinct from spasms and other episodic events seen in relaxation, which appear as interference patterns, made up of composite motor unit activity. The occurance of "spasms" or multi-muscle sequenced activation patterns that are not annotated as volitional movements can take the general form of the reinforcement response (Figure I–4). The other such "spasm" that is commonly seen in the relaxation segment presents with a multi-muscle pattern and clinical movement resembling the cutaneomuscular reflex that brings whole-limb flexion (Figure I–5). This event can occur randomly or with great regularity, as if pacemaker timed, as seen in the illustration. When this

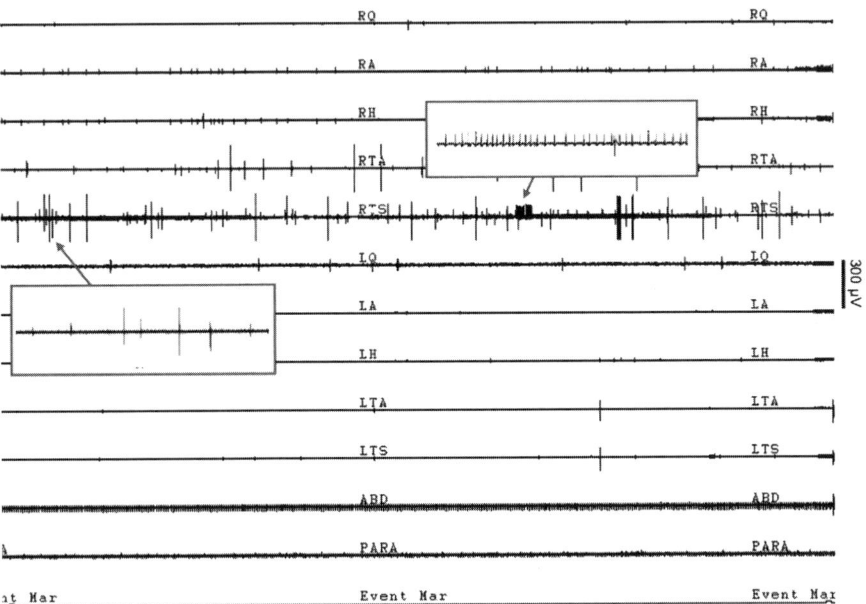

Appendix Figure I–3 Examples of sEMG recording taken from the "scrolling stripchart" display showing the full five minutes of relaxation with time-expanded insets (*boxes*). Although most subjects are able to achieve sEMG silence during the five-minute relaxation period, numerous electrical events can be seen. This stripchart segment was taken from a T12 incomplete SCI subject with a partial cauda equina lesion. The random spontaneous activity seen here is thought to be the surface-recorded version of the denervation potentials seen in needle EMG testing.

pattern is present, the examiner should reposition the subject to change and reduce the peripheral input to the spinal cord that drives the event. These repeating "spasms" can persist beyond the relaxation period and can produce inaccurate results in quantification when not recognized.

5. REINFORCEMENT MANEUVERS

The cuing tone or light and event mark with a preset duration of three seconds is used for this section (Figure I–6). The first instruction given is to wait for the tone before beginning any of the motor tasks. *The test subject is told: "In a moment, you will hear a tone (or see a light). When you do, please take a deep breath. At the end of the tone blow it out forcefully and relax. Please be sure to wait for the tone before you start and relax after it ends. Do you understand?"* Verbal encouragement from the examiner during reinforcement and voluntary movement attempts is appropriate, especially if there is no sEMG activity seen. If errors are made that suggest inadequate understanding of the instructions or cognitive confusion, trials should be repeated with additional instruction. Notes should be entered into the recorded file describing the reason for repeating the trials.

The Relaxation Standard: sEMG channels must achieve complete electrical silence, or 30 seconds is allowed to pass before the next trial or task is begun. It is appropriate

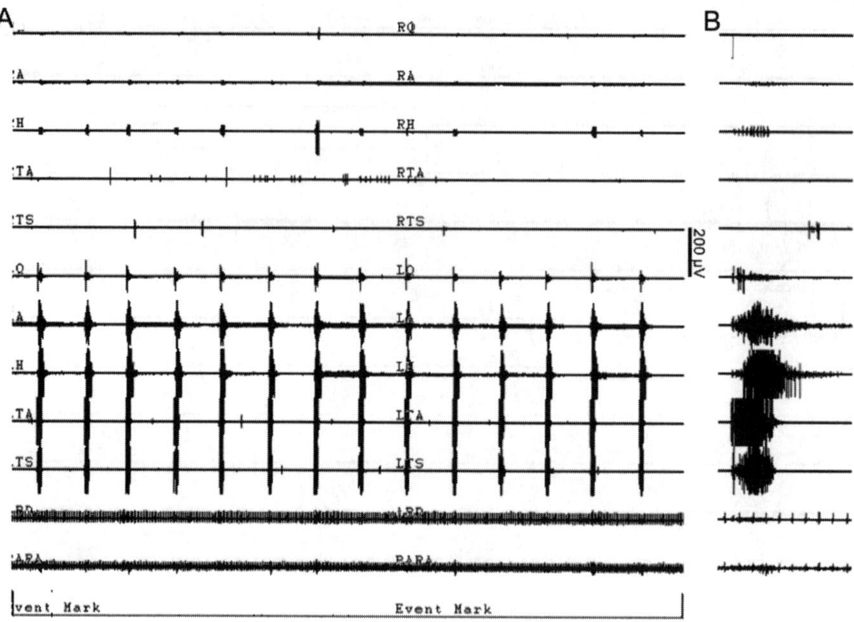

Appendix Figure I–4 Episodic events recorded during the five-minute relaxation period (*A*) can include regularly-repeating flexion events (*B*). Note that the Left Tibialis Anterior (LTA) activates before the Left Hamstrings (LH) helps to produce ankle dorsiflexion and knee flexion. Furthermore, it can be seen that the event "irradiates" to involve muscles of the contralateral limb. Since this pattern resembles the cutaneomuscular reflex seen with plantar surface stimulation, it is important for the examiner to reposition the limbs in an attempt to reduce peripheral input to the spinal cord.

to instruct the test subject to relax, and to be specific about which muscle or muscles need relaxing. For purposes of post-recording data reduction, at least five seconds must pass before another trial is attempted. And each reinforcement maneuver is repeated three times. It is common for these maneuvers to elicit long-lasting activity in many muscles that will appear clinically as flexion and extension spasms.

The other reinforcement maneuvers are: neck flexion against resistance; Jendrassik; and shoulder shrug. Subject instructions are similar. For neck flexion, the subject is asked to lift their head against resistance applied at their forehead by the examiner. To perform the Jendrassik maneuver, the subject is asked to grasp their hands together and pull strongly without releasing their grip. The shoulder shrug maneuver is performed when the test subject "lifts" their shoulders (toward their ears in the supine position). For all of these reinforcement maneuvers, the subject is instructed to begin when they hear the tone and continuing to hold until the tone ends, at three seconds.

The presence of reinforcement task responses in paralyzed individuals is indicative of a "discomplete" lesion in which some long-tract fibers remain functional. In incomplete paralysis or paresis, such responses can indicate other aspects of control, including the impairment of inhibitory control, as responses are absent in neurologically intact people.

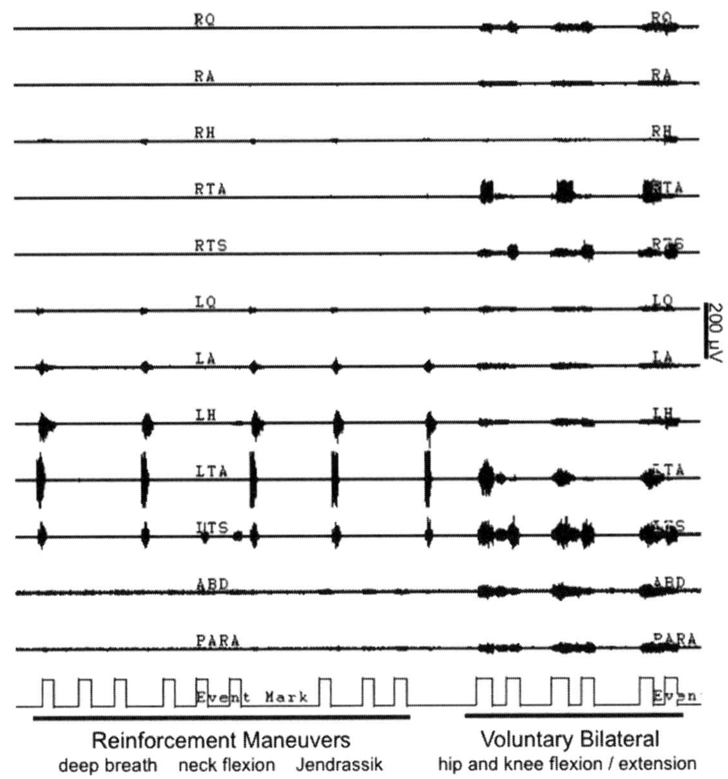

Appendix Figure I–5 Repeating episodic bursts of withdrawal-patterned activity (Figure I–4) continue past the end of relaxation, do not synchronize with reinforcement maneuver attempts, but were suppressed by voluntary movement task attempts. If unrecognized as a spontaneously repeating event, this activity would have been quantified and represented as a response to reinforcement, and if not ended by volitional attempts, would be erroneously counted when analyzing other segments of the recording.

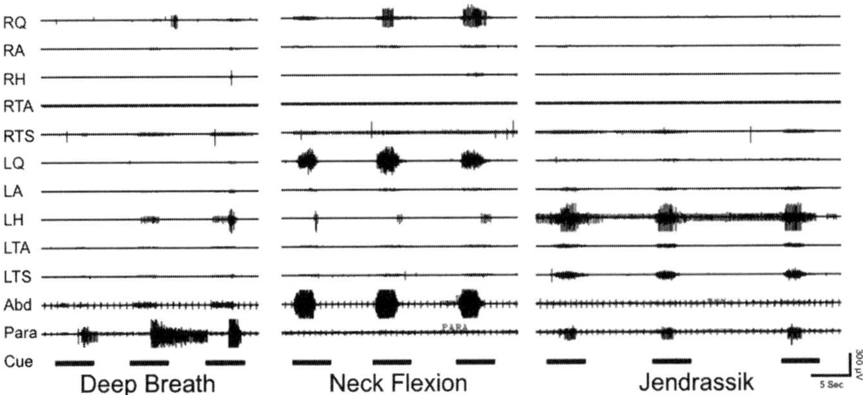

Appendix Figure I–6 Multiple-muscle lower-limb activity, reinforcement maneuver responses (RMR) recorded from a motor-complete chronic spinal cord injured subject. Note that all tasks are performed three times.

6. VOLUNTARY MOVEMENT

Using the same criteria for cuing as with the preceding reinforcement maneuvers, one bilateral and two unilateral voluntary motor tasks are presented (Figure I–7). All voluntary tasks in the BMCA protocol have two phases, flexion and extension, with the first phase held until the cuing tone ends and the second phase and cue presented following a brief pause, less than one second. For this and following manually marked events, both the cuing tone and marker length are controlled by the examiner. This allows the examiner to mark the end of the movement for each phase by releasing the marker button. This also provides feedback to the subject that the hold phase of the two-phase task has been reached. This hold phase duration and the beginning of the second phase of the task can be adjusted by the examiner to allow for different performance speeds while allowing the recorded data to meet processing criteria for analysis window lengths of at least five seconds after a command tone begins. Analysis of this segment of the BMCA quantifies parameters of motor control that include the recruitment rate of the agonist muscle and co-activation of antagonistic and muscles not activated by neurologically intact subjects for the presented tasks.

For the purpose of limiting the length of this manual, only selected representative tasks from the lower-limb protocol will be described from this point onward. Bilateral hip and knee flexion and extension are paired to form the first two-phase task tested. *The test subject is told: "As before, please wait for the tone to begin what will be a series of voluntary movements that we will ask you to attempt. Please try your best even though you may not feel any movement. Remember that we can pick up very small muscle activation. Each movement will be repeated three times, and the first one is to lift both of your knees to your chest, hold them there until you hear second tone, and then push them out straight, and relax when the tone ends. Do you have any questions? All right,* (tone), *lift both of your knees to your chest, hold them there, hold them . . .* (second tone), *push them out straight* (tone ends), *and relax.*" Note that there is no instruction with regard to whether or not to dorsiflex the ankles at the same time as they flex the hips and knees. The analysis of this task allows either strategy to be used.

Again, re-instructing and repeating first trials when instructions appear to have been misunderstood by the subject/patient is recommended. The parallel instruction and tone cue delivery during performance of the task is recommended as it provides encouragement and confirms the task to the subject/patient. The second and third voluntary tasks are unilateral hip and knee flexion and extension, right side three times followed by the left side three times. Ankle dorsiflexion and plantar flexion tasks also begin with a bilateral series and then moves to the right side. *The test subject is told: "With the tone, please pull your toes up, bending only the ankle. Hold that position until you hear the second tone. With the second tone, please push your toes down, and relax when the tone ends."*

Analysis of this section of the BMCA quantifies the co-activation of antagonistic and inappropriate muscles during each of the tasks to characterize the degree of disordered motor control in comparison with healthy subject controls. Movement sensors and video recordings can serve to prove that movement has occurred, and measure the range and rate of movement. However, no standards have been published for such sensors or the analysis of the data they produce. The multi-muscle patterns recorded will range from no spinal motor output as in paralysis, through the

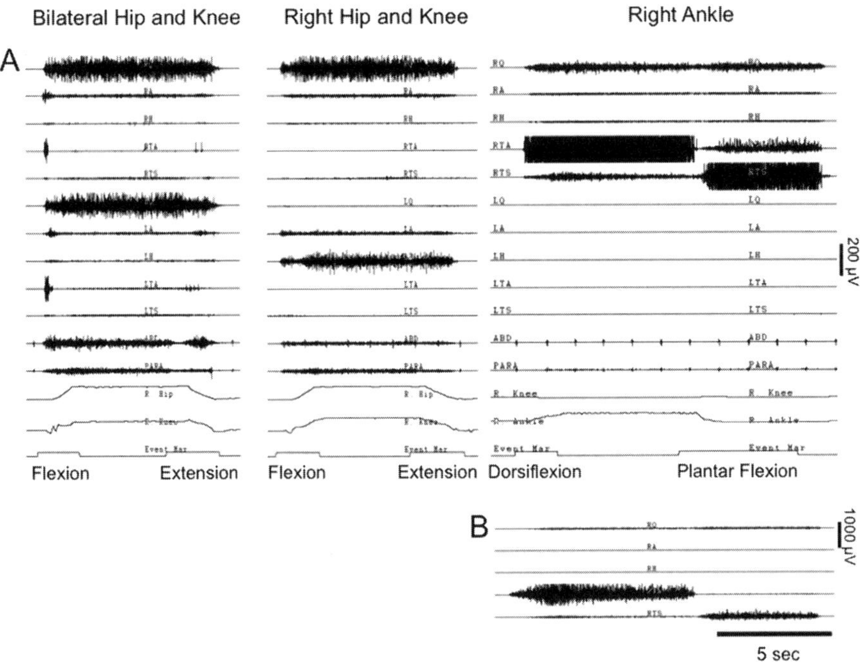

Appendix Figure I–7 Voluntary motor tasks performed by a healthy subject. (*A*) Bilateral and unilateral hip and knee flexion and extension and unilateral ankle dorsi- and plantar flexion showing the typical multi-muscle patterns recorded for these simple, self-paced motor tasks. (*B*) Decreased amplification shows the envelope shape of the agonist muscle for the ankle dorsal and plantar flexion tasks. During the recording session, a sensitive display is maintained to monitor recording quality changes and recognize low-amplitude events.

co-activation of multiple muscles antagonistic or usually uninvolved in performing the requested motor task (Figure I–8), to properly sequenced reciprocal activation needed for controlled single- and multi-joint movement (Figure I–9). However, in contrast to neurologically intact subjects who perform these voluntary tasks by producing multi-muscle patterns that are quite similar across trials and individuals, patients present for testing with relatively individualized degrees of disrupted motor control and wide variety of multi-muscle patterns. However, even in those with damaged control, patterns for each task should be quite similar to oneanother across three trials within each individual (Figure I–10).

7. PASSIVE STRETCH

At this point in the recording, the cuing tone is turned off. Silent event-marking will be used for the remainder of the protocol. The unilateral motor tasks presented in the previous segment of the BMCA protocol are repeated passively. Again, three trials of each task are collected in the same sequence as above. *The test subject is told: "Please relax as completely as you can and allow me to do all of the work. I am going to move*

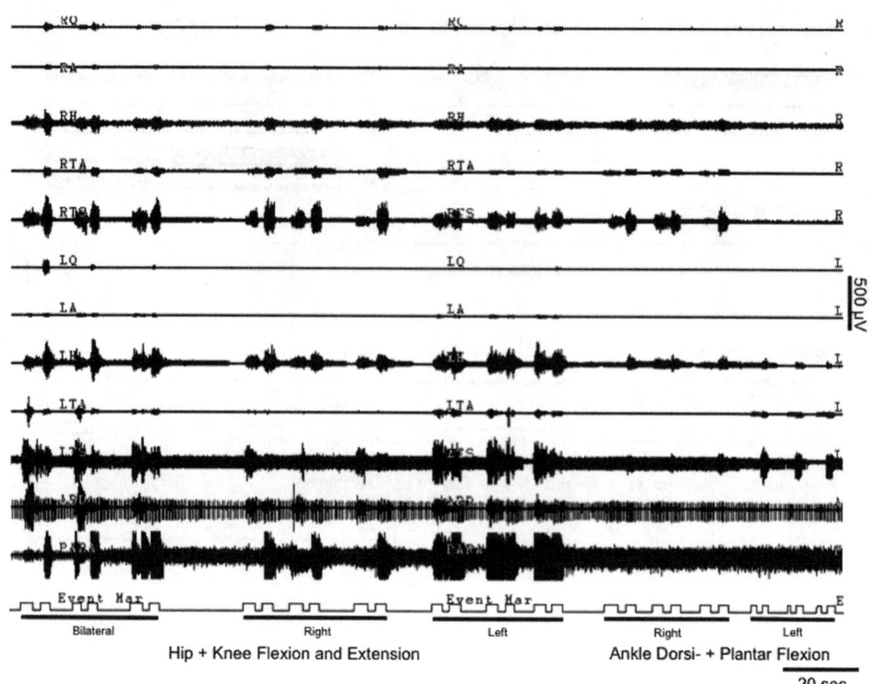

Appendix Figure I–8 Nearly four minutes of stripchart display showing the voluntary motor task segment of a BMCA recorded from a C5 AIS-C SCI subject. Seen is the typical lower amplitude sEMG and lack of appropriate multi-muscle patterning characteristic of altered motor control. Note the generally similar patterns recorded for the very different motor tasks attempted. Also, background activity seen here was verified during the recording to be sEMG. This individual was clinically spastic, showing dystonia-like continuous activity and considerable co-activation of inappropriate muscles for each of the tasks.

your legs through the same movements you did or attempted a few minutes ago." Touch of the leg can bring activation of spasm activity in many patient categories, so the BMCA standards include waiting after the initial touch while monitoring the sEMG for a response. If a response occurs, it must dissipate before the trial can begin. Also, if the examiner perceives "help" from the subject, re-instruction and retrial is necessary, but only for the first trial of each task. Again, it is important to achieve sEMG silence between trials and the two phases of each task.

In persons with altered motor control, passive stretch can elicit spinal motor output patterns that range from activation of the muscle stretched to complex combinations of muscles (Figure I–11). Healthy subjects are able to relax completely and suppress spinal motor output during this passive manipulation (Figure I–12). If activity is recorded during this section in healthy subjects, it can take the spatiotemporal pattern of voluntary activation assisting with the task. The examiner will perceive assistance with the movement and must re-instruct the subject and repeat. Such a pattern is clinically termed a "shortening response" and is exaggerated and uncontrollable in patients with Parkinson's disease or other movement disorders (Figure I–11), and can occur on the so-called unaffected side in stroke patients.

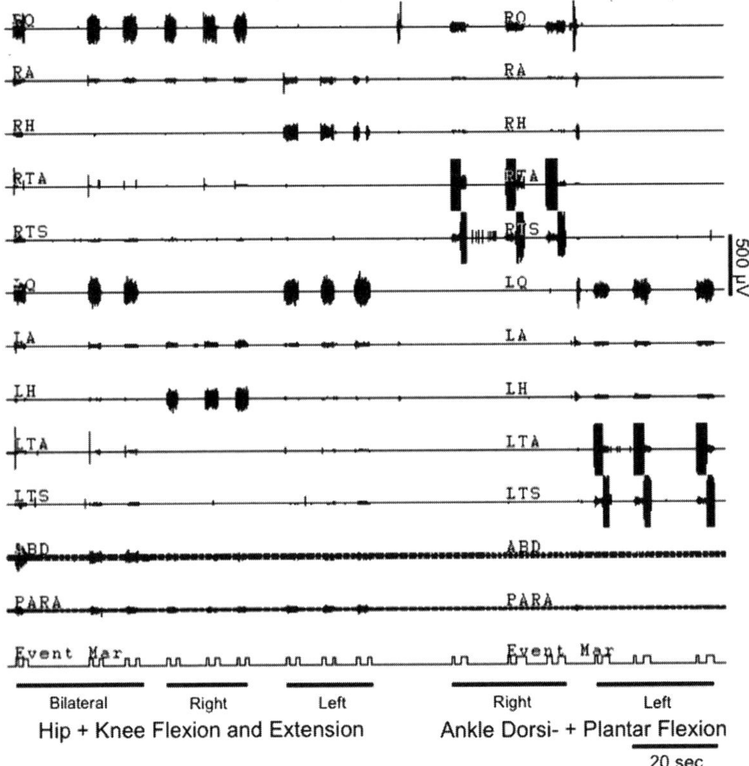

Appendix Figure I–9 Records of all voluntary motor task trials the healthy subject illustrated in the previous Figure I–7—showing three repetitions of for each of the five "paired" tasks. Note the highly repeatable multi-muscle patterns within each task.

8. TENDON TAP REFLEXES

The right and left patellar (lower pole) and Achilles tendons are tapped manually, ten times each at a rate of approximately 1 Hz in the lower-limb protocol. Taps should be delivered by a standard clinical hammer, preferably instrumented with an accelerometer to mark the recording event channel with a pulse of preset amplitude or one that represents its force.

This segment of the protocol confirms the presence of a functioning stretch reflex arc and indicates peripheral nerve sparing. In addition to the elicited t-waves, after-discharge characteristics are recorded from the muscle tapped and other ipsilateral and contralateral muscles (Figure I–13). Irradiation to other muscles and the presence of after-discharging are uncommon in neurologically intact subjects.

9. MANUAL CLONUS ELICITATION

The subject is instructed to relax before three attempts to manually elicit patellar and Achilles clonus are made with manual event-marking held for the duration of any clonic response (8 Hz to 13 Hz) that may appear (Figure I–14). Once elicited, the

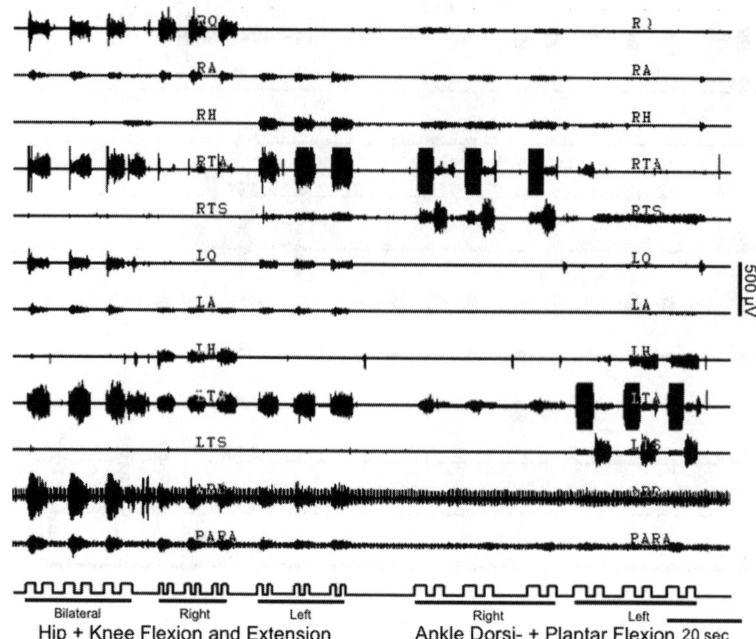

Appendix Figure I–10 sEMG activity during three minutes of standard BMCA voluntary movement tasks taken from an AIS-D subject (ASIA Impairment Scale) whose main motor control finding was asymmetrical hip and knee control. Note that more muscles, spinal motor nuclei, are activated by the attempts in this incomplete SCI example than in healthy subjects (*previous figure*).

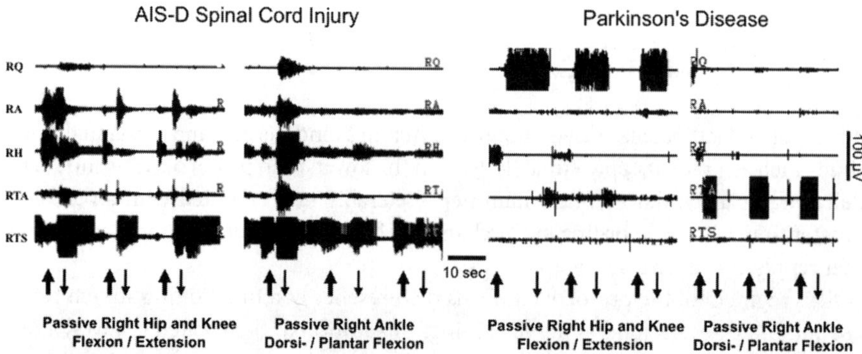

Appendix Figure I–11 Passive flexion (*up arrow*) and extension (*down arrow*) movements elicit complex "stretch" responses from subjects with incomplete SCI (*left*) and "shortening" responses from a person with Parkinson's disease (*right*). Note that more than the muscle stretched activates with passive movement in the AIS-D SCI subject on the left. Also, see that continuous, dystonia-like motor unit activity can be seen in both SCI and Parkinson's disease subjects. The Parkinson's disease subject shows the classic "shortening response" in which the muscle stretched remains inactive, but the muscle shortened is activated. Dotted lines are offered as guides for the visualization of repeating patterns to differentiate between stretched-induced and "spontaneous" spinal motor output.

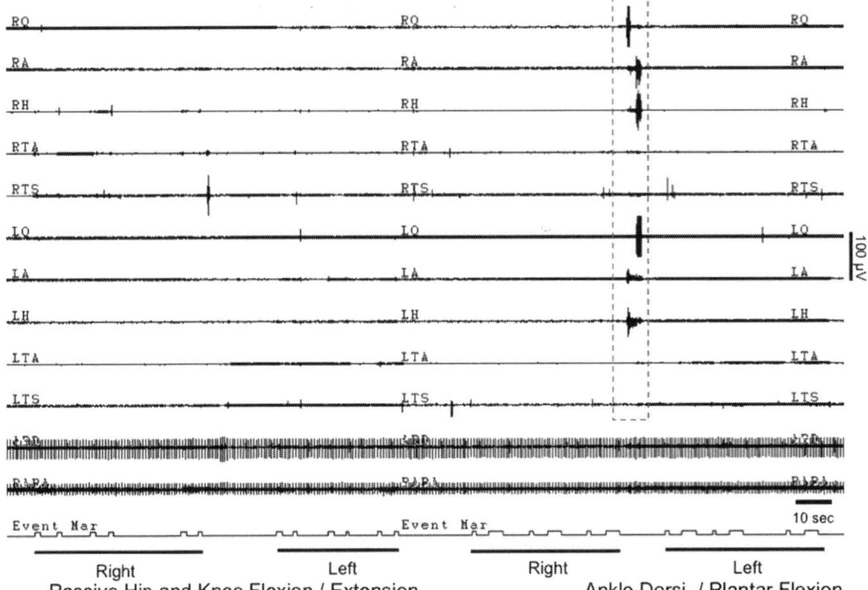

Appendix Figure I–12 Passive movement segment of BMCA performed in a neurologically intact healthy subject. Subject voluntarily moved to adjust position for comfort (*box*). Note the lack of spinal motor response to passive manipulation of the legs. This is typical of healthy subjects. A possible normal variation is low-amplitude spinal motor output to the muscles shortened by the movement.

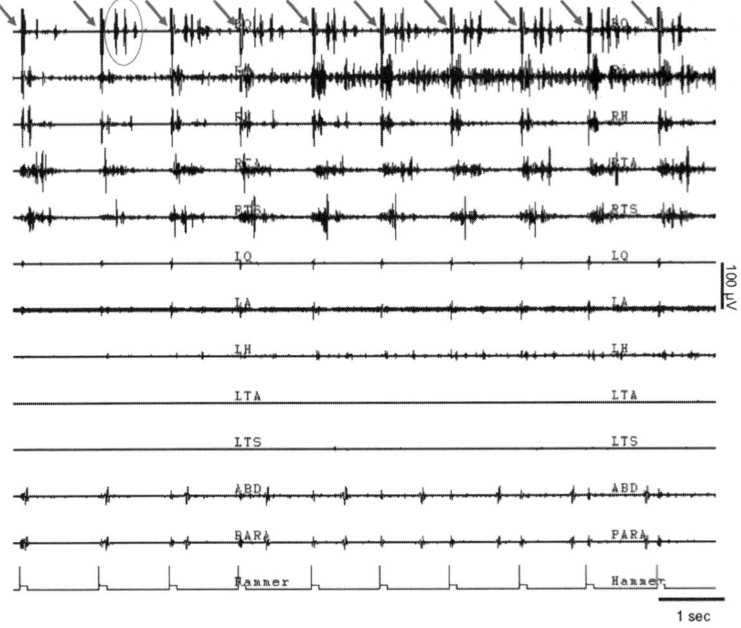

Appendix Figure I–13 Right patellar tendon taps elicited large-amplitude responses that irradiated to ipsilateral distal-muscles and contralateral proximal-muscle spinal motor nuclei. Also present are phasic after-discharge patterns (*circle*).

Appendix Figure I–14 Manually-elicited right ankle clonus in a clinically motor-complete SCI subject showing that there remains some translesional connections that support spinal motor excitability and a repetitive-stretch response.

examiner maintains the stretch for up to 30 seconds if the response persists. When the response lasts 30 seconds, it is considered to be evidence of supraspinal facilitation of the spinal motor neurons in persons who are clinically paralyzed.

10. TONIC VIBRATORY RESPONSE (TVR)

This segment requires the availability of compressed air and a pneumatic vibrator with which to strongly vibrate muscles or tendons. For the lower-limb protocol, the patellar (upper pole) and Achilles tendons are vibrated for 20 seconds each (Figure I–15). Again, instructions to the subject/patient are to relax. The examiner

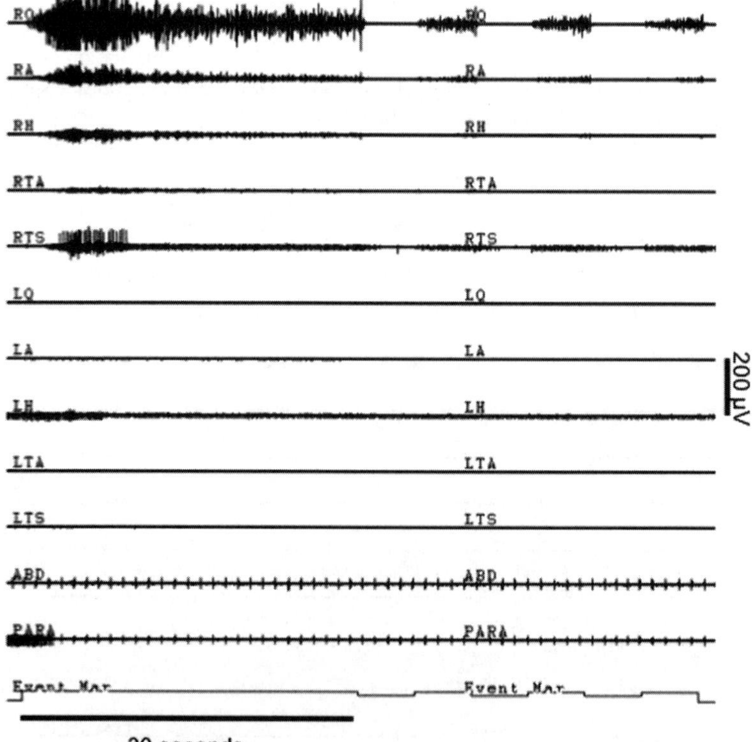

Appendix Figure I–15 Strong vibration to the upper pole of the patellar tendon induced a sustained tonic vibratory response (TVR) in a motor-complete SCI subject. BMCA protocol standards require that five-second periods of on and off vibration follow sustained responses to test habituation. Note the irradiation of activity to other muscles of the same limb.

manually marks the delivery of vibration, or the vibrator can be equipped with a sensor to indicate when it is running. Response duration in the vibrated muscle is used as an indicator of "central state" modification by the brain in the face of clinical paralysis. When the response is absent in the muscle vibrated or disappears before 30 seconds have elapsed, the subject/patient is instructed to perform the Jendrassik reinforcement maneuver as they did earlier in the BMCA.

It should be noted here that the vibrator used for this segment of the BMCA is custom-constructed from a pneumatic hand-grinder fitted with an offset weight and protective barrel that produces 60 Hz to 120 Hz vibration, depending upon driving air pressure. Electrical vibrators have difficulty developing adequate force and always cause artifacts in the sEMG channels.

11. WITHDRAWAL SUPPRESSION (PLANTAR-STIMULATION RESPONSE SUPPRESSION–PRS)

This section of the BMCA protocol is stimulus-response based. It uses the manual stroking of the plantar surface as is done to elicit the classic clinical Babinski sign. The stimulus is delivered with the sharp end of a neurological hammer placed on the heel and drawn along the plantar surface toward the fifth toe, turning and traveling medially across the ball of the foot. For three trials on each side, the test subject is instructed to relax and allow the leg to jump, should it do so. Rate of stimulus delivery is determined by background activity and requires at least five seconds between trials. After three trials on each side, *the test subject is told: "Relax to prevent the leg from jumping. Do not tense as if to oppose the response but rather relax to prevent it."* This parameter, the ability to actively inhibit spinal reflex response, is another indicator of residual brain influence over the central state of excitability in paralyzed persons (Figure I–16).

12. OPTIONAL SEGMENT FOR ALL PROTOCOLS

Transcranial magnetic stimulation (TMS) of the motor cortex to elicit a motor evoked response (MEP) can be used to assess threshold and conduction times within the corticospinal system. The best results are obtained in the supine position, because sitting (even reclining) or standing increases the resting excitability of the system. Important information obtained includes the threshold or minimum stimulus strength at which a response can be elicited. Also, the conduction time from the motor cortex to the muscle can be measured. MEPs can be obtained from all skeletal muscles in neurologically intact subjects. Delayed or high-threshold responses are indicative of damage to the corticospinal system. In neurologically intact persons, TMS is usually not considered to be uncomfortable at motor threshold levels. However, a caution must be issued here: stimuli will become uncomfortable at some intensity in all people with clinically complete or incomplete paralysis.

For lower limb muscles, TMS is delivered through a 110-degree double-cone coil (9 cm diameter each). For the upper limb muscles, a flat 9 cm diameter coil is used. In both cases, they are placed centered over the scalp vertex (Cz using the International 10–20 system for EEG electrode placement). The dual-cone coil is oriented so that

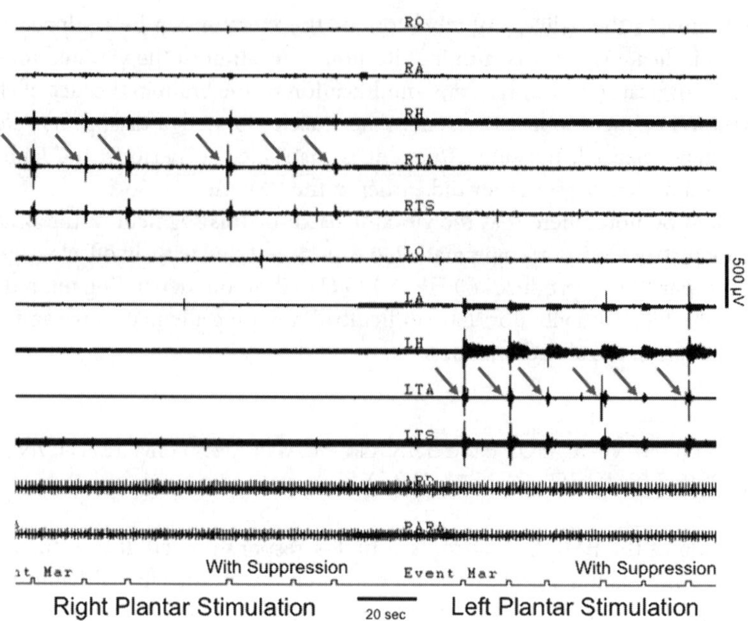

Appendix Figure I–16 Right and left plantar-stimulation withdrawal reflex response in a spinal cord injured individual during three repetitions without, and then with, instructions to suppress movement through relaxation. Note the asymmetry in the number of muscles activated and their amplitude of activation. The plantar response suppression (PRS) marker of incompleteness is present but better on the right than the left in this AIS-D example.

current flow inside the brain is counterclockwise in the left hemisphere and clockwise in the right hemisphere. The posterior-to-anterior current flow from the two coils overlaps in the region of the lower limb muscle representations of the motor cortex. For upper-limb muscles, the flat coil will produce high flux density at its edge, which is over the motor cortex hand representations for the right and left hemispheres. As with other segments of the BMCA protocol, pre-stimulus relaxation is required. The process begins with single pulses at minimum stimulator output. Each intensity is tested three times. In paralyzed persons, a paired-pulse paradigm using an inter-stimulus interval of 15 msec to 25 msec may be required (Figure I–17). Stimulus intensity is advanced in 10% increments until maximum single-pulse output is reached. If MEPs are not observed by the examiner, the second stimulus is added, beginning again at 40% for both stimulators. Both pulses are increased together until all recorded muscles respond or maximum stimulator output is reached. The delivery of single or paired stimuli must be separate by at least five seconds.

Finally, to complete the TMS section of the protocol, voluntary activation against a 2 kgm load will increase the MEP amplitude in those with incomplete lesions and allow the recording of TMS-induced silent periods under standard conditions. Stimulus intensity will be threshold, determined earlier, plus 10% of stimulus output. The duration of the silent period has been linked to corticospinal system dysfunction and can be used as an indicator of recovery.

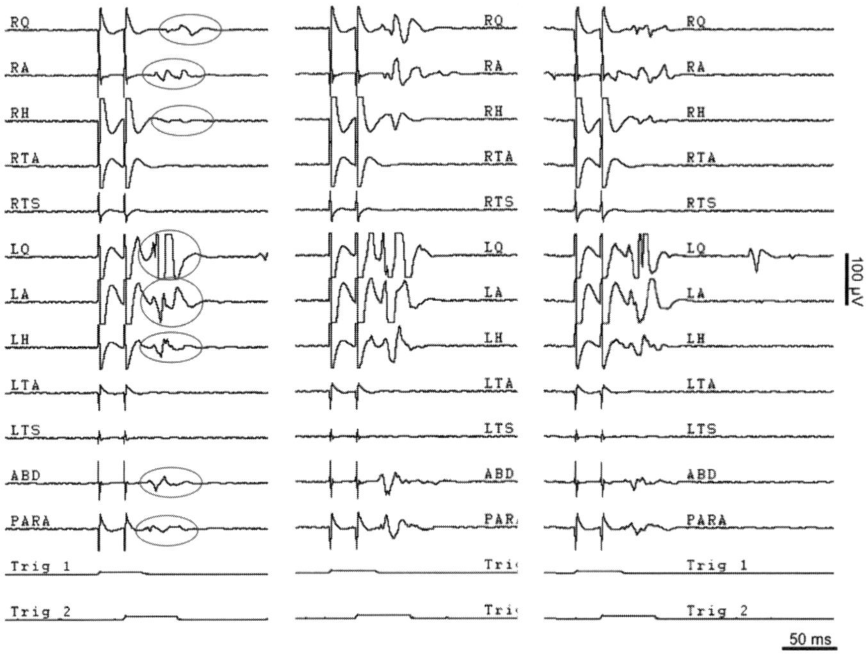

Appendix Figure I–17 Examples of records during three repetitions of paired-pulse transcranial magnetic motor cortex stimulation (TMS). Display scale should be adequate to recognize a 5 μV p/p response. Single-pulse stimulation was not adequate to evoke motor evoked potentials; however, paired pulses with 25 ms inter-stimulus interval successfully elicit motor evoked potentials (MEPs) in the right and left quadriceps, adductor, and hamstrings muscles (*circled*). Also note the MEPs in the abdominal and paraspinal muscles. This AIS-D individual was capable of voluntary hip and knee flexion and extension but could not voluntarily move either ankle.

13. SITTING AND STANDING

The standard trunk protocol includes sitting and standing sections in which 30 seconds of quiet sitting and three minutes of quiet standing are followed by 10-second periods of leaning forward, back, right, and left. When standing, gait initiation and stepping in place are recorded. All of these tasks are cued with beginning and ending tones and event marks and are repeated three times each. Analysis of these segments is focused on asymmetrical activation of muscles, slow or absent responses to position changes, and instability within the multi-muscle activation patterns. Initiation of gait and stepping provide insight into the control of sequenced activation within multi-muscle patterns.

Data collection is ended with the removal of electrodes, cleaning of the skin, examination for skin irritation, and treatment of any irritation with antibiotic ointment. The examiner should express gratitude to the subject for their cooperation and explain to them how they may obtain results from the testing. Different laboratories have different policies regarding who may tell patients the results of testing that must be observed. Regardless, the subject should be told that quantitative results will only be available after some time for analysis.

Appendix II

Academic Environment for the Development of Human Motor Control in Ljubljana

ZVONKA ZUPANIČ SLAVEC

CONTENTS

1. The Beginnings of Neurophysiology in the World
2. The Beginnings of Neurophysiology in Slovenia
3. Promoters of Neurophysiology among Slovenes
4. Milan R. Dimitrijević
5. Dr. Janez Faganel (1943–1984) and Faganel's Memorial Meetings
6. Conclusion
References

1. THE BEGINNINGS OF NEUROPHYSIOLOGY IN THE WORLD

Neurophysiology started to develop in the twentieth century, when the human nervous system could be observed without damage to the health of the patient. The beginnings of clinical neurophysiology go back to before World War II, when electrophysiological methods began to spread from zoophysiology laboratories to the clinical environment. Individual investigation methods were first developed separately. By electroencephalographs (EEG) it was possible to perceive very low waves generated in the human brain. With electromyography (EMG) it became possible to detect electrical activity in muscles. And with the use of electronic computers, the weakest responses to visual, auditory, and tactile stimuli can now be perceived, by *sensory encephalography* (Janko, 1991).

Clinical electroencephalography was initially developed in the context of neurology and psychiatry. The first data on human EEG activity were published in 1935, which rapidly increased the number of academic and clinical researchers of the central nervous system (Wallace, 2002). In 1949 they began to study children with epilepsy and in 1951 started the brain operation for epilepsy. Research was conducted primarily in conjunction with EEG. In 1957, they developed the first intraoperative

EEG recording of the carotid artery, and in 1965, they recorded the first EEG during flight through space.

Electromyography (EMG) was the first established clinical pathway in physical and rehabilitation medicine, and its main function was examining the actions of individual muscles in normal and pathological movements. The importance of EMG today is mostly in a rehabilitation setting, where the functional aspect of the study of movement disorders is very important for the treatment of disabled persons. In the context of a more focused diagnostic clinical neurology, such use of EMG was not established as it was not contributing to a better diagnosis of neurological diseases. In the field of neurology, other electrophysiological investigation techniques were developed, which have demonstrated their diagnostic utility and have been indispensable in daily clinical work, especially in the diagnosis of diseases and injuries of peripheral nerves and muscles: for example, the analysis of potentials of motor units with a coaxial needle electrode; measuring peripheral nerve conductive velocity; micro-electromyography; analysis of neuromuscular transmission; electroneurography.

Clinical neurophysiology began its development in Scandinavia and then spread throughout Europe. Combining methods and laboratories in the new discipline has strengthened the development of test methods, with increased detection and irritation so as to increase the excitability and conductivity of the central nervous system. Clinical neurophysiology and its development of test methods made a huge step toward improving identification of neurological disorders, their nature and their location. The instrumental diagnostic investigations may diagnose important functional nervous system disorders that do not cause symptoms or clinical signs of impairment. "Therefore not only clinical and anatomical diagnosis is important, it is also important to evaluate the type and severity of functional impairment accurately, reliably, and quantitatively" (Gregorič, 1994).

Investigative techniques of clinical neurophysiology are useful in clinical diagnosis, localization of impairment, detection of clinically silent defects, monitoring of disease progress and recovery, and evaluation of treatment effect. Of particular importance is the detection of nerve damage in the early periods of acute illness or traumatic injuries with the neurophysiological investigations when the patient can not participate in the investigation. At that time the clinical picture is still unclear. In patients with brain damage, somatosensory evoked potentials may be used to determine the degree to which the central nervous system is affected, specific areas of disability, and a prognosis of functional performance. Multiple sclerosis is one of the diseases studied by this technique.

Motor impairments are the most obvious and can be detected in a general examination. They can be confirmed with electromyographic survey. Because of this, sensory neurology remained in the shadow of a more developed and already established "motor" neurophysiology for a long time. One part of the sensory investigation was established by the development of evoked responses. There are many disorders that affect hearing, smell, sight, taste, and touch. With appropriate devices, which are the input of the successful development of neurophysiology, it is possible to document these changes and to follow the deterioration or improvement of the affected sense through the course of therapy. On the other hand, on the basis of these studies it is possible to determine the correct diagnosis of the disease and consequently to define the proper treatment. Also, Slovenian neurophysiology has already employed a few methods for the quantitative evaluation of perception. Such an assessment allows the alert investigator with sufficient knowledge of sensory physiology to assess reliably the perception and evaluation of abnormal operation.

Technological developments over the past two decades have improved equipment and meters exploring the brain and spinal cord. There are many opportunities to improve these devices. Scientists are trying to make a noninvasive apparatus that would measure action potentials of even a single neuron in a randomly selected part of the brain, which is perhaps impossible now, but will no doubt be successful in the future.

2. THE BEGINNINGS OF NEUROPHYSIOLOGY IN SLOVENIA

The basis of Slovenian neurophysiology was established in 1947 when Aleš Strojnik, at that time an assistant at the Institute of Physics, Faculty of Medicine, made the first electroencephalograph (Strojnik, 1947). Clinical electroencephalography in Slovenia, however, started at the Pediatric Clinic in Ljubljana, which received a commercial electroencephalograph in 1954. The machine was entrusted to child neurologist Professor Jože Jeras (born 1920) (Jeras, 1973). The initial interest in the new profession of neurophysiology was triggered by the first postwar teachers at the Ljubljana School of Medicine; some among them were erudite and cosmopolitan, open to innovation, capable of unconventional thinking. Unencumbered by the knowledge of that time, they were able to look at things from other angles, and that way develop their work, which brought different and new results. These led to new trends in neurophysiology and gave new perspectives on it. Among the individuals of the Ljubljana Faculty of Medicine who influenced the development of neurophysiology in Ljubljana with their ideas were: Professor of Physiology, biologist and chemist Albin Seliškar (1896–1973); Professor of Biology, biologist and physician Hubert Pehani (1900–1994); Professor of Pathological Physiology, physician Andrej O. Župančič (1916–2007); and Medical Professors of Neurology and Neuropsychiatry Janez Plečnik (1875–1940), Alfred Šerko (1889–1938), Ivan Robida (1871–1941), and Ivan Marinčič (1892–1970) (Prevec & Vodušek, 1994).

3. PROMOTERS OF NEUROPHYSIOLOGY AMONG SLOVENES

Professor Alfred Šerko (1889–1938), B.Sc., a philosopher and physician, was among the founders of the Ljubljana Faculty of Medicine, the first professor of anatomy and physiology of the nervous system, a philosopher, physician, and free thinker. As a humanist and natural scientist, he contributed significantly to the development of the first Medical Faculty of Ljubljana, founded in 1919, and influenced its first teachers. He acquired his philosophical and psychological knowledge and his knowledge of logic from the most prestigious teachers of that time in Vienna (promoted 1904) with Professor Richard von Krafft-Ebing (1840–1902), who studied the border fields of psychiatry—forensics and sexual psychopathology, and Sigmund Freud (1856–1939), who had a significant impact on Šerko's development. In Vienna, he enrolled also in the Medical School and completed his studies in 1909 (Felc, 2003). Then he went to Munich to study under Emil Kraepelin (1856–1926), a professor of clinical psychiatry who was a pioneer in experimental psychiatry. Here Šerko was involved in differential diagnosis of paranoid states, and he gathered hundreds of inventories of paranoid psychosis in different psychiatric hospitals in Bavaria. As a result of this study, he settled the naming of paranoid psychoses, and in 1912 he published the first discussion about it. By this time he had completed his system of psychosis disorders and set up a new medical unit of paraphrenia. After that he went to work in Vienna and became an assistant (1912–1914) to a psychiatrist and a Nobel Prize winner, Wagner von Jauregg (1857–1940). After a few months he took over the leadership of neurology. In 1914 he went to Trieste, Italy, where he performed forensic work. During the war, he was habilitated to become an assistant professor of neurology in Prague, Czechoslovakia. After the war he became a teacher of neuroanatomy at the newly established Medical School in Ljubljana. In 1928, he took over the position of head in the Ljubljana Hospital for Mental Illness. He was studying the still-unknown impact of alkaloid mescaline on himself and got valuable information on the phenomena of the psychopathology of mescaline. He wrote *Im Mescalinrausch* (In Mescaline Ecstasy) (Šerko, 1913), the most important work in the field of psychopathology states, which is quoted even by Karl Jaspers (1883–1969) in his famous book *Allgemeine Psychopatologie* (General Psychopathology) (Jaspers, 1948). He wrote many other works (Šerko, 1924–25; Šerko, 1934).

Professor Albin Seliškar (1896–1973) had a penchant for research, which is proved by his life—after studying chemistry and biology in Vienna (promoted in 1923) he was invited to join the biological experimental research unit (*Biologische Versuchsanstalt)* of the Vienna Academy of Science and its clinical chemistry laboratories. The findings from his thesis were published in the prestigious international journal *Zoologischer Anzeiger* (Biological Magazine) (Seliškar, 1923). At the end of the year 1923, he became an assistant at the Institute of Physiology, Faculty of Medicine. In the autumn of 1924–1925, he received a Rockefeller Foundation scholarship to study experimental physiology in Cambridge University (Great Britain) and at the pharmacological institute of the University of London. There Seliškar demonstrated his creative spirit, and published four debates in the reputable *Journal of Physiology* (Župančič, 1997). With his new knowledge he became an assistant professor of physiology in Ljubljana in 1927, and at the same time he was working as a teacher on the Faculty of General and Comparative Animal Physiology. After 1939, he was working as an associate, and after 1945 as a full university professor; he was the head of the Physiological-Chemical Institute. As a professor he was always encouraging young and curious medical students (Zupanič Slavec, 2010).

Academician Andrej O. Župančič (1916–2007) was a doctor and pathophysiologist, but also an anthropologist, researcher, and recognized scientist. He was a charismatic personality with broad knowledge from many fields and a sparkling spirit. He took his study inspiration from Central Europe (Ljubljana; Prague, Czechoslovakia), and in 1945 he obtained the position of assistant professor of pathological physiology on the medical faculty in Ljubljana, where he studied under the mentorship of Professor Albin Seliškar. Župančič also studied abroad at institutes in Leningrad, London, and the United States (Konjajev, 2008). An excellent researcher, he led a newly created department of the Faculty for Postgraduate Studies from

1967 on. Later this department became a part of the university's doctoral studies in biomedicine. Župančič was a mentor to many young researchers, including M. Dimitrijević. He led the Yugoslavian project to investigate neurotransmitters. In 1951, Župančič published his striking theory of receptor enzymes for biological agents. This theory was a powerful initiative for the expansion of research work, and Professor Župančič gathered many different researchers and teachers who (under his leadership) created the first strong core of research of the nervous system in Slovenia. After 1970, Župančič and his colleagues designed a study of the active center of AChE. Academician Župančič and his original way of thinking and infectious enthusiasm for research and his sense for humor were a magnet for many young doctors oriented toward scientific research. He supported them in their advanced professional and research efforts, and by doing this he also contributed significantly to the development of another core of neuroscience in Slovenia, the current Institute of Clinical Neurophysiology, and the University Medical Center, Ljubljana (Bögel, 1991; Sketelj, 2001).

A significant impact on the development of neuropsychiatry in Ljubljana was also made by the great intellectual, scientist, doctor, psychiatrist, polyhistorian, and writer Ivan Robida (1871–1941). As a student at the Vienna and Graz Medical Faculty (promoted 1897), Robida also specialized in neuropsychiatry in the former Austria and also in Germany, Switzerland, and France. With all his fresh knowledge, he (unfortunately unsuccessfully) tried to modernize psychiatry in Slovenia, but he was successful in managing the new Neurology Department of the Hospital in Ljubljana (Department for Nervous and Mental Diseases) until his retirement in 1937. With a wealth of knowledge and personal ambition, he was habilitated as private assistant professor of neurology at the University of Krakow, Poland. Throughout his life, Robida was an avid writer of fiction, and he also wrote popular science articles. In his scientific work, he was clearing a path for neurological-psychiatric science in Slovenia. Robida was a witty, unique, and free-thinking interlocutor (Milčinski, 1996).

Where the neuropsychiatric work of Assistant Professor Robida stopped, it was continued by his professional successor Ivan Marinčič (1892–1970), who was an exceptional man, an intellectual, an excellent writer, a lover of culture and art, predisposed to successful research and leadership. He studied medicine in Prague and Zagreb (promoted 1929), and after graduation he worked at the Neurological Clinic in Ljubljana. Head Assistant Professor Robida had realized the significant potential of young Marinčič and sent him to specialize in Paris, which was the world's leading center of neuroscience between the world wars. Marinčič was educated at Charcot's famous Salpêtrière Hospital with professors George Guillaino (1876–1961) and Ivan Bertrand (1893–1965). He was in on the beginning of a new neurological science, and he was infected by the creative research thinking, which he transferred to the Neurological Clinic in Ljubljana. In 1945, now an outstanding clinical neurologist, Ivan Marinčič became the first Slovenian Professor of Neurology on the Ljubljana Faculty of Medicine, and was a dedicated educator of several generations of students at the Ljubljana Faculty of Medicine, doctors, and specialists in neurology. For many years he was also the chief editor of the central Slovenian medical journal (*Zdravniški vestnik*). One of his students was Milan Dimitrijević (Marinčič, 1962).

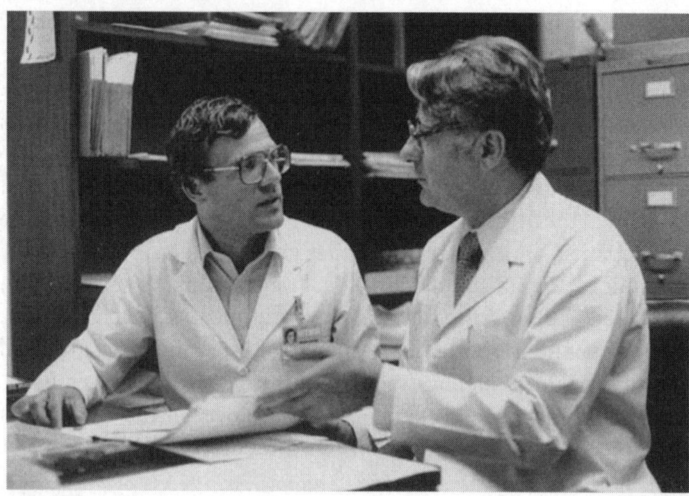

Appendix Figure II–1 Milan R. Dimitrijevic, M.D., D.Sc. (*right*) and Janez Faganel, M.D. (*left*) working in the office of the Department of Clinical Neurophysiology in the Institute for Rehabilitation and Research in Houston, Texas, in 1974.

4. MILAN R. DIMITRIJEVIĆ

Milan R. Dimitrijević was born in Niš (Serbia) on January 27, 1931. After high school he came to Ljubljana to study medicine. Already as a student at the medical school he carried out a four-year research study with Professor of Physiology Albin Seliškar, Professor of Biology Hubert Pehani (1900–1994) and Assistant Professor of Biophysics Engineer Ladislav Jenček. In 1955 Dimitrijević was promoted and soon recruited by the Neurological Clinic in Ljubljana, where his creativity was encouraged by his direct specialization supervisor and Head of Clinics Professor Ivan Marinčič (Dimitrijević & Dimitrijević, 1959). In 1962 he completed his specialization in neuropsychiatry (Janko, 1988). Milan Dimitrijević wanted to be interdisciplinary and chose pathophysiologist Professor Andrej O. Župančič as co-mentor for his Ph.D. dissertation. Župančič was familiar with the methodology of excellent research work and guided Dimitrijević's development to become a doctor—a researcher of the human nervous system (human neuroscientist) (Pohar & Dimitrijević, 1961). The idea for the dissertation came to Milan's mind one morning before the morning rounds, when Professor Marinčič asked him if he thought it would ever be possible to determine whether the tendon reflex response is present even when it does not appear visibly. This quite early question, in the years 1958 and 1959, aroused Milan's curiosity about the subclinical responses, at a time when neurology was still primarily structural. The questions of physiology, functions, and the relationship between structure and function developed rapidly only in the last decades of the twentieth century. The development of Dimitrijević's research work was strongly influenced also by the orthopedist Professor Bogdan Brecelj (1906–1986) from Ljubljana, who was a Slovenian pioneer of modern rehabilitation medicine (Moody & Dimitrijević, 1964). Brecelj purchased the necessary research equipment, organized seminars with neurophysiological themes, and argued for the usefulness of clinical neurophysiology in orthopedics. In 1958, Milan Dimitrijević, who was interested in cerebral circulation, won a scholarship of the nuclear commission and went to the neurological clinic in Karolinska University in Stockholm, Sweden, to study under Professor Erik Klas Henrik Kugelberg (1913–1983). Professor Kugelberg was one of the founders of clinical electromyelography and was thinking about the functional aspects of neurology and became a pioneer of clinical neurophysiology. But this name was actually given by the Swedish Professor of neurology Lars-Erik Larsson.

In 1959 the first neurophysiological laboratory was founded at the Orthopedic Clinic, and in 1963 it was moved to a Neurological Clinic (Vodovnik et al., 1966). The laboratory became an independent unit in the 1969. The laboratory evaluated cerebral functions, muscle functions, and nerve functions in health and disease (Zidar & Dimitrijević, 2010).

Dimitrijević's postgraduate education in 1963 at the National Hospital for Neurology and Neurosurgery, Queen Square, London, was important. There he met Peter Nathan (1914–2002), a well-recognized neurologist and researcher. They found the common language in the area of spasticity, which connected them. Peter Nathan then came over to Slovenia for a period of several years for occasional work at the Neurophysiological Institute. With Milan Dimitrijević he published some high-quality research in international scientific journals (Dimitrijević & Nathan, 1969). The articles were published in the years from 1967 to 1973 in several volumes, under the title *Study of Spasticity in Man* (Dimitrijević & Nathan, 1967; Dimitrijević & Nathan, 1968; Dimitrijević & Nathan, 1970; Dimitrijević & Nathan, 1971; Dimitrijević & Nathan, 1973).

In 1960, getting funds for research work was quite difficult in Yugoslavia. In the American embassy in Yugoslavia, there was the "cereal fund for health services," through which it was agreed that researchers from Ljubljana would get funding for neurophysiological research if they would share the results with relevant American experts. At the World Congress of Neurology in Vienna in 1965, Milan Dimitrijević, who had already completed his thesis at the time (Dimitrijević, 1965), was invited by Richard Masland (1910–2003) from the National Institute of Health in Bethesda, Maryland, to come lecture on neurophysiology and neurophysiological methods for studying spasticity, spinal reflexes, and neurocontrol of movements in American medical schools for three months.

Milan Dimitrijević carefully combined clinical and research programs. He knew that a clinical question is at the same time a research question; therefore, his team studied patients with muscular dystrophy, stroke, and spinal cord injury. They settled research questions such as: Is it possible that the outcomes after spinal cord injury or a progressive neuromuscular disease or a stroke can vary and may have different clinical picture at the same structure?

Dimitrijević managed to create a pleasant working atmosphere at the Institute of Clinical Neurophysiology in Ljubljana with his own organizational talents. He provided the necessary apparatus and other equipment and selected the right employees for the right working places: Tine Prevec was dealing with the cortical sensory system (Larsson & Prevec, 1969); Jože Trontelj (born 1939) was dealing with muscle neuromuscular transmission (Trontelj & Stålberg, 1983); Janez Faganel (1943–1984) with sensory-motor functions of the spinal cord (Faganel & Dimitrijević, 1982); Milan Gregorič (born 1941) with the brain stem (Gregorič et al., 1981); and Martin Janko (1942–2003) with the sensory function of peripheral nerves (Janko & Trontelj, 1980).

Besides spasticity, Milan Dimitrijević also studied the neurophysiological mechanisms of functional electrical stimulation. Experts in other fields joined him in this effort: neurosurgeon Vinko Dolenc (born 1940) (Halter et al., 1983); psychiatrist Jože Lokar (1939–1996) (Vodušek et al., 1982); orthopedist Fedor Pečak (Trontelj & Pečak, 1979); doctor of rehabilitation medicine Franjo Gračanin (Dimitrijević & Gračanin, 1966); engineers Marinček and Lojze Vodovnik (born 1933) (Vodovnik et al., 1978); and computer specialists Ludwig Gergek and Janez Trontelj (Drinovec, 2007). A group of engineers also participated. They were the first faculty at the clinic to have a computer, and they developed their own system of research and clinical work. They also collaborated with other, similar institutions: the Institute for Rehabilitation, Neurosurgical Clinic, Clinic for Plastic and Reparative Surgery.

During this hard work, all the researchers began to realize how extensive the structural and functional nerve recovery is and how axon growth is dependent on its envelope. Peripheral axons eventually find a new way through the peripheral myelin sheath, whereas central axons do not. They are also incompatible, because one has dopamine, while the other has a cholinergic transmitter system. The central nervous system is even more complex, and neurophysiologists see it, from a functional point of view, as a highly integrated system that combines a variety of regional processing systems, which can be put together in different ways. Regeneration plays an important role as during the regeneration new links are formed and the function is resumed. A nice example of this is the correction of the functioning of a patient after a stroke (Janko, 1993).

Despite many administrative obstacles, research in Ljubljana was making progress due to the enthusiasm of researchers, who also started publishing in reputable scientific journals. They successfully carried out research and became experts on the damaged spinal cord, neuromuscular disease, and the restoration of functions after a stroke. They were successful in their work because they had the needed equipment, knowledge, good staff, and a clear idea of how to restore the functions. They were learning from others who had had the needed equipment and knowledge before them. At the Institute they had been dealing with focal spasticity, pain, and treatment. There was never a difference between clinical and research work. All their methods have been substantiated, verified, and published.

In 1968, Milan Dimitrijević visited the Texas Institute for Rehabilitation and Research (TIRR), the Department of Rehabilitation of the Baylor College of Medicine, in Houston (Texas, USA), and later was appointed as a visiting professor. In 1972, he established the Department for Clinical Neurophysiology within TIRR. He traveled frequently between Houston and Ljubljana and brought clinical scientists to Houston to contribute to the development of new neurophysiological methods. In 1975, he left Ljubljana permanently but continued a strong relationship with the members of the Institute of Clinical Neurophysiology, which remains active today. With continued development, the TIRR department became the Division of Restorative Neurology and Human Neurobiology within Baylor Medical School in 1987. Milan Dimitrijević became its first professor.

The scientific interest that drove Milan Dimitrijević at the time of his specialization is still alive. He remains an active researcher and has authored about 50 articles in SCI journals, and co-authored another 70 scientific articles. He has written over 50 chapters in foreign professional books and organized nine symposia about restorative neurology. As part of these symposia he published a series of books entitled

Recent Achievements in Restorative Neurology, issued by Karger Publishing House, the first one in 1985, the second in 1986, and the third one in 1990 (Dimitrijević et al., 1986). Dimitrijević is a member of the editorial boards of most well-known neurological journals, committees, and associations. He has received a series of awards, honorary doctorates, and memberships in various associations and academies. Among the most important ones are: honorary doctor of the Polish Medical Academy in Warsaw, honorary doctor of Medical Faculty of Linköping in Sweden, and corresponding member of the Slovenian Academy of Sciences and Arts. For his work he received in Slovenia in 1975 the Boris Kidrič Fund Award, and in 1986 the Boris Kidrič Award for outstanding achievements in the field of study of spasticity in humans (Zupanič Slavec, 2000).

Professor Dimitrijević has played a very important role in the development of clinical neurophysiology and neurology at the Ljubljana Medical Center and at the Ljubljana Medical Faculty, especially between 1960 and 1970. With his help, the Institute of Clinical Neurophysiology at University Medical Center–Ljubljana has become a well-recognized and respected clinical research institution, known both in Europe and the United States. He has also developed an international project for the "Recovery of Movement" with the support of the Foundation for Movement Recovery (Oslo, Norway). This program has spread via Vienna to the rest of Europe, the United States (Atlanta, Georgia), Asia (Taiwan), and Australia.

In Dimitrijević's first generation of collaborators trained in Ljubljana, in his second generation from Houston, in the third of collaborators from Asia, Europe, and the United States, with the support of the Vivian Smith Foundation for Restorative Neurology. In Houston he trained 185 professionals in 10 years; most of them are scattered all over the world. A part of this program is also being developed in Los Angeles. A fourth generation of younger members of this growing network come from Vienna, Atlanta, and Taipei. In Vienna, seven institutions joined in the "Vienna Program for Restoration of Locomotion" to implement clinical and neuroscience research.

Professor Dimitrijević is an international pioneer of restorative neurology. His main interest is in the neurophysiology of movement and human motor control. He has described the subclinical features of neurocontrol that can exist in those with upper motor neuron paralysis, and through this research, he was able to advance the understanding of neurocontrol in people with peripheral and central neurological conditions. Regardless of the future of biological treatment of neurological conditions with different varieties of movement impairment, knowledge on motor control will be essential for recovery and repair of the CNS.

Modern bio-neurology will most probably be based on new solutions that take place through interventions that target genetic, molecular, membrane, cellular, synaptic, neural networks, and other yet-to-be-discovered biological mechanisms. New gene technology for the treatment of neurological diseases contributes mainly to the diagnosis and differentiation of various neurological disorders, particularly degenerative disorders. On the other hand, we are still differentiating phenotype from genotype poorly, although the achievements of Professor Vrbová from London are very promising (Vrbová & Hausmanowa-Petrusewitcz, 2004). With electrostimulation, we may be able to alter the relationship between the phenotypes and also affect the growth of denervated muscle. Research is based on well-defined hypotheses and solid methodologies that provide a functional outcome.

5. DR. JANEZ FAGANEL (1943–1984) AND FAGANEL'S MEMORIAL MEETINGS

Janez Faganel (1943–1984) was the fifth young physician to join (in 1968) Professor Milan R. Dimitrijević in the Ljubljana Laboratory for Clinical Neurophysiology of the Neurology Department, which—a year later—became an independent institution. Clinical neurophysiology at that time was more research than routine, and Dr. Faganel immediately joined the group in research, first, on neurophysiological parameters of human spinal reflexes (his M.Sc. thesis, 1971), and, later, on the propriospinal interneuronal system of the human spinal cord (Ph.D., 1977). In 1975 he founded, at the Institute, the Slovenian Neuromuscular Diseases Center, and started the registry of patients. When the founder of the Ljubljana Institute, Professor Dimitrijević, moved to the United States, Janez Faganel spent much time with him in research on spasticity and the mechanisms of motor control. Janez Faganel was an enthusiastic researcher, a kind-hearted colleague, and a knowledgeable clinician, much appreciated by his patients and coworkers. In his forty-first year he died from complications of hemophilia. He was married and the father of four children. One year after his death, to promote further development of clinical neurophysiology in Slovenia and neighboring countries, Professor Dimitrijević started a now traditional series of annual lectures, devoted to the memory of our colleague and friend Janez Faganel (Anon, 1984).

The Institute of Clinical Neurophysiology still organizes the annual symposium of clinical neurophysiology for educational purposes, with a lecture in memory of Janez Faganel. In 1985, on the initiative of the founder and first Head of the Institute of Clinical Neurophysiology, Professor Dimitrijević, at the satellite symposium on head injuries, there was a lecture dedicated to the memory of his colleague and friend Janez Faganel, who had passed away the year before. In 1986 the Institute of Clinical Neurophysiology started hosting independent lectures, which have since grown into annual neurophysiological educational, professional, and research meetings. The last meeting, in October 2010, was already the twenty-sixth in the series.

The symposium is traditionally held in Ljubljana in the autumn and lasts for a day or two. Although it is a regional event, in addition to domestic expert lecturers, eminent foreign lecturers are always invited to present new clinical and research findings with neurophysiology and related fields. For the younger researchers in these disciplines, the symposium is an opportunity to show their research work.

Every year, in the context of this symposium, the memorial lecture of Janez Faganel, after which the symposium is named, is also organized. The course content usually comprises a wider context of issues than the topic of the symposium that year. The lecturers are almost exclusively renowned foreign experts in their respective areas. Through all of the 26 symposia, the memorial meeting was cancelled only once, in 1998. On that occasion, the Slovenian symposium was merged with the European Congress of Clinical Neurophysiology, which was organized in Slovenia that year.

The meeting soon outgrew the bare framework of neurology and neurophysiology, and the links have begun with other areas such as genetics, otorhinolaryngology and maxillofacial surgery, neurosurgery, and ophthalmology in 2010. The traditional organizer of the symposium is the Institute of Clinical Neurophysiology, Neurological Clinic of the University Medical Center–Ljubljana. Over the years, the latter invited different associations and clinical departments to participate, such as the Section for Clinical Neurophysiology of the Slovenian Medical Society, the Muscular Dystrophy Association of Slovenia, the Association League Against Epilepsy of Slovenia, the Slovenian Association for the Treatment of Pain, the Association of Ophthalmologists of Slovenia, the Clinical Department of Otorhinolaryngology and Maxillofacial Surgery, the Orthopedic Clinic in Ljubljana, the Clinical Department of Traumatology, the Clinic of Neurosurgery, the Clinical Department of Anesthesiology, and the Ophthalmic Clinic in Ljubljana.

A couple of times in the history of the "Faganel Days Symposium," it was merged with the organization of a major international congress: the first time in 1987, when the second Yugoslav Symposium of Neurology and Urodynamics was organized in Ljubljana, and then in 1998 with the above-mentioned ninth European Congress of Clinical Neurophysiology. The collection of lectures at this meeting was published as a supplement of the *Journal of the International Federation of Clinical Neurophysiology*. In 2001, "extraordinary" Faganel's Days were organized by the EC-IFCN (European Chapter of the International Federation of Clinical Neurophysiology), Ljubljana 2001 Regional EMG Refresher Course, and also in 2005 as the International Danube Symposium for Neurological Sciences and Continuing Education, organized by International Association Of Neurology Of East Central Europe—Collaborating Society of the EFNS, and the Institute of Clinical Neurophysiology, with the Association of Neurologists of Slovenia and the Section of Clinical Neurophysiology, Slovenian Medical Association. In 2008, a symposium was entitled Symposium on Amyotrophic Lateral Sclerosis. A collection of lectures of this meeting was published as a supplement to the magazine *Rehabilitacija*. A year later a new meeting was organized, the First Congress of the Slovenian Association for the Treatment of Pain; it was organized as an associate congress to the Symposium of Clinical Neurophysiology. It was organized by the Slovenian Association for the Treatment of Pain, Section of Clinical Neurophysiology, Slovenian Medical Association, Institute of Clinical Neurophysiology at Neurological Clinic of the University Medical Center–Ljubljana.

Over nearly three decades, the Faganel's Days have brought together Slovenian and international experts in the field of neurophysiology and other related medical fields. They bring global innovations in this area to Slovenian doctors and their colleagues and are connecting local knowledge with international. They encourage further development of different clinical neurological disciplines, and they contribute a lot to Slovenian neurological ideas (Zidar, 1993).

6. CONCLUSION

Volitional movement of the hand, arm, or lower limb is based on rather complex neurocontrol. Neurocontrol is supposed to provide coordination between bones, joints, peripheral nerves, muscles, and chains of neuronal circuits of the brain, brain stem, cerebellum, and spinal cord. In the past 50 years, by application of human neurophysiological studies of motor control, we have had the opportunity to learn how the complexity of motor control provides conditions for implementing motor tasks with different purposes.

At present we are aware of a variety of alternatives that can be applied to achieve the recovery of movement in spinal cord injury, stroke, head injury, and other brain motor disorders. This knowledge acquired in the past 20 years has opened a new avenue of treatment of neurological conditions. This is illustrated in this book: and by learning how to assess movement disorders in neurological conditions and how to upgrade motor control performance by application of interventional procedures, we can see the future of restorative neurology. Restorative neurology is not the practice of biological repair of an injured nervous system, but knowledge of how to apply interventional procedures in order to advance existing motor control. Briefly, the control of movement is the result of a multi-hierarchical and multi-parallel organization of the motor structures, and our understanding of this and how such organization can become part of a newly established nervous system integrated for improved function through the application of the principles and interventions of restorative neurology. That is the challenge for today and tomorrow of restorative neurology and the treatment of neurological disorders.

References

Anonymous. "Dr. Janez Faganel, 1943–1984." *Zdravniški Vestnik* 53 (1984): 475–476.

Bögel, M. "Župančič Andrej O." In *Slovenski biografski leksikon* [Slovenian Biographical Lexicon], edited by Munda, J, 278–280. Ljubljana, Slovenia: Slovenska akademija znanosti in umetnosti, 1991.

Dimitrijević, M. R. "*Študij elektrofizioloških značilnosti spinalne refleksne aktivnosti pri perifernih nevropatijah in njihov klinični pomen*" [Study of electrophysiological mechanisms of spinal reflex activity in peripheral neuropathies and their clinical importance]. Ph.D. diss., University of Ljubljana, 1965.

Dimitrijević, M. R., Dimitrijević, M. M. "Electromyography in kinesiology." *Medical Professional Rehabilitation* 2 (1959): 57–58.

Dimitrijević, M. R., Gračanin, F. "Differential involvement of tibialis anterior, gastrocnemius and soleus in muscular dystrophy." *Journal of the Neurological Sciences* 6 (1968): 105–115.

Dimitrijević, M. R., Nathan, P. W. "Studies of spasticity in man. 1. Some features of spasticity." *Brain* 90 (1967a): 1–30.

Dimitrijević, M. R., Nathan, P. W. "Studies of spasticity in man. 2. Analysis of stretch reflexes in spasticity." *Brain* 90 (1967b): 233–258.

Dimitrijević, M. R., Nathan, P. W. "Studies of spasticity in man. 3. Analysis of reflex activity evoked by noxious cutaneous stimulation." *Brain* 91 (1968): 349–368.

Dimitrijević, M. R., Nathan, P. W. "Changes in the flexion reflex with repetitive cutaneous stimulation in spinal man." *Electroencephalography and Clinical Neurophysiology* 27 (1969): 721–722.

Dimitrijević, M. R., Nathan, P. W. "Studies of spasticity in man. 4. Changes in flexion reflex with repetitive cutaneous stimulation in spinal man." *Brain* 93 (1970): 743–768.

Dimitrijević, M. R., Nathan, P. W. "Studies of spasticity in man. 5. Dishabituation of the flexion reflex in spinal man." *Brain* 94 (1971): 77–90.

Dimitrijević, M. R., Nathan, P. W. "Studies of spasticity in man. 6. Habituation, dishabituation and sensitization of tendon reflexes in spinal man." *Brain* 96 (1973): 337–354.

Dimitrijević, M. R., Kakulas, B. A., Vrbová, G. *Recent Achievements in Restorative Neurology*. Basel, Switzerland: Karger Publishing House, 1986.

Drinovec, J. "Aktualni pogovor s Prof. Dr. Milanom Dimitrijevićem" [Actual interview with Professor Milan Dimitrijević]. *Zdravniški vestnik* 76 (2007): 266–270.

Faganel, J., Dimitrijević, M. R. "Study of propriospinal system in man. Cutaneous exteroceptive conditioning of stretch reflexes." *Journal of the Neurological Sciences* Division 56 (1982): 155–172.

Felc, J. "Alfred Šerko." In *Medicinska fakulteta Univerze v Ljubljani: 1919–1945: Zgodovinski Zbornik*. [Medical Faculty of University of Ljubljana: 1919–1945: Historical Almanac], edited by F. Urlep, M. Kališnik, P. Borisov, 107–124. Ljubljana, Slovenia: Inštitut za zgodovino medicine Medicinske Fakultete: Zdravniška zbornica Slovenije, 2003.

Gregorič, M. "Pomen klinične nevrofiziologije in kineziologije v rehabilitaciji" [The importance of clinical neurophysiology and kinesiology in rehabilitation]. In *Klinična nevrofiziologija in kineziologija v rehabilitacij*, edited by M. Gregorič, 3–11. Ljubljana, Slovenia: Inštitut Republike Slovenije za rehabilitacijo, 1994.

Gregorič, M., Pečak, F., Trontelj, J. V., Dimitrijević, M. R. "Postural control in scoliosis. A statokinesimetric study in patients with scoliosis due to neuromuscular disorders and in patients with idiopathic scoliosis." *Acta Orthopaedica Scandinavica* 52 (1982): 59–63.

Halter, J., Dolenc, V., Dimitrijević, M. R., Sharkey, P. C. "Neurophysiological assessment of electrode placement in the spinal cord." *Applied Neurophysiology* 46 (1983): 124–128.

Janko, M. "Dimitrijević, Milan." In *Enciklopedija Slovenije*, vol. 2, 260. Ljubljana, Slovenia: Mladinska knjiga, 1988.

Janko, M. "Klinična nevrofiziologija" [Clinical neurophysiology]. In *Enciklopedija Slovenije*, vol. 5, 101. Ljubljana, Slovenia: Mladinska knjiga, 1991.

Janko, M. "Profesor Milan R. Dimitrijević." *Zdravniški Vestnik* 62 (1993): 339–340.

Janko, M., Trontelj, J. V. "Transcutaneous electrical nerve stimulation: A microneurographic and perceptual study." *Pain* 9 (1980): 219–230.

Jaspers, K. *Allgemeine Psychopatologie* [General Psychopathology], 5th edition. Berlin & Heidelberg, 1948.

Jeras, J. "Pedonevrologija in splošna zdravstvena služba" [Pediatric neurology and general health service]. *Zdravniški Vestnik* 42 (1973): 287–290.

Konjajev, Z. "Akademik Andrej O. Župančič—partizanski zdravnik Dr. Mike" [Academician Andrej O. Župančič—partisan Dr. Mike]. *Zdravniški Vestnik* 77 (2008): 163–168.

Larsson, L. E., Prevec, T. "Evoked responses to slight taps, recorded in the somatosensory region." *Electroencephalography and Clinical Neurophysiology* 26 (1969): 339–340.

Marinčič, I. "Ob Nevrološki Številki Zdravniškega Vestnika" [To Neurological Volume of Slovenian Medical Journal]. *Zdravniški Vestnik* 31 (1962): 47–49.

Milčinski, L. "Ivan Robida." In *Enciklopedija Slovenije*, vol. 10, 248. Ljubljana, Slovenia: Mladinska knjiga, 1996.

Moody, J. R., Dimitrijević, M. R. "An electromyographic study of tendon reflexes in progressive muscular dystrophy in man." *Brain* 87 (1964): 511–520.

Pohar, E., Dimitrijević, M. R. "Study of the function of the biceps brachii muscle." *Medical Professional Rehabilitation* 4 (1961): 1–8.

Prevec, T., Vodušek, D. B. "*25 let Inštituta za klinično nevrofiziologijo (1969–1994)*" [Twenty-five Years of Institute of Clinical Neurophysiology (1969–1994)]. Ljubljana, Slovenia: Klinični center, 1994.

Seliškar, A. "Die männlichen Duftorgane der Höhlenheuschrecke Troglophilus" [The male scent organs of the cave locust *Troglophilus*]. *Zoologischer Anzeiger* 57 (1923): 253–268.

Sketelj, J. "Akademik Andrej O. Župančič, 90-letnik" [Academician Andrej O. Župančič, 90th anniversary]. *Delo*, January 26, 2001.

Strojnik, A. "Protitaktni ojačevalnik s katodno cevjo za elektroencefalografske registracije" [Antitactile multiplier with cathode tube for electroencephalographic registration]. *Zdravniški Vestnik* 16 (1947): 393–399.

Šerko, A. "Im Mescalinrausch" [In mescaline ecstasy]. *Jahrbuch für Psychiatrie und Neurologie* 34 (1913): 355–366.

Šerko, A. *O psihoanalizi* [About Psychoanalysis]. Ljubljana, Slovenia: Medicinska fakulteta, 1934.

Šerko, A. *Živčevje človeka za zdravnike in medicince* [Human Nervous System for Physicians and Medical Students]. Ljubljana, Slovenia: Zvezna tiskarna, 1924–1925.

Trontelj, J., Stålberg, E. "Responses to electrical stimulation of denervated human muscle fibres recorded with single fibre EMG." *Journal of Neurology, Neurosurgery and Psychiatry* 46 (1983): 305–309.

Trontelj, J. V., Pecak, F., Dimitrijević, M. R. "Segmental neurophysiological mechanisms in scoliosis." *Journal of Bone and Joint Surgery* (British) 61-B (1979): 310–313.

Vodovnik, L., Dimitrijević, M. R., Prevec, T., Lokar, M. "Electronic walking aids for patients with peroneal palsy." Brighton, England, Sept. 28–Oct. 1, 1965. *World Medical Instruments* 61 (1966): 58–61.

Vodovnik, L., Kralj, A., Stanič, U., Ačimović, R., Gros, N. "Recent applications of functional electric stimulation to stroke patients in Ljubljana." *Clinical Orthopaedics and Related Research* (1978): 64–70.

Vodušek, D. B., Janko, M., Lokar, J. "EMG, single fibre EMG and sacral reflexes in assessment of sacral nervous system lesions." *Journal of Neurology, Neurosurgery and Psychiatry* 45 (1982): 1064–1066.

Vrbová, G., Hausmanowa-Petrusewitcz, I. "Biology of some neuromuscular disorders." *Zdravniški Vestnik* 73 Suppl. II (2004): 3–10.

Wallace, B. A. "*Toward a New Science of Consciousness*." New York: Oxford University Press, 2002.

Zidar, J. "Spominska predavanja Dr. Janez Faganel" [Memorial lectures of Dr. Janez Faganel]. *Zdravniški Vestnik* 62 Suppl I (1993): 2.

Zidar, J., Dimitrijević, M. D. "Štirideset let Inštituta za klinično nevrofiziologijo in 50 let klinične nevrofiziologije v Sloveniji" [Forty years of the Ljubljana Institute of Clinical Neurophysiology and 50 years of clinical neurophysiology in Slovenia]. *Zdravniški Vestnik* 79 (2010): 375–382.

Zupanič Slavec, Z. "Milan Dimitrijević: zdravnik, nevrolog (1931): vabila iz širnega sveta" [Milan Dimitrijević: doctor, neurologist (1931): the invitations from the wide world]. In *Znameniti Slovenci* [Famous Slovenians], edited by N. Brun, 64–65. *Ljubljana Forma* 7, 2000: 64–65.

Zupanič Slavec, Z. "Prva učitelja fiziologije in mikrobiologije na popolni Medicinski fakulteti, Albin Seliškar in Milica Petrović Valentinčič" [First professors of physiology and microbiology on the completed medical faculty of Ljubljana, Albin Seliškar and Milica Petrović Valentinčič]. *Isis* 9 (2010): 33–39.

Župančič, O. A. "Nekaj drobcev o fragmentih" [Couple of particles about fragments]. In M. Seliškar, *Fragmenti o Očetu*. [Fragments About Father]. Ljubljana, Slovenia: Prirodoslovno društvo Slovenije, 1997.

INDEX

Page numbers followed by "*f*" refer to figures.

ablative procedures for spasticity, 146–47
abnormal involuntary movements, 136
active function, 157
afferent influences, locomotion after SCI and, 78–80
AIS. *See* ASIA impairment scale
aldynoglia, 102
American Spinal Injury Association (ASIA), 172
anatomically discomplete SCI, 15
anatomy
  new, sublesional segment, 141, 142*f*
  reduced, sublesional segment, 141, 142*f*
animal models
  cat, locomotion after SCI, 71–74
  grafting, 99
  of locomotion, 70, 70*f*
    after SCI, 71–78
  MEP, 203–4, 209
  rat, locomotion after SCI, 74–78
  SCI, 65–66, 170
    experimental, 209
    locomotion and, 71–78
  SEP, 203–4, 209
ASIA. *See* American Spinal Injury Association
ASIA impairment scale (AIS), 12
  SCI classification, 190, 192*f*
axons
  of grafted motoneurones, skeletal muscles and connecting to, 113–14
  macrophages and growth of, 103
  peripheral nerve grafts and regenerating, 95–97, 96*f*
axons, CNS
  activity of residual, 5–6
  bridge for regeneration of, 107–8
  encouraging regeneration of, 95–106
    isolated cell population implantation and, 97–106
    macrophage implantation and, 102–4
    OEC implantation and, 100–102
    peripheral nerve grafts to support, 95–97, 96*f*
    Schwann cell implantation and, 97–100, 98*f*
    stem cell implantation and, 104–6
    unfavorable environment and, 95
  macrophages and, 103

baclofen, 44
  intrathecal drug delivery system
    pumps, 58–60
    for spasticity, 145
BBB scale, 76–77
biological interventions for SCI repair, 169–79
  acute phase, 176–77
  clinical application of, 177–78
  established SCI and, 177
  fictive, 178
biomechanical effects, 15
Bischof myelotomy, 147
BMCA. *See* brain motor-control assessment

body-weight-supported treadmill training (BWSTT), 47
bone marrow stromal cells (MSCs), 105
botulinum toxin (Botox), 44
  spasticity treatment with, 60, 158
brain influence, residual motor control below SCI and
  suprasegmentally induced motor unit activity in paralyzed muscles, 34–35, 34*f*
  tendon jerks in spastic SCI, 28–30, 29*f*
  vibratory tonic reflex in complete SCI syndrome, 31, 32*f*
  withdrawal flexor plantar reflex volitional suppression, 31–33, 33*f*
brain motor control, 2
  of locomotion
    residual motor control below SCI and, 37–40, 39*f*
    SCI and, 71–78
    spinal cord network and, 66–68, 67*f*
    supraspinal control and, 68–71, 71*f*
    transcutaneous SCS modification of neural circuit activity and, 247, 248*f*
brain motor-control assessment (BMCA), 28, 185, 190–92. *See also* motor control
  fEMG, protocols for, 262–67, 265*t*, 266*f*, 268*t*
    electrode, 262–63
    study setup and, 265–67, 267*f*
  sEMG and, 262
  transcutaneous SCS and, 244
  voluntary tasks in, 274
brain stem, embryonic, 115–16
Brecelj, Bogdan, 290
BWSTT. *See* body-weight-supported treadmill training

cat animal models, locomotion after SCI, 71–74
cauda equina, transcutaneous SCS applied over, 237–39, 237*f*, 238*f*, 239*f*
central nervous system (CNS)
  axons
    bridge for regeneration of, 107–8
    macrophages and, 103
    residual activity, 5–6
  axons, encouraging regeneration of
    isolated cell population implantation and, 97–106
    macrophage implantation and, 102–4
    OEC implantation and, 100–102
    peripheral nerve grafts to support, 95–97, 96*f*
    Schwann cell implantation and, 97–100, 98*f*
    stem cell implantation and, 104–6
    unfavorable environment and, 95
  embryonic grafts for replacing damaged tissue in, 109–16
    motoneurones and, 111–14
    spinal cord grafts, embryonic, 110–11, 110*f*
  motor control and, 258
  motor organization, 189
  SCI and, ix
central pattern generator (CPG)
  activity modulation and, 69
  spinal cord, 39–40, 66–68
cerebellum, locomotion and, 69
cervicomedullary glioma, KEEP and, 217
clonidine, locomotion and, 70, 81
clonus elicitation, manual, 277–80, 280*f*
CMAPs. *See* compound motor action potentials
CNS. *See* central nervous system
complete motor clinical syndrome, 12–14
complete SCI, 12–14
  neurologically, 205, 208*t*
  vibratory tonic reflex in, 31, 32*f*
compound motor action potentials (CMAPs), 141
compression injuries, spinal, 77–78
continuous motor events, 270, 271*f*, 272*f*, 273*f*
contusion injuries, spinal, 77–78
cortical SEPs (cSEPs), 215–16

CPG. *See* central pattern generator
cSEPs. *See* cortical SEPs
cutaneo-muscular reflex organization
  residual motor function after SCI and, 25–27, 26*f*, 27*f*
  tiring and, 27
cyproheptadine
  locomotion, 81
  spasticity, 151

dantrolene, spasticity, 145
DC. *See* dorsal column
deficits
  neurological motor, ix–x
  sensory, nerve transfer, 157, 160*f*
diazepam, spasticity, 145
Dimitrijević, Milan R., 289–93, 290*f*
  achievements, 292–93
  collaborators, 293
  education, 290–91
  at Institute of Clinical Neurophysiology in Ljubljana, 291–92
  Marinčič and, 290
  Seliškar and, 290
discomplete motor clinical syndrome, 11, 14, 186
discomplete SCI, 11, 14, 256
  anatomically, 15
DLF. *See* dorsolateral funiculus
dorsal column (DC), 76
dorsal rhizotomy, OEC transplantation after, 101
dorsolateral funiculus (DLF), 78
dysfunction
  functional neurosurgery for, 136
  LMN, 138
    IM pathology and, 139
    nerve transfer surgery, 153–55, 158*f*
  UMN, 138
    IM pathology and, 139
    nerve transfer surgery, 153–55, 158*f*

EEG. *See* electroencephalography
electrical stimulation
  after SCI, 49–50
  spasticity, 143–45, 146*f*
electroencephalography (EEG), 285–86
electromyography (EMG), 194, 285–86. *See also* functional electromyography
  PRM reflex, 233–34, 233*f*, 234*t*
  spasticity, focal, 157, 160*f*
electrophysiology, PRM reflexes and
  double stimulation and, 235–36, 235*f*
  tendon vibration and, 236, 236*f*
embryonic brain stem, 115–16
embryonic grafts
  CNS tissue, damaged replaced by, 109–16
    motoneurones and, 111–14
    spinal cord grafts, embryonic, 110–11, 110*f*
  intraspinal, spinal cord circuitry and serotoninergic, 115–18, 116*f*
  motoneuron replacement by, 111–14
  for SCI repair, 109–14
eMEPs. *See* epidural MEPs
EMG. *See* electromyography
encephalography, sensory, 285
epidural MEPs (eMEPs), 204–5, 214
epidural SCS (ESCS), 146, 227–29, 230*f*
  locomotor activity enhancement and, 243
  transcutaneous SCS and, 243
epidural SEPs (eSEPs), 204, 215
epilepsy, functional neurosurgery, 136
episodic motor events, 270, 271*f*, 272*f*, 273*f*
ESCS. *See* epidural SCS
eSEPs. *See* epidural SEPs

Faganel, Janez, 290*f*, 291, 294–95
  "Faganel Days Symposium," 294–95
  at Institute of Clinical Neurophysiology in Ljubljana, 294
fEMG. *See* functional electromyography
FES. *See* functional electrical stimulation
foot-drop stimulator, clinical program for fitting, 49
Freud, Sigmund, 287
functional augmentation, spasticity
  function recovery and, 152–60
  nerve transfers and, 152–60

functional augmentation, spasticity (*Cont'd*)
  pathological input optimization and, 148–51, 150*f*
  pathological input reduction and, 148
functional electrical stimulation (FES), 47–49. *See also* electrical stimulation
  for impaired functional movement of single muscle group, 52
functional electromyography (fEMG), 261
  BMCA, protocols for, 262–67, 265*t*, 266*f*, 268*t*
    electrode, 262–63
    study setup and, 265–67, 267*f*
  motor control measured with, 182–83
functional neurosurgery
  current state of, 136–37
  for dysfunction, 136
  for epilepsy, 136
  for impaired motor control, 136
  for neuroendocrine disorders, 136
  for pain, 136
  for psychiatric disorders, 136
  for spasticity, 136, 143–47
  sublesional segment, 143–47
functional procedures, 135
functional recovery
  of IM, 140
  reconstructive neurosurgery focal interventions for, 152–60
    tendon transfer surgery, 152–53, 154*f*
  of SCI lesion, 175
  of spasticity, 152–60
    focal, 157–60, 160*t*

gait, after SCI, 37–38
gate theory of pain, 242
glial fibrillary acidic protein (GFAP), 100
glioma, cervicomedullary, 217
glutamatergic system, 82
grafts
  animal models, 99
  embryonic, 116*f*
    CNS tissue, damaged replaced by, 109–16, 110*f*
    motoneuron replacement by, 111–14
    for SCI repair, 109–14
    serotoninergic, spinal cord circuitry and, 115–18, 116*f*
  intraspinal, 115–18, 116*f*
  monoaminergic cells and intraspinal, 114–18
  motoneurones
    axons of, connected to skeletal muscles, 113–14
    survival of, 112
  noradrenergic cells, 117
  peripheral nerve
    axon regeneration and, 95–97, 96*f*
    in paraplegic patients, 108–9
    SCI bypassing lesion site by, 106–9, 107*f*
  Schwann cells, 98–99
  serotonergic cells, 117
  of spinal cord, embryonic, 110–11, 110*f*
  stem cell, umbilical cord, 105–6
  timing, 99
Gregorič, Milan, 291

half-center, 66
Hoffman reflex (H reflex)
  multiple muscle studies, PRM reflexes and, 241–42, 241*f*, 242*f*
  PRM reflexes and, 239–42, 240*f*, 241*f*, 242*f*
  studies, 241–42, 241*f*, 242*f*
5-hydroxytryptophan (5-HT), 81–82
hyperreflexia, 172
hypertonia, muscle, 51

ILS. *See* infralesional segment
IM. *See* injured metamere
immunobased therapy for SCI, 102–4
impaired functional movement, FES for, 52
impaired motor control, functional neurosurgery, 136
incomplete motor clinical syndrome, 11–14
incomplete SCI, 11–14
  neurologically, 205–6, 210*t*, 213*f*
individual stereotype response, residual motor function after SCI, 22
infralesional segment (ILS), 137–38, 137*f*

classification, 141, 142*f*
peripheral inputs, 143, 144*f*
injured metamere (IM), 137–38, 137*f*
consequences of pathological changes in, 139
functional recovery, 140
intervention at, 139–41
complications of, 140
surgical, 140
LMN dysfunction and, 139
nerve roots affected by, 141
pathology of, 138–41
SCI reconstructive neurosurgery and, 138–41
UMN dysfunction and, 139
innervation, serotoninergic, 114–15
Institute of Clinical Neurophysiology in Ljubljana
Dimitrijević at, 291–92
Faganel at, 294
intracerebral transplantation, 94
intrathecal drug delivery systems
baclofen
pumps, 58–60
for spasticity, 145
locomotion and, 81
in vitro OEC experiments, 101
in vivo OEC experiments, 101

Janko, Martin, 291
Jaspers, Karl, 288
Jeras, Jože, 287

killed-end potential (KEEP), 216–20
ASIA, 219–20, 219*f*
cervicomedullary glioma and, 217
Kraepelin, Emil, 288
Kugelberg, Erik Klas Henrik, 291

L-dihydroxyphenylanine (L-DOPA), 80
lesions
ILS, 137–38, 137*f*
classification, 141, 142*f*
peripheral inputs, 143, 144*f*
SCI
acute, 171–73, 172*f*
established, 173–76, 173*f*, 174*f*
functional recovery of, 175
spinal cord
bridge construction and, 96, 96*f*
preoperative determination and level of, 217
sublesional segment
classification of injuries, 141, 142*f*
functional neurosurgery and, 143–47
lesion severity, 142
pathology, 141–52
reconstructive neurosurgery of SCI and, 141–52
spasticity reduction and, 143–47
Ljubljana
Institute of Clinical Neurophysiology
Dimitrijević, at, 291–92
Faganel at, 294
motor control development in, academic environment for, 285–96
Dimitrijević and, 289–93, 290*f*
Faganel and, 294–95
Yugoslav Symposium of Neurology and Urodynamics, 295
LMN dysfunction. *See* lower motor neuron dysfunction
locomotion
animal models, 70–78, 70*f*
cerebellum and, 69
clonidine, 70
cyproheptadine, 81
drugs and, 70, 81
intrathecal drug delivery systems, 81
neurocontrol of, 65–82
residual motor control below SCI and, 37–40, 39*f*
SCI and, 71–78
spinal cord network and, 66–68, 67*f*
supraspinal control and, 68–71, 71*f*
transcutaneous SCS modification of neural circuit activity and, 247, 248*f*
after SCI, 69–70
afferent influence and, 78–80
cat animal model of, 71–74
changes in, 71–78
compression injuries and, 77–78
contusion injuries and, 77–78
neurotransmitter roles and, 80–82
rat animal model of, 74–78

locomotion (*Cont'd*)
spinal cord network, 66–68, 67*f*
spinal cord transection and, 71–78
supraspinal control of, 68–71, 71*f*
yohimbine, 81
locomotor activity, epidural SCS enhancement of, 243
locomotor movement, neurotransmitter roles in, 80–82
locomotor patterns after SCI, 38
lower motor neuron (LMN) dysfunction, 138
IM pathology and, 139
nerve transfer surgery, 153–55, 158*f*
lumbar spine. *See* transcutaneous lumbar posterior root stimulation
lumbosacral spine, transcutaneous SCS and, 237–39, 237*f*, 238*f*
PRM reflexes elicited by, 233–34, 233*f*, 234*t*

macrophages
autologous, 104
axonal growth and, 103
CNS axon regeneration and implanting, 102–4
transplantation, 104
manual muscle testing, 2
Marinčič, Ivan, 287, 289
Dimitrijević and, 290
MEPs. *See* motor evoked potentials
mesencephalic locomotor region (MLR), 66. *See also* locomotion
mMEPs. *See* muscle MEPs
mobility-oriented recovery after SCI, 49–50
monoaminergic cells
intraspinal grafting of, 114–18
spinal cord, 116
motoneurones
embryonic grafts and replacement of, 111–14
grafted
axons of, connected to skeletal muscles, 113–14
survival of, 112
host, depletion of, 112–13
motor activity
SCI, above and below, 11
after SCI, transcutaneous lumbar posterior root stimulation for, 226–49
motor clinical syndromes, SCI
complete, 12–14
discomplete, 11, 14
incomplete, 11–14
motor control, xii–xiii
brain, 2
residual motor control below SCI and, 37–40, 39*f*
SCI and, 71–78
spinal cord network and, 66–68, 67*f*
supraspinal control and, 68–71, 71*f*
transcutaneous SCS modification of neural circuit activity and, 247, 248*f*
in chronic SCI, characteristic patterns of, 184–87, 185*f*, 186*f*, 187*f*, 188*f*
CNS and, 258
fEMG measurement of, 182–83
impaired, functional neurosurgery for, 136
in Ljubljana, academic environment for development of, 285–96
Dimitrijević and, 289–93, 290*f*
Faganel and, 294–95
neurological motor deficits and, ix–x
neurophysiological assessment of, 181–97
clonus elicitation, manual, 277–80, 280*f*
fEMG BMCA recording protocols and, 262–67, 265*t*, 266*f*, 268*t*
manual for, 261–83
motor task sequence and, 268*t*, 270
passive stretch and, 275–76, 278*f*, 279*f*
protocols, optional segment for all, 281–83, 283*f*
reinforcement maneuvers and, 271–72, 273*f*
relaxation and, 270–71, 271*f*, 272*f*, 273*f*
results of, 195–97, 196*f*
sitting and, 283

standing and, 283
tendon tap reflexes and, 277, 279*f*
TVR and, 280–81, 280*f*
voluntary movement, 273*f*, 274–75, 275*f*–278*f*
withdrawal suppression and, 281, 282*f*
non-injured, characteristics of, 183, 184*f*
patterns, 189–90
recovery, after SCI, 6–7, 8*f*
SCI
characteristic patterns of, 184–87, 185*f*, 186*f*, 187*f*, 188*f*
data analysis of, 190–95, 193*t*
neurophysiological assessment of, 181–97
results of, 195–97, 196*f*
after SCI, restorative neurology of, 43–60
baclofen for, intrathecal, 58–60
botulinum toxin treatment of spasticity, 60
electrical stimulation after SCI, 49–50
FES, 47–49
FES for impaired functional movement of single muscle group, 52
foot-drop stimulator, clinical program for fitting, 49
interventions for, 46–54
motor performance assessment and, 45–46
muscle hypertonia and, 51
neurocontrol, externally electrically induced modification of altered, 52, 53*f*, 54*f*
NMS, 47–50
patterns of movement, NMS for modification of, 51
physiotherapy, 46–47
recommendation for, 52–54
SCS and movement augmentation, 55–57, 55*f*
SCS and movement elicitation, 57–58, 59*f*
spinal cord, 258
neurological evaluation principles, 12–20
neurophysiological assessment of, 11–12, 13*f*
studies, transcutaneous lumbar posterior root stimulation for, 226–49
subclinical, residual motor function and, 3–6, 3*f*, 4*f*, 6*f*
volitional activity and, 4–5, 4*f*
motor control, residual
below SCI
brain influence and, 28–35
central state of spinal cord, 22–23, 23*f*
cutaneo-muscular reflex organization and, 25–27, 26*f*, 27*f*
individual stereotype response, 22
neurocontrol of locomotion and, 37–40, 39*f*
neurophysiological evaluation principles, 20–27
neurophysiological principles of, 10–40
phasic stretch reflex and, 16–17, 18*f*
repetitive tendon jerks and, 27
spasticity and spasms, 21–22, 22*f*
spinal cord CPG and, 39–40
summary and recommendation for, 19–20, 20*f*
suprasegmentally induced motor unit activity in paralyzed muscles, 34–35, 34*f*
tendon jerk afterdischarge and, 23–25, 24*f*
tendon jerks in spastic SCI, 28–30, 29*f*
testing paradigms for, 15, 16*f*
tonic stretch reflex and, 16–17, 18*f*
vibratory tonic reflex in complete SCI syndrome, 31, 32*f*
volitional motor activity and, 19
volitional motor task output and, modification of, 35–37, 36*f*, 37*f*
withdrawal flexor plantar reflex volitional suppression, 31–33, 33*f*
withdrawal reflex and, 19
preservation of, 44

motor events, 270, 271*f*, 272*f*, 273*f*
motor evoked potentials (MEPs), 281–82
  animal models, 209
  epidural, 204–5, 214
  intraoperative, 203, 209–12
motor function, residual
  restorative neurological intervention and, 2
  after SCI, 1–10
    clinical and subclinical function of, 1–2, 2*f*
    cutaneo-muscular reflex organization and, 25–27, 26*f*, 27*f*
    motor control recovery and, 6–7, 8*f*
    neurophysiological assessment and, 2–3
    restoration of function and, 2–3
    subclinical motor control and, 3–6, 3*f*, 4*f*, 6*f*
motor impairments, 286–87
motor organization, CNS, 189
motor performance assessment, restorative neurology of motor control after SCI, 45–46
motor tasks
  output, volitional, 36*f*, 37*f*
    modification of, residual motor control below SCI and, 35–37, 36*f*, 37*f*
  sequence, 268*t*, 270
motor unit activity
  features of, 35–36, 36*f*
  in paralyzed muscles, suprasegmentally induced, residual motor control below SCI and, 34–35, 34*f*
motor unit potentials (MUP), 33
movement
  abnormal involuntary, 136
  augmentation, SCS for, 55–57, 55*f*
  elicitation, SCS and, 57–58, 59*f*
  FES for impaired functional, 52
  locomotor, neurotransmitter roles and, 80–82
  patterns, 51
  voluntary
    disrupted by SCI, 187–90, 189*f*, 190*f*, 191*f*
    neurophysiological assessment of motor control and, 273*f*, 274–75, 275*f*–278*f*
MSCs. *See* bone marrow stromal cells
multi-parallel system injury, 3
multipulse stimulation techniques, 201, 202*f*
MUP. *See* motor unit potentials
muscle MEPs (mMEPs), 204–5, 214–15
muscles
  FES for impaired functional movement of single muscle group, 52
  H reflex studies and multiple, 241–42, 241*f*, 242*f*
  hypertonia, nerve/NMS and modification of, 51
  paralyzed, suprasegmentally induced motor unit activity in residual motor control below SCI and, 34–35, 34*f*
  passive stretch, 275–76, 278*f*, 279*f*
  skeletal, axons of grafted motoneurones and connecting to, 113–14
  SMMT, 153
  testing, manual, 2
  trophic state of, 50
myelotomies, 147

nerves
  hypertonia, muscle and, 51
  innervation, serotoninergic, 114–15
  roots, IM and affected, 141
  sciatic, bridge construction and, 96, 96*f*
  stimulation, 51
nerve transfers
  LMN, 153–55, 158*f*
  reconstructive neurosurgery and, 152–60
  surgery, 153–57, 156*f*
  tendon transfers compared with, 153–54
  UMN, 153–55, 158*f*
neural circuit activity, transcutaneous SCS modification of, 242–47
  neural control of locomotion augmentation and, 247, 248*f*

spasticity control and, 244–47, 245*f*, 246*f*
neural plasticity, SCI and, 175
neurobiology, 171
neurocontrol, 295–96
altered, externally electrically induced modification of, 52, 53*f*, 54*f*
of locomotion
residual motor control below SCI and, 37–40, 39*f*
SCI and, 71–78
spinal cord network and, 66–68, 67*f*
supraspinal control and, 68–71, 71*f*
transcutaneous SCS modification of neural circuit activity and, 247, 248*f*
of spinal reflex activity, 21
neuroendocrine disorders, functional neurosurgery, 136
neurological evaluation principles, residual motor control after SCI and, 12–20
neurological motor deficits, SCI and, ix–x
neurology
restorative, x
clinical practice of, 15
of motor control after SCI, 43–60
SCI, 176, 258–59
Yugoslav Symposium of Neurology and Urodynamics, 295
neuromuscular stimulation (NMS), 47–50. *See also* stimulation
of muscle hypertonia, 51
neuronal circuitry
pattern generators, 257
of spinal cord, 257
neurons, corticospinal tract, 201
neuropathology, SCI, 256
neurophysiological assessment
methods, ix
of motor control, 181–97
clonus elicitation, manual, 277–80, 280*f*
fEMG BMCA recording protocols and, 262–67, 265*t*, 266*f*, 268*t*
manual for, 261–83
motor task sequence and, 268*t*, 270
passive stretch and, 275–76, 278*f*, 279*f*
protocols, optional segment for all, 281–83, 283*f*
reinforcement maneuvers and, 271–72, 273*f*
relaxation and, 270–71, 271*f*, 272*f*, 273*f*
results of, 195–97, 196*f*
sitting and, 283
spinal cord, 11–20, 13*f*
standing and, 283
tendon tap reflexes and, 277, 279*f*
TVR and, 280–81, 280*f*
voluntary movement, 273*f*, 274–75, 275*f*–278*f*
withdrawal suppression and, 281, 282*f*
motor function, residual and, 2–3
of SCI-caused changes, 181–97
results of, 195–97, 196*f*
of spinal cord motor control, 11–12, 13*f*
principles of, 12–20
neurophysiological evaluation, residual motor function after SCI, 20
central state of spinal cord, 22–23, 23*f*
cutaneo-muscular reflex organization and, 25–27, 26*f*, 27*f*
individual stereotype response, 22
repetitive tendon jerks and, 27
spasticity and spasms, 21–22, 22*f*
tendon jerk afterdischarge and, 23–25, 24*f*
neurophysiological interventions, 259
neurophysiological markers, paraplegia, 201–2, 203*f*
neurophysiological monitoring
corticospinal tract neuron, 201
of spinal cord, 200–220
cSEPs, 216
discussion of, 207–12
eMEPs, 214
eSEPs, 215
intraoperative, 202–16
mMEPs, 214–15
paraplegia markers and, 201–2, 203*f*
protocol for, 204–5
results of, 205–7, 206*f*, 207*f*, 209*f*, 211*f*, 212*f*
safety and, 216

neurophysiological principles of residual motor control below SCI, 10–40
neurophysiology
  beginnings, 285–87
  clinical
    beginnings of, 286
    investigative techniques, 286
  intraoperative, protocol for, 204–5
  of SCI, traumatic, 202–16
    cSEPs, 216
    discussion of, 207–12
    eMEPs, 214
    eSEPs, 215
    mMEPs, 214–15
    protocol for, 204–5
    results of, 205–7, 206*f*, 207*f*, 209*f*, 211*f*, 212*f*
    safety and, 216
  SCI site determination with, 216–20
  in Slovenia
    beginnings of, 287
    promoters of, 287–89
neurosurgery
  functional
    current state of, 136–37
    for dysfunction, 136
    for epilepsy, 136
    for impaired motor control, 136
    for neuroendocrine disorders, 136
    for pain, 136
    for psychiatric disorders, 136
    spasticity, 143–47
    for spasticity, 136, 143–47
    sublesional segment, 143–47
  reconstructive, 136*t*
    functional procedures, 135
    function recovery, focal interventions for, 152–60, 154*f*
    nerve transfers and, 152–60
    of SCI, 134–61, 161*t*
neurotransmitters, locomotor movement and roles of, 80–82
new anatomy, sublesional segment, 141, 142*f*
NMDA, 82
NMS. *See* neuromuscular stimulation
noradrenergic cells grafts, 117
olfactory ensheathing cells (OECs)
  CNS axon regeneration and implanting, 100–102
  in vitro experiments, 101
  in vivo experiments, 101

pain
  functional neurosurgery, 136
  gate theory, 242
paralyzed muscles, suprasegmentally induced motor unit activity in, 34–35, 34*f*
paraplegia
  neurophysiological markers for, 201–2, 203*f*
  peripheral nerve grafts in, 108–9
  permanent, neurophysiological markers for, 201–2, 203*f*
  transient, neurophysiological markers for, 201–2, 203*f*
Parkinson's disease, 276, 278*f*
partial-weight-bearing therapy (PWBT), 149
passive function, 157
passive stretch, neurophysiological assessment of motor control and, 275–76, 278*f*, 279*f*
pattern generators, 257
patterns of movement, NMS for modification of, 51
Pehani, Hubert, 287
peripheral nerve grafts
  axon regeneration and, 95–97, 96*f*
  in paraplegic patients, 108–9
  SCI bypassing lesion site by, 106–9, 107*f*
peripheral nervous system (PNS), 102. *See also* central nervous system
persistent inward currents (PICs), 142
phasic stretch reflex, 16, 18*f*
  threshold, 17
phenomena of absence, 157
phenomena of presence, 157
physiological inputs, spasticity and, 148–51, 150*f*
physiotherapy, restorative neurology, 46–47
PICs. *See* persistent inward currents
plantar stimulation, 264

Plečnik, Janez, 287
PNS. *See* peripheral nervous system
posterior root-muscle (PRM) reflexes. *See also* reflexes
  asymmetries, 233*f*, 234
  electrophysiological characteristics
    double stimulation and, 235–36, 235*f*
    tendon vibration and, 236, 236*f*
  epidural spinal cord stimulation of, 227–28
  H reflex and, 239–41, 240*f*
    multiple muscle, 241–42, 241*f*, 242*f*
  transcutaneous lumbosacral SCS and, 233–34, 233*f*, 234*t*
Prevec, Tine, 291
PRM. *See* posterior root-muscle reflexes
ProCord™, 104
Propofol, 204
psychiatric disorders, functional neurosurgery, 136
PWBT. *See* partial-weight-bearing therapy

quipazine, locomotion and, 81

rat animal models, locomotion after SCI, 74–78
reconstructive neurosurgery, 136*t*
  functional procedures, 135
  function recovery, focal interventions for, 152–60
    tendon transfer surgery, 152–53, 154*f*
  nerve transfers and, 152–60
    surgery, 153–57
  of SCI, 134–61, 161*t*
    IM and, 138–41
    sublesional segment pathology and, 141–52
reconstructive surgery, 258
reduced anatomy, sublesional segment, 141
reflexes
  cutaneo-muscular, organization
    residual motor function after SCI and, 25–27, 26*f*, 27*f*
    tiring and, 27
  H-reflex
    multiple muscle studies, PRM reflexes and, 241*f*, 242*f*
    PRM reflexes and, 239–42, 240*f*, 241*f*, 242*f*
    studies, 241–42, 241*f*, 242*f*
  neurocontrol of spinal reflex activity, 21
  phasic stretch, 16–17, 18*f*
    threshold of, 17
  PRM
    asymmetries, 233*f*, 234
    electrophysiological characteristics, 235–36, 235*f*, 236*f*
    epidural spinal cord stimulation of, 227–28
    H reflex and, 239–41, 240*f*, 241–42, 241*f*, 242*f*
    transcutaneous lumbosacral SCS and, 233–34, 233*f*, 234*t*
  spinal
    activity, neurocontrol of, 21
    responses, 2
  stretch, 16–17, 18*f*
  tendon tap, neurophysiological assessment of motor control and, 277, 279*f*
  vibratory tonic, in complete SCI, 31, 32*f*
  withdrawal, 19
  withdrawal flexor plantar, residual motor control below SCI and, 31–33, 33*f*
reinforcement maneuver response (RMR), 34
reinforcement maneuvers, neurophysiological assessment of motor control and, 271–72, 273*f*
reinforcement tasks, 264
relaxation
  motor events during, 270, 271*f*, 272*f*, 273*f*
  neurophysiological assessment of motor control and, 270–71, 271*f*, 272*f*, 273*f*
  standard, 271–72
Remifentanil, 204

residual motor control
below SCI
brain influence and, 28–35
central state of spinal cord, 22–23, 23*f*
cutaneo-muscular reflex organization and, 25–27, 26*f*, 27*f*
individual stereotype response, 22
neurocontrol of locomotion and, 37–40, 39*f*
neurophysiological evaluation principles, 20–27
neurophysiological principles of, 10–40
phasic stretch reflex and, 16–17, 18*f*
repetitive tendon jerks and, 27
spasticity and spasms, 21–22, 22*f*
spinal cord CPG and, 39–40
summary and recommendation for, 19–20, 20*f*
suprasegmentally induced motor unit activity in paralyzed muscles, 34–35, 34*f*
tendon jerk afterdischarge and, 23–25, 24*f*
tendon jerks in spastic SCI, 28–30, 29*f*
testing paradigms for, 15, 16*f*
tonic stretch reflex and, 16–17, 18*f*
vibratory tonic reflex in complete SCI syndrome, 31, 32*f*
volitional motor activity and, 19
volitional motor task output and, modification of, 35–37, 36*f*, 37*f*
withdrawal flexor plantar reflex volitional suppression, 31–33, 33*f*
withdrawal reflex and, 19
preservation of, 44
restorative neurology, x
clinical practice of, 15
interventions
electrical stimulation after SCI, 49–50
FES, 47–49
FES for impaired functional movement of single muscle group, 52
foot-drop stimulator, clinical program for fitting, 49
muscle hypertonia and, 51
neurocontrol, externally electrically induced modification of altered, 52, 53*f*, 54*f*
NMS, 47–50
patterns of movement, NMS for modification of, 51
physiotherapy, 46–47
recommendation for, 52–54
motor control, residual and, 2
of motor control after SCI, 43–60
baclofen for, intrathecal, 58–60
botulinum toxin treatment of spasticity, 60
interventions for, 46–54
motor performance assessment and, 45–46
SCS and movement augmentation, 55–57, 55*f*
SCS and movement elicitation, 57–58, 59*f*
of SCI, 176, 258–59
treatment issues in, 44
rhizotomy, dorsal, 101
RMR. *See* reinforcement maneuver response
Robida, Ivan, 287, 289

Schwann cells
CNS axon regeneration and implanting, 97–100, 98*f*
grafted, 98–99
SCI. *See* spinal cord injury
sciatic nerve, bridge construction and, 96, 96*f*
SCS. *See* spinal cord stimulation
Seliškar, Albin, 287, 288
Dimitrijević and, 290
sEMG. *See* surface EMG
sensory deficits, nerve transfer, 157, 160*f*
sensory encephalography, 285
SEPs. *See* somatosensory evoked potentials
Šerko, Alfred, 287–88
serotonergic cell grafts, 117
serotonergic system, 81

embryonic grafts, intraspinal, spinal cord circuitry and, 115–18, 116*f*
serotonic system, locomotion and, 81
serotoninergic innervation, 114–15
shock, spinal, 172
shortening response, 276
sitting, neurophysiological assessment of motor control and, 283
skeletal muscles, axons of grafted motoneurones and connecting to, 113–14
SLR. *See* subthalamic locomotor region
SLS. *See* supralesional segment
SMMT. *See* stimulated manual muscle test
soluble NSF attachment protein receptor (SNAP), 60
somatosensory evoked potentials (SEPs)
  animal models, 209
  epidural, 204, 215
  intraoperative, 203, 209–12
spasms, residual motor function after SCI, 21–22, 22*f*
spasticity
  ablative procedures, 146–47
  baclofen, 145
  Botox, 60
  botulinum toxin treatment of, 60
  cyproheptadine, 151
  dantrolene, 145
  diazepam, 145
  focal, function recovery and managing, 157–60, 160*t*
  functional augmentation: restorative approach, 148–52
    pathological input optimization and, 148–51, 150*f*
    pathological input reduction and, 148
  functional neurosurgery, 136, 143–47
  functional recovery of, 152–60, 160*t*
  myelotomies, 147
  pharmacological interventions, 145–46, 151
  prevalence, 246–47
  reduction, sublesional segment and, 143–47
  residual motor function after SCI, 21–22, 22*f*
  SCS for, 55–57, 55*f*
  stimulation, 143–45, 146*f*
  suppression, 247
  tendon transfer surgery, 159–60
  therapy, 143, 145*f*
  tizanidine, 145
  transcutaneous SCS modification of neural circuit activity and control of, 244–47, 245*f*, 246*f*
  treatment, neurolytic, 158–59
spastic SCI, tendon jerks in, 28–30, 29*f*
sPEMG. *See* surface electrode polyelectromyography
spinal cord
  central state of
    cutaneo-muscular reflex organization and, 25–27, 26*f*, 27*f*
    repetitive tendon jerks and, 27
    residual motor function after SCI and, 22–23, 23*f*
    tendon jerk afterdischarge and, 23–25, 24*f*
  circuitry, 67, 67*f*
    SCI repair and activation of existing, 114–18
    serotoninergic embryonic cell intraspinal grafting and, 115–18, 116*f*
    serotoninergic innervation and, 114–15
  CPG, 39–40, 66–68
  grafts of embryonic, 110–11, 110*f*
  locomotion and, 66–68, 67*f*, 71–78
  monoaminergic cells, 116
  motor control, 258
    neurological evaluation principles, 12–20
    neurophysiological assessment of, 11–12, 13*f*
  neuronal circuitry, 257
  neurophysiological monitoring, 200–220
    cSEPs, 216
    discussion of, 207–12
    eMEPs, 214
    eSEPs, 215
    intraoperative, 202–16
    mMEPs, 214–15
    paraplegia markers and, 201–2, 203*f*

spinal cord (*Cont'd*)
neurophysiological monitoring (*Cont'd*)
protocol for, 204–5
results of, 205–7, 206*f*, 207*f*, 209*f*, 211*f*, 212*f*
safety and, 216
shock, 172
stimulation, 39–40
epidural, 227–28
transection, 70
locomotion in cats and, 71–74
locomotion in rats and, 74–78
partial, in cats, 72–74
partial, in rats, 75–77
total, in cats, 71–72
total, in rats, 74–75
traumatized, 137–38, 137*f*
spinal cord injury (SCI)
acute phase, biological interventions in, 176–77
AIS classification, 190, 192*f*
animal models, 65–66, 170
biological interventions, 176–77
clinical application of, 177–78
fictive, 178
central nervous system and, ix
changes caused by
neurophysiological assessment of, 181–97
results of, 195–97, 196*f*
chronic stage, 178
characteristic patterns of motor control in, 184–87, 185*f*, 186*f*, 187*f*, 188*f*
clinical pathophysiology
acute SCI lesion and, 171–73, 172*f*
established lesion and, 173–76, 173*f*, 174*f*
subacute stage, 173
complete, 12–14
neurologically, 205, 208*t*
vibratory tonic reflex in, 31, 32*f*
compression, 77–78
contusion, 77–78
damage caused by, 257–58
discomplete, 11, 14, 256
anatomically, 15
effects, 65
established, biological interventions in, 177
gait after, 37–38
immunobased therapy, 102–4
incidence, ix
incomplete, 11–14
neurologically, 205–6, 210*t*, 213*f*
incomplete lesion with distinct biomechanical characteristics, 14–15, 15*f*
lesion
acute, 171–73, 172*f*
established, 173–76, 173*f*, 174*f*
functional recovery of, 175
locomotion after, 69–70
afferent influence and, 78–80
cat animal model of, 71–74
changes in, 71–78
compression injuries and, 77–78
contusion injuries and, 77–78
neurotransmitter roles and, 80–82
rat animal model of, 74–78
mobility-oriented recovery after, 49–50
motor activity above and below, 11
motor activity after, transcutaneous lumbar posterior root stimulation for, 226–49
motor clinical syndrome in, 11–12
motor control
characteristic patterns of, 184–87, 185*f*, 186*f*, 187*f*, 188*f*
data analysis of, 190–95, 193*t*
neurophysiological assessment of, 181–97
results of, 195–97, 196*f*
motor control, residual below
brain influence and, 28–35
central state of spinal cord, 22–23, 23*f*
cutaneo-muscular reflex organization and, 25–27, 26*f*, 27*f*
individual stereotype response, 22
neurocontrol of locomotion and, 37–40, 39*f*
neurophysiological evaluation principles, 20–27
neurophysiological principles of, 10–40

phasic stretch reflex and, 16–17, 18*f*
repetitive tendon jerks and, 27
spasticity and spasms, 21–22, 22*f*
spinal cord CPG and, 39–40
summary and recommendation for, 19–20, 20*f*
suprasegmentally induced motor unit activity in paralyzed muscles, 34–35, 34*f*
tendon jerk afterdischarge and, 23–25, 24*f*
tendon jerks and, 28–30, 29*f*
testing paradigms for, 15, 16*f*
tonic stretch reflex and, 16–17, 18*f*
vibratory tonic reflex in complete SCI syndrome, 31, 32*f*
volitional motor activity and, 19
volitional motor task output and, 35–37, 36*f*, 37*f*
withdrawal flexor plantar reflex volitional suppression, 31–33, 33*f*
withdrawal reflex and, 19
motor control after, restorative neurology of, 43–60
baclofen for, intrathecal, 58–60
botulinum toxin treatment of spasticity, 60
electrical stimulation after SCI, 49–50
FES, 47–49
FES for impaired functional movement of single muscle group, 52
foot-drop stimulator, clinical program for fitting, 49
interventions for, 46–54
motor performance assessment and, 45–46
muscle hypertonia and, 51
neurocontrol, externally electrically induced modification of altered, 52, 53*f*, 54*f*
NMS, 47–50
patterns of movement, NMS for modification of, 51
physiotherapy, 46–47
recommendation for, 52–54
SCS and movement augmentation, 55–57, 55*f*
SCS and movement elicitation, 57–58, 59*f*
motor function after, residual, 1–10
clinical and subclinical function of, 1–2, 2*f*
cutaneo-muscular reflex organization and, 25–27, 26*f*, 27*f*
motor control recovery and, 6–7, 8*f*
neurophysiological assessment and, 2–3
restoration of function and, 2–3
subclinical motor control and, 3–6, 3*f*, 4*f*, 6*f*
motor neuron activity in, upper, 15, 16*f*
neural plasticity, 175
neurologically complete, 205, 208*t*
neurologically incomplete, 205–6, 210*t*, 213*f*
neurological motor deficits and, ix–x
neuropathology, 256
pathophysiology, 170
clinical, 171–76
peripheral nerve grafts and bypassing lesion site of, 106–9, 107*f*
reconstructive neurosurgery of, 134–61, 161*t*
function recovery and, 152–60
IM and, 138–41
nerve transfers and, 152–60
sublesional segment pathology and, 141–52
repair
axon regeneration and, 93–106
biological interventions for, 169–79
embryonic grafts for, 109–14
peripheral nerve grafts and, 106–9, 107*f*
spinal cord circuitry activation and, 114–18
strategies used to, summary of, 93–118
restorative neurology and, 176, 258–59
site, neurophysiological determination of, 216–20
spastic, tendon jerks in, 28–30, 29*f*
suprasegmental influences in, 15
therapeutically-oriented recovery after, 49–50

spinal cord injury (SCI) (*Cont'd*)
traumatic, 94
neurophysiology of acute, intraoperative, 202–16
voluntary movement disrupted by, selective control of, 187–90, 189*f*, 190*f*, 191*f*
spinal cord lesions
bridge construction and, 96, 96*f*
preoperative determination and level of, 217
spinal cord stimulation (SCS), 39–40. *See also* stimulation
for movement augmentation, 55–57, 55*f*
for movement elicitation, 57–58, 59*f*
sites, 56–57
for spasticity control, 55–57, 55*f*
transcutaneous
biophysics, 231–33, 232*f*
continuous, 245–46
electrode placement, 244
epidural SCS and, 243
transcutaneous lumbosacral, PRM reflexes elicited by, 233–34, 233*f*, 234*t*
spinal reflexes
activity, neurocontrol of, 21
responses, 2
sPMG. *See* surface polyelectromyography
standing, neurophysiological assessment of motor control and, 283
stem cells
CNS axon regeneration and implanting, 104–6
embryonic, 105
sources, 105
umbilical cord, 105–6
grafts, 105–6
stimulated manual muscle test (SMMT), 153
stimulation
double, 235–36, 235*f*
electrical
after SCI, 49–50
spasticity, 143–45, 146*f*
multipulse techniques, 201, 202*f*
nerve, muscle hypertonia, 51
plantar, 264
PRM reflexes and double, 235–36, 235*f*
spasticity, 143–45, 146*f*
spinal cord, 39–40
epidural, 227–28
transcutaneous lumbar posterior root, 230*f*
advantages, 228–29
electrode placement, 230, 231*f*
methodology, 229–31, 231*f*
motor activity after SCI, 226–49
for motor control studies, 226–49
stimulus-response paradigms, 16
stretch reflex
phasic, 16–17, 18*f*
tonic, 16–17, 18*f*
Strojnik, Aleš, 287
sublesional segment
classification of injuries, 141, 142*f*
functional neurosurgery and, 143–47
lesion severity, 142
pathology, 141–52
reconstructive neurosurgery of SCI and, 141–52
spasticity reduction and, 143–47
subthalamic locomotor region (SLR), 68. *See also* locomotion
supralesional segment (SLS), 137–38, 137*f*
suprasegmental influences
motor unit activity in paralyzed muscles and, 34–35, 34*f*
in SCI, 15
supraspinal control of locomotion, 68–71, 71*f*
surface electrode polyelectromyography (sPEMG), 21
of tendon jerk afterdischarge, 23–25, 24*f*
surface EMG (sEMG), 194, 262
BMCA and, 262
relaxation standard, 271–72
surface polyelectromyography (sPMG), 15
surgery
nerve transfer, 153–57, 156*f*
tendon transfer, 152–53, 154*f*
nerve transfer surgery compared with, 153–54
for spasticity, 159–60

surgical interventions
functional integrity during, 200–220
neurophysiology of acute traumatic SCI, 202–16
for IM, 140
symtomatic improvement, 157

tendon jerks
afterdischarge, residual motor function after SCI and, 23–25, 24*f*
exaggerated, 28–30, 29*f*
repetitive, residual motor function after SCI and, 27
in spastic SCI, 28–30, 29*f*
tendon taps, 264
reflexes, neurophysiological assessment of motor control and, 277, 279*f*
tendon transfer surgery, 152–53, 154*f*
nerve transfer surgery compared with, 153–54
for spasticity, 159–60
tendon vibration, PRM reflexes and, 236, 236*f*
TENS. *See* transcutaneous electrical neural stimulation
therapeutically-oriented recovery after SCI, 49–50
tiring, 27
tizanidine, spasticity, 145, 151
TMS. *See* transcranial magnetic stimulation
T-myelotomy, 147
tonic stretch reflex, 16–17, 18*f*
position for examination of, 16
tonic vibratory response (TVR), 280–81, 280*f*
transcranial magnetic stimulation (TMS), 281–82
transcutaneous electrical neural stimulation (TENS), 230. *See also* stimulation
transcutaneous lumbar posterior root stimulation, 230*f*. *See also* stimulation
advantages, 228–29
electrode placement, 230, 231*f*
methodology, 229–31, 231*f*
motor activity after SCI, 226–49
for motor control studies, 226–49
transcutaneous lumbosacral SCS
application of, 237–39, 237*f*, 238*f*
PRM reflexes elicited by, 233–34, 233*f*, 234*t*
transcutaneous SCS
biophysics, 231–33, 232*f*
cauda equina and, 237–39, 237*f*, 238*f*, 239*f*
continuous, 245–46
electrode placement, 244–45
epidural SCS and, 243
neural circuit activity modification with, 242–47
neural control of locomotion augmentation and, 247, 248*f*
spasticity control and, 244–47, 245*f*, 246*f*
transection, spinal cord, 70
locomotion and, 71–78
partial
locomotion in cats and, 72–74
locomotion in rats and, 75–77
total
locomotion in cats and, 71–72
locomotion in rats and, 74–75
traumatic SCI, 94
traumatized spinal cord, 137–38, 137*f*
Trontelj, Jože, 291
TVR. *See* tonic vibratory response

upper motor neuron (UMN)
activity, in SCI, 15, 16*f*
dysfunction, 138
IM pathology and, 139
nerve transfer surgery, 153–55, 158*f*
syndrome, 172

ventral column (VC), 76
ventrolateral funiculus (VLF), 76
vibratory tonic reflex in complete SCI, 31, 32*f*
volitional activity, 4–5, 4*f*
volitional motor activity after SCI, 19
voluntary movement, neurophysiological assessment of motor control and, 273*f*, 274–75, 275*f*–278*f*

von Jauregg, Wagner, 288
von Krafft-Ebing, Richard, 287

wave recording technique, 201
withdrawal flexor plantar reflex, residual motor control below SCI and, 31–33, 33*f*
withdrawal reflex, 19
withdrawal suppression, neurophysiological assessment of motor control and, 281, 282*f*

yohimbine, locomotion, 81
Yugoslav Symposium of Neurology and Urodynamics, 295

zone of partial preservation (ZPP), 12
Župančič, Andrej O., 287, 288–89